Oxford Specialist Handbook of
Community Paediatrics

Edited by

Srinivas Gada

Consultant Community Paediatrician
Oxford University
Hospitals NHS Trust
Honorary Senior
Clinical Lecturer
University of Oxford, UK

OXFORD
UNIVERSITY PRESS

OXFORD
UNIVERSITY PRESS

Great Clarendon Street, Oxford, OX2 6DP,
United Kingdom

Oxford University Press is a department of the University of Oxford.
It furthers the University's objective of excellence in research, scholarship,
and education by publishing worldwide. Oxford is a registered trade mark of
Oxford University Press in the UK and in certain other countries

© Oxford University Press 2012

The moral rights of the author have been asserted

First Edition published in 2012

Impression: 1

British Library Cataloguing in Publication Data

Data available

Library of Congress Cataloging in Publication Data

Data available

ISBN 978-0-19-969695-6

Printed in Italy by
L.E.G.O. S.p.A - Lavis TN

Foreword

In 1976, Professor Donald Court's inquiry into child health services was published. The report identified a range of failures in the way in which care is delivered in the UK, with poor mortality data compared to our European counterparts. The report also identified fragmentation and poor communication between primary and secondary care, and a lack of paediatric competence amongst many staff looking after children. Court made a series of radical proposals, only a few of which were implemented. Perhaps unsurprisingly not all of the problems he identified were solved; indeed recent data still demonstrate that our all-cause child mortality remains unacceptably high compared to that of much of Western Europe. However, one recommendation which was followed through was for a group of paediatricians to work in community settings with a remit—among other things—to look after children with disabilities and to support a range of health promotion activities.

Contemporary child health needs and demographics within the UK have changed considerably since Court's time, and there is now an even greater demand for paediatricians to be trained in social and behavioural paediatrics, care of children with disabilities, child health promotion and child protection. Arguably we now need even more paediatricians to work outside of traditional hospital settings and boundaries.

Dr Gada's book provides an excellent overview of this critically important area of paediatrics. The book combines clear and concise notes on the full range of community paediatric topics, along with a wealth of pragmatic and practical information. The topics are brought alive with case vignettes, and importantly samples reports (for example, a court report) and letters (for example, a 'leaving care' letter). Complex legal and statutory procedures are explained clearly and in straightforward language, and there are numerous lists of useful resources and contacts.

This comprehensive book will provide an invaluable reference text to health care professionals working either wholly or partly in the community, including paediatricians, GPs, therapists, nurses, health visitors, trainees, medical students and indeed to the many generalists who also play a part in the essential aspects of care outlined within these pages.

Hilary Cass
Neurodisability Consultant
Evelina Children's Hospital
President
Royal College of Paediatrics and Child Health, UK
2012

Preface

My inability to refer trainees to a single source of up-to-date information on community paediatrics and the need for me to carry multiple folders each filled with milestones, guidelines, diagnostic checklists, growth charts, etc., motivated me to write this book.

Community paediatrics encompasses a wide range of subspecialities, each covering a range of conditions managed in a variety of settings, i.e. primary, secondary, and specialist tertiary settings. Despite this challenge I have endeavoured to cover all aspects of the speciality into this small pocket book.

Naturally, this book has been organized into chapters each covering a subspeciality or an aspect of community paediatrics. You will find that the information on a topic is in a readily accessible format with extensive use of bullet points, tables, boxes, etc. The focus is on presenting clinically relevant information with less emphasis on theory or background information. Further reading and references have been intentionally limited and all topics have been cross-referenced with other relevant aspects of the book. Readers are encouraged to refer to BNFC for further details on drug doses.

Hence this book is a practical guide that can quickly be referenced in the clinic. Its practicality, portability, and well-laid out information will enable the reader to deliver clinically effective and child/family-centred care on the go!

This book has been written for anyone who manages children in the community, i.e. out-of-hospital. Therefore this book can serve as an essential companion and a first point of reference to undergraduates, paediatric trainees, general practitioners, doctors, professionals from allied specialities, and members of community nursing and multidisciplinary teams.

I have been fortunate to be able to bring together the expertise of contributors (who are experts in their fields) from a wide variety of disciplines. In close collaboration with them I have managed to present their expertise into concise clear summaries on each topic. Consequently this book encourages you to work collaboratively with other professionals enabling you to provide holistic care to the child and family.

Community paediatrics is intriguing and I hope this book makes it more exciting and rewarding. I would welcome your constructive suggestions for improvement.

S. Gada
Oxford
March 2012

Dedication

To

My Family

*For their numerous sacrifices, generous support,
endless encouragement, & abundant love.*

&

You (the reader)

*For using the information contained in this book, to make a
positive difference in the lives of children & their families, you serve.*

Acknowledgements

As in life, the journey of this book has seen numerous successes, some failures, near misses, computer crashes, delays in getting responses, staff vacancies, and relocations in the department. All of these have played their part in its prolonged gestation! This book would not have come into being without the support and assistance of the editorial team at OUP in particular patience of Helen Liepman, the commissioning editor, and Tessa Eaton, the production editor.

As a working community paediatrician much of the information that has shaped the book was gleaned during the course of my clinical practice. Therefore my utmost thanks go to all the children and their families who have shared their everyday challenges, with me.

I would like to extend my sincere gratitude to all the contributors for their hard work and for offering their invaluable time and expertise. My special appreciation is here for their patience with numerous revisions. Their dedication was crucial for the conclusion of this project.

My special thanks to following individuals for their assistance in reviewing/ revising the following: Michele McCoy (Public health), Dave Long (Clinical engineering and PIMS), Fiona Ryan (Bone health), T. Girish (Gynaecological care), Jeremy Hull (Respiratory care), Anupam Chakrapani (Inherited metabolic diseases), Denise Challis (Development), Meg Buckingham (Orthopaedic line diagrams), Sarah Lang (Immunisation Advisor, HPA), Noel McCarthy (Consultant in Communicable Diseases, HPA), Nicole Bigler (OT), Lesley Bucke (SLT), Linda Luxon (Audiology), Minoo Irani (Chapter 4), and Neal Thurley (help with literature searches).

I am indebted to Jen Nutt (my secretary) for her seamless service.

S. Gada
2012

Contents

Contributors

Rachel Buckingham
Consultant in Paediatric
Orthopaedics,
Nuffield Orthopaedic Centre,
Oxford, UK

Robert Chapman
Consultant Child & Adolescent
Psychiatrist,
Oxford Health NHS Foundation
Trust;
Honorary Senior Clinical Lecturer,
University of Oxford, UK

Srinivas Gada
Consultant Community
Paediatrician,
Oxford Children's Hospital;
Honorary Senior Clinical Lecturer,
University of Oxford, UK

Praveen Goyal
Consultant Community
Paediatrician,
Department of Community
Paediatrics,
Oxford Children's Hospital, UK

David Henderson Slater
Consultant in Neurological
Disability and Rehabilitation
Medicine,
Oxford Centre for Enablement,
Nuffield Orthopaedic Centre,
Oxford, UK

Julia Hyde
Children's Community
Physiotherapist,
Department of Community
Paediatrics,
Oxford Children's Hospital, UK

Minoo Irani
Consultant Community
Paediatrician,
Upton Hospital, Slough, UK

Christine Ireland
Highly Specialist Speech and
Language Therapist,
Department of Community
Paediatrics,
Oxford Children's Hospital, UK

Georgia Jackson
Consultant Community
Paediatrician,
Royal Berkshire Hospital,
Reading, UK

Sandeep Jayawant
Consultant Paediatric Neurologist,
Honorary Senior Clinical Lecturer,
Oxford Children's Hospital,
Oxford, UK

Dominic Kelly
Consultant Paediatrician,
Oxford University Hospital NHS
Trust; Senior Clinical Lecturer,
University of Oxford, UK

Usha Kini
Consultant Clinical Geneticist,
Oxford University Hospitals NHS
Trust;
Honorary Senior Lecturer,
University of Oxford, UK

Sue King
Associate Specialist,
Department of Community
Paediatrics,
Oxford Children's Hospital,
Oxford, UK

Graham Mackenzie
Consultant in Public Health,
NHS Lothian, Edinburgh, UK

Chris Morris
Senior Research Fellow in Child
Health,
Peninsula Medical School,
University of Exeter, UK

Manoj Parulekar
Consultant Ophthalmic Surgeon,
Birmingham Children's Hospital,
UK

Anne Peake
Educational Psychologist,
Educational Psychology Service,
Oxfordshire Local Education
Authority,
Oxford, UK

Clare Robertson
Consultant Community
Paediatrician, Department of
Community Paediatrics,
Oxford Children's Hospital, UK

Richard Scott
Consultant Clinical
Neuropsychologist,
John Radcliffe Hospital,
Oxford, UK

Doug Simkiss
Associate Clinical Professor in
Child Health,
Division of Mental Health and
Wellbeing,
Warwick Medical School,
Coventry, UK

Peter Sullivan
Honorary Consultant
Paediatrician,
Oxford University Hospitals NHS
Trust, UK

Clare Wallace
Lead Children's Community
Occupational Therapist,
Oxford Health NHS Foundation
Trust, UK

Symbols and Abbreviations

📖	cross-reference
❶	warning
▶	important
🕮	website
◐	telephone
~	approximately
↑	increased
↓	decreased
→	leading to
♂	male
♀	female
1°	primary
2°	secondary
A&E	Accident and Emergency (department)
AA	amino acids
AABR	automated auditory brainstem response
AAC	augmentative and alternative communication
AASA	alpha amino adipic succinylaldehyde
ABR	auditory brainstem response
ACE	angiotensin converting enzyme
ACTH	adrenocorticotrophic hormone
AD	autosomal dominant
ADD	attention deficit disorder
ADEM	acute disseminated encephalomyelitis
ADHD	attention-deficit hyperactivity disorder
ADI	Autism Diagnostic Interview
ADL	activities of daily living
ADOS-G	Autism Diagnostic Observation Schedule
AED	antiepileptic drugs
AFO	ankle foot orthoses
AFP	alphafetoprotein
AHA	assisting hand assessment
AN	anorexia nervosa
ANSD	auditory neuropathy spectrum disorder
AOM	acute otitis media
AOS	apraxia of speech
AP	action potential

AP	antero-posterior
APA	American Psychiatric Association
APD	auditory processing disorder
AR	autosomal recessive
AS	Asperger's syndrome
ASD	autistic spectrum disorder
ASSA	adoption support service advisor
ASSR	auditory steady state response
AT	ataxia telangiectasia
ATRX	alpha thalassaemia/mental retardation syndrome
BAAF	British Association for Adoption and Fostering
BAAP	British Association of Audiological Physicians
BAHA	bone anchored hearing aid
BAPA	British Association of Paediatricians in Audiology
BAS	British Ability Scales
BC	bone conduction
BCECT	benign childhood epilepsy with centrotemporal spikes
BCG	Bacille Calmette–Guérin
BMD	bone mineral density
BN	bulimia nervosa
BOR	branchio-oto-renal syndrome
BP	blood pressure
BP1	blind and partial sight registration form 1
BPVC	benign paroxysmal vertigo of childhood
BPVS	British Picture Vocabulary Scales
BSA	British Society of Audiologists
BSID	Bayley Scale of Infant Development
BSL	British Sign Language
BTE	behind-the-ear
C&YP	children and young people
CaF	Contact a Family (charity)
CAMHS	Child and Adolescent Mental Health Service
CBC	child behaviour checklist
CBT	cognitive behaviour therapy
CCN	children's community nurse
CCTV	closed circuit TV
CD	conduct disorder
CDC	child development centre
CDOP	child death overview process
CDT	child development team
CEA	carcinoembryonic antigen

CELF	clinical evaluation of language fundamentals
CERA	cortical evoked response audiometry
CFS	chronic fatigue syndrome
CGH	comparative genomic hybridization
CHARGE	choanae, heart, anal, growth and ear anomalies
CHL	conductive hearing loss
CIMT	constraint-induced movement therapy
CK	creatine kinase
CLD	chronic lung disease
CM	cochlear microphonic
CMAP	compound motor action potential
CMT	Charcot–Marie–Tooth
CNS	central nervous system
COGMED	Cogmed working memory training
CONI	care of next infant
CP	cerebral palsy
CPA	care programme approach
CRS	congenital rubella syndrome
CSA	child sexual abuse
CSF	cerebrospinal fluid
CSWS	continuous spike wave discharge in slow sleep
CT	computed tomography
CTEV	congenital talipes equino varus
CVI	certificate of vision impairment
CVS	cardiovascular system
CXR	chest X-ray
DAMP	deficit in attention motor control and perception
DBT	dialectic behaviour therapy
DCD	developmental coordination disorder
DD	developmental delay
DDH	developmental dysplasia of the hip
DDK	diadochokinesis
DDST	Denver Development Screening Test
DEAP	diagnostic evaluation of articulation and phonology
DGE	delayed gastric emptying
DIDMOAD	diabetes insipidus, diabetes mellitus optic atrophy deafness
DLA	disability living allowance
DMD	Duchenne muscular dystrophy
DNA	deoxyribonucleic acid
DNA	did not attend
DOB	Date of Birth

DPOAEs	distortion product otoacoustic emissions
DRB	deaf resource base
DRPLA	dentatorubropallidoluysian atrophy
DS	Down syndrome
DSH	deliberate self-harm
DSM	Diagnostic and Statistical Manual
DSM-IV	Diagnostic and Statistical Manual Version 4
DT	distraction testing
DTaP	Diphtheria tetanus pertussis
DTI	diffusion tensor imaging
DXA	dual-energy x-ray absorptiometry
EAC	external auditory canal
EAL	English as an additional language
ECG	electrocardiogram
ECHO	echocardiogram
ECM	'Every Child Matters'
ECU	environmental control units
ED	eating disorder
EDNOS	eating disorder not otherwise specified
EDS	Ehler–Danlos syndrome
EEG	electroencephalogram
EF	executive functioning
EHC	eye–hand coordination
EMG	electromyogram
ENT	ear, nose, throat
EP	educational psychology
EPO	emergency protection order
EPODE	Ensemble, Prévenons l'Obésité des Enfants
EPS	evoked potential studies
ERG	electroretinogram
ERIC	education and resource for improving continence
ESR	erythrocyte sedimentation rate
EUA	examination under anaesthesia
EYSENIT	early years special educational needs inclusion team
FASD	fetal alcohol spectrum disorder
FBC	full blood count
FES	functional electrical stimulation
FGM	female genital mutilation
FH_x	Family history
FII	fabricated or induced illness
FISH	fluorescent *in situ* hybridisation

FM	fine motor
FRAXTAS	fragile X tremor ataxia syndrome
FTT	failure to thrive
FVC	forced vital capacity
GA	gestational age
GABA	gamma amino butyric acid
GCSE	general certificate of secondary education
GDD	global developmental delay
GI	gastrointestinal
GM	gross motor
GMDS-ER	Griffiths Mental Development Scales-Extended Revised
GMFCS	gross motor function classification system
GMFM	gross motor function classification
GOR	gastro-oesophageal reflux
GOS	general ophthalmic services
GP	general practitioner
GSD	glycogen storage disease
GT	gastrostomy tube
GUM	genito-urinary medicine
HA	hearing aid
HELLP	haemolytic anaemia elevated liver enzymes low platelets
HEP	hepatitis
HES	hospital eye service
HGPRT	hypoxanthine guanine phosphoribosyl transferase
HI	hearing impairment
Hib	*Haemophilus influenzae* b
HIE	hypoxic ischaemic encephalopathy
HIU	hearing impaired unit
HIV	human immunodeficiency virus
HL	hearing loss
HMSN	hereditary motor sensory neuropathy
HPA	health protection agency
HPV	human papilloma virus
HSQ	home screening questionnaire
HSV	herpes simplex virus
Ht/Wt	Height/weight
HV	health visitor
Hx	history
IADLs	instrumental activities of daily living scales
ICD	International Classification of Diseases

ICD-10	International Classification of Diseases Version 10
ICF	International Classification of Functioning Disability and Health
ICH	intracranial haemorrhage
ICO	interim care order
ICP	intracranial pressure
ICU	intensive care unit
ID	intellectual disability
Id	Identification
IEM	inborn error of metabolism
IEP	individual educational plan
Ig	immunoglobulin
IMD	inherited metabolic disorder
INO	internuclear ophthalmoplegia
IPT	interpersonal psychotherapy
IPV	inactivated polio vaccine
ITE	in-the-ear
IUGR	intrauterine growth retardation
IVDU	Intravenous drug user
IVF	*in vitro* fertilization
JIA	juvenile idiopathic arthritis
KS	key stage
LA	local authority
LAC	looked after children
LD	learning disability
LE	lower extremity
LFT	liver function test
LI	language impairment
LRTI	lower respiratory tract infection
LSCB	local safeguarding childrens board
LSD	lysosomal storage disease
M-ABC	movement assessment battery for children
MACE	mitrofanoff for antegrade colonic enema
MAP	minimum auditory percept
MCAD	medium chain acyl coenzyme A dehydrogenase
MCADD	medium chain acyl-coenzyme A dehydrogenase deficiency
ME	middle ear
ME	myalgic encephalitis
MEE	middle ear effusion
MELAS	mitochondrial encephalopathy lactic acidosis stroke-like episodes

Men B	meningococcal serogroup b
Men C	meningococcal serogroup c
MERRF	myoclonic epilepsy ragged red fibres
MLPA	multiplex ligation-dependent probe amplification
MMR	measles, mumps, and rubella
MPH	methylphenidate
MPNST	malignant peripheral nerve sheath tumours
MPS	mucopolysaccharidoses
MRA	magnetic resonance angiogram
MRC	Medical Research Council
MRI	magnetic resonance imaging
MRS	magnetic resonance spectroscopy
MRSA	meticillin resistant *Staphylococcus aureus*
MSE	Mental State Examination
MTHFR	methyl tetrahydrofolate reductase
MVP	mitral value prolapse
N/PICU	neonatal/paediatric intensive care unit
NAHI	non-accidental head injury
NAI	non-accidental injury
NARP	neuropathy ataxia retinitis pigmentosa
NBM	nil by mouth
NCL	neuronal ceroid lipofuscinosis
NCMP	National Child Measurement Programme
NEPSY	neuropsychological assessment
NF-1	neurofibromatosis type 1
NF-2	neurofibromatosis type 2
NG	nasogastric
NGT	nasogastric tube
NHS	National Health Service
NHSP	Newborn Hearing Screening Programme
NICE	National Institute for Health and Clinical Excellence
Nm	Neisseria meningitidis
NSC	(UK) National Screening Committee
OA	organic acids
OAE	otoacoustic emission
OCD	obsessive–compulsive disorder
OCE	Oxford Centre of Enablement
ODD	oppositional defiant disorder
OFC	occipitofrontal circumference
OMD	oromotor dysfunction
OME	otitis media with effusion

OPD	outpatient department
OSA	obstructive sleep apnoea
OT	occupational therapist
P scales	assessing progress of children with SEN
PA	postero-anterior
PCHI	permanent childhood hearing impairment
PCHR	parent-held child record
PCR	polymerase chain reaction
PCT	Primary Care Team
PDA	pathological demand avoidance
PDD	pervasive developmental disorder
PDD-NOS	pervasive developmental disorder-not otherwise specified
PECS	picture exchange communication system
PEG	percutaneous endoscopic gastrostomy
PEP	post-exposure prophylaxis
Perf	performance
PHU	partial hearing unit
PIMS	posture independence mobility service
PKAN	pantothenate kinase associated neurodegeneration
PKU	phenylketonuria
PM	post mortem
PMHx	past medical history
PNS	peripheral nervous system
POLG	polymerase gamma
PR	parental responsibility
PS	personal social
PSCHE	Personal Social Health and Citizenship Education
PSG	polysomnography
PT	physiotherapist
PTA	pure tone audiometry/audiogram
PTH	parathyroid hormone
PTSD	post-traumatic stress disorder
PVL	periventricular leucomalacia
PWMI	periventricular white matter injury
PWS	Prader–Willi syndrome
RAS	reflex asystolic syncope
RCFT	Rey complex figure test
RCPCH	Royal College of Paediatrics and Child Health
RD	reading disability
RDS	respiratory distress syndrome
RNIB	Royal National Institute of Blind People

ROM	range of movements
ROP	retinopathy of prematurity
RS	respiratory system
RTA	road traffic accident
Rx	Treatment
SA	sexual abuse
SA	school action/school action plus
SARC	sexual assault referral centre
SATS	standard attainment tests
SCA	spinocerebellar ataxia
SCIE	Social Care Institute for Excellence
SCN1A	sodium channel 1 alpha
SCR	serious case review
sd	standard deviation
SDQ	Strengths and Difficulties Questionnaire
SE	side effects
SEGA	subependymal giant cell astrocytoma
SEN	special educational needs
SENCO	SEN coordinator
SFEMG	single fibre electromyogram
SHUEE	Shriners Hospital Upper Extremity Evaluation
SLT	speech and language therapist
SMA	spinal muscular atrophy
SMART	Specific Measurable Achievable Relevant Time specific
SMEI	severe myoclonic epilepsy of infancy
SMN	survival motor neuron
SMO	supramalleolar orthoses
SNHL	sensorineural hearing loss
SNR	signal-to-noise ratio
SOGS	schedule of growing skills
SP	summating potential
Sp	Streptococcus pneumoniae
SPD	sensory processing disorder
SPECT	single photon emission computed tomography
SpLD	specific learning disabilities
SQCP	severe quadriplegic cerebral palsy
SS	Social Services
SSE	sign-supported English
SSEN	statement of special educational needs
SSPE	subacute sclerosing panencephalitis

SSRI	selective serotonin reuptake inhibitor
SSQ	social support questionnaire
SSS	sensory support services
ST4	specialist trainee 4
STAP	South Tyneside Assessment of Phonology
STASS	South Tyneside Assessment of Syntactic Structures
STD	sexually transmitted disease
STI	sexually transmitted infection
SUDI	sudden unexpected death in infancy
SW	social worker
T&A	tonsillectomy and adenoidectomy
TA	teaching assistant
TAC	team around child
TAM	transient abnormal myelopoiesis
TBI	traumatic brain injury
Td	tetanus diphtheria
TFT	thyroid function test
TLSO	thoracolumbar sacral spine orthoses
TM	tympanic membrane
TOAEs	transient evoked otoacoustic responses
ToD	teacher of the deaf
TORCH	toxoplasmosis, other infections, rubella, cytomegalovirus, herpes
TROG	test for reception of grammar
TS	tuberous sclerosis
TS	Tourette's syndrome
TSC	tuberous sclerosis complex
TSH	thyroid stimulating hormone
U&E	urea and electrolytes
UE	upper extremity
UNCRC	United Nations Convention on the Rights of the Child
UNCRPD	United Nations Convention on the Rights of People with Disabilities
UPD	uniparental disomy
VACTERL	vertebral anal cardiac tracheal esophageal renal limb anomalies
VEMP	vestibular evoked myogenic potential
VEP	visual-evoked potential
VI	vision impairment
VI team	vision impairment team
VLCFA	very long chain fatty acids

VOCA	voice output communication aid
VOR	vestibulo-ocular reflex
VRA	visual reinforcement audiometry
WAIS	Wechsler Adult Intelligence Scales
WHO	World Health Organization
WHO	wrist hand orthoses
WISC	Wechsler Intelligence Scale for Children
WPPSI	Wechsler Preschool and Primary Scale of Intelligence
WRAMA	wide range assessment of visual motor abilities
WRAML	wide range assessment of memory and learning
XLD	X-linked dominant
XLR	X-linked recessive

Introduction to community paediatrics

The soul is healed by being with children.

English proverb

Community paediatrics and roles of the community paediatrician

- Until 1974, community child health services in UK were administered by local authorities; thereafter, they were provided within the National Health Service (NHS), but were distinct from hospital paediatric services as well as general practitioner (GP) services.
- The current model of working of community paediatricians in delivering community child health services was largely determined by the recommendations of the working party set up by the government in 1973, under the chairmanship of Professor Donald Court (see 📖 Foreword) .

Definition of community paediatrics (American Academy of Paediatrics)

- A perspective that enlarges the paediatrician's focus from one child to all children in the community.
- A recognition that family, educational, social, cultural, spiritual, economic, environmental, and political forces act favourably or unfavourably, but always significantly, on the health and functioning of children.
- A synthesis of clinical practice and public health principles directed toward providing healthcare to a given child and promoting the health of all children within the context of the family, school, and the community.
- A commitment to use a community's resources in collaboration with other professionals, agencies, and parents to achieve optimal accessibility, appropriateness, and quality of services for all children, and to advocate especially for those who lack access to care because of social or economic conditions or their special healthcare needs.
- An integral part of the professional role and duty of the paediatrician.

Community-based paediatrician and community paediatrician

- Paediatric medical care in the UK is broadly provided in two settings—hospital-based paediatrics (inpatient and outpatient services) and 'out-of-hospital' paediatric care (community-based general paediatric outpatient clinics, community child health services, and, occasionally, medical care in the child's home).
- It is not uncommon for the same paediatrician to provide both hospital-based and out-of-hospital paediatric care.
- The roles of a community-based paediatrician and community paediatrician are quite distinct.
- The community-based paediatrician ('ambulatory paediatrician') is a paediatrician whose practice is focused on providing paediatric medical care outside the hospital environment, often with additional duties in the hospital service.
- The community paediatrician, on the other hand, focuses practice on all children and young people in a defined population, in addition to those who come to the clinic.
- The community paediatrician aims to strike a balance between the medical and social models of healthcare delivery, working in partnership with a range of professionals in health, education, and social care (see 📖 p20 and p23).

Roles of the community paediatrician
- Community paediatrics provides opportunities for paediatricians to develop an interest in one or more of the specialist areas of the discipline (see below).
- While an individual may not be able to contribute to every area of community paediatrics in day-to-day work, it is required that a community paediatrician has the awareness, training, and skills for the majority of these specialist areas.

Developmental paediatrics and childhood disability
- Developmental assessment (see 📖 p35) and identification of developmental disorders (see 📖 Chapter 4: Neurodevelopmental disorders).
- Assessment, care, and management of the child with a disability:
  - Physical disability.
  - Learning disability.
  - Sensory disability (see 📖 p269 and p295)
  - Autism spectrum disorders (see 📖 p107 and p327).

Social paediatrics
- Safeguarding children and young people (see 📖 p473).
- Adoption and fostering (see 📖 p479).
- Children looked after by local authorities.
- Health and well-being of immigrant children (see 📖 p495).
- Services for 'children in need'.

Child public health
- Coordination of the Healthy Child Programme (see 📖 p550 and p557).
- School-based health promotion programmes (see 📖 p542).
- Health needs assessment.

Child mental health
- Assessment and management of behavioural difficulties in children (see 📖 p210).
- Assessment and management of attention deficit hyperactivity disorder (ADHD) in children (see 📖 p126).

Partnership working
- Providing medical advice to education authorities and schools (see 📖 p524).
- Providing medical advice to social services, courts, and other statutory bodies (see 📖 p465).
- Advising health organizations (strategic health authorities, primary care trusts, GP surgeries) about health and care needs of children (see 📖 Chapter 16).

Training
- Medical students, paediatric specialty trainees.
- Other professional groups who support children's services.

The future
- For the vast majority of community paediatricians, supporting the most vulnerable children and families in society provides a high level of professional satisfaction.
- The low profile of this specialty in the healthcare arena, its low popularity among paediatric specialty trainees, variable service delivery models, recruitment difficulties for career grade community paediatrician posts, and perceived low profitability in healthcare markets are factors which pose a threat to the long-term viability of this discipline.
- There remains an urgent need for modernization of this important service for safeguarding the health and well-being of the nation's children (see 📖 Foreword).

Consultation in community

- Large majority of clinical work in community child health is carried out in an outpatient setting.
- Most appropriate management plan and adequate provision of support services requires detailed understanding of not only the child's health problems but in-depth information about family structure and social circumstances.
- Working in close partnership and effective communication between a child's parents and various professionals is vital (see 📖 p18).

Considerations before consultation

- Adequate time provisions: consultations generally take longer in a community clinic than in a hospital-based setting.
- Try to collect available information regarding a referral prior to clinic except when a second opinion is requested, e.g. information from teachers, nursery staff, health visitor (HV), etc.
- Appointment letter should have clear instructions, e.g. reporting to reception, parking, etc. and practical information regarding encouraging parents to bring, e.g. parent-held child record (PCHR), any medical records, etc.
- Copy appointment letter to social worker (SW) or HV to facilitate attendance, e.g. help with transport especially for some disadvantaged families.
- Consider need for interpreter/language line. Try to avoid using family or friend for interpretation.

Consultation settings in community

- Development clinic: a new referral or a follow-up appointment (see 📖 p36).
- Breaking news: following investigations, e.g. Duchenne muscular dystrophy (DMD) following creatine kinase (CK), test result, etc.
- Clinical assessments: could be in an outpatient clinic, school clinic, or a multidisciplinary setting, i.e. child development centre (CDC) with family (see 📖 p22).
- Home visit: for a severely disabled child or palliative care (see 📖 p105).
- Specialist clinics, e.g. looked after children (LAC) clinic with SW & foster carer, adoption and fostering clinic, Down syndrome (DS) clinic, epilepsy clinic, etc.
- Child protection assessment and assessments for allegations of child sexual abuse (CSA) (see 📖 p455).
- Special school clinics (see 📖 p534).

Key principles and considerations for a consultation in community

- Information about routine history taking (see 📖 p6) and clinical examination (see 📖 p9) can also be found in many available texts.
- Appropriate private and comfortable setting without interruption.
- Facilities and equipment for examination and detailed assessment.
- Awareness of parental concerns and fears and checking their expectations from consultation.

- Not to make assumptions.
- Treating families with respect, dignity, empathy, and insight and involving them in decision-making.
- Acknowledging the fact that disabled children can communicate.
- Starting with open questions and allowing parents to talk without interruption, at least for few minutes.
- Chaperone if and when required, especially for CSA examinations.
- Honest and appropriate summary and explanation of findings and opinion at the end of consultation.
- Clear further actions and follow-up plan.
- Copy of written letter to supplement verbal discussion.

Good practice points
- Calling parents and child personally from waiting area may provide an opportunity to observe child's activity during free play.
- Don't ignore index child for a normal sibling.
- In children with behavioural/emotional problems talking to parents privately may facilitate free exchange of information.
- Introduce colleagues/trainee and obtain permission for them to stay.
- Provision of appropriate toys in the clinic.
- Clinic room set up to ensure an active child's safety:
  - Handles high on doors.
  - Cupboard locks.
  - High shelves and taps with stopcocks.

Difficult consultation—some tips
- Could be due to a very hyperactive child distracting parents and clinician.
- Try a joint observation with a colleague/trainee while other person is keeping child engaged.
- In an ideal world, there would be 2 adjacent rooms with one-way mirror in between to provide an opportunity to observe child's behaviour without being noticed (available in very few centres).
- Observe both parents playing and interacting with the child.
- If everything else fails, arrange a further appointment without child.

Non-attendance
- Leads to wastage of professional time (frustrating) and lost opportunity for the child.

Causes
- Parents not convinced that there is anything wrong with the child.
- Denial or fear of a serious diagnosis.
- Need for more time after initial assessment to adjust to the diagnosis before further review.
- Dissatisfaction with opinion.
- Muddled appointment timings.
- Difficulty in taking time off work.
- Problem with transportation etc.

History taking

- A good history can provide most of the information needed to make a clinical assessment and formulate a management plan.
- It needs enough time, and clinician's willingness and ability to help.
- History taking should convey an attitude of empathy, concern, and interest. It could be therapeutic.
- To make the best use of limited time in a busy clinic, a pro-forma for collecting information may be sent to the family beforehand so that attention can be focused on assessment and discussing important issues.
- General principles of history taking are similar to those in other clinical situations. The following additional points may be helpful.

Remember

- Proper introduction and greeting child by name
- Explaining the reasons for the referral.
- Use of tact and discretion when taking history in child's presence.
- Behavioural problems like enuresis, encopresis, and temper tantrum needs sensitive questioning.
- Some parents may want to speak without the child being present, especially if an adopted child or has very traumatic past.
- Some teenagers may speak freely without their parents and they should be offered this opportunity.

Style

Can vary according to individual preference. The author found the following useful:

Presenting features

- Open-ended questions at the start and closed questions later to elicit more details.
- Active and attentive listening with clarification as required.
- Information/opinion from child if appropriate.
- Ascertaining the family's perception of the problem.
- Use of appropriate language and avoiding medical jargon.
- Summarize and reflect on the information obtained at various times during interview.
- Ascertainment of associated symptoms and their functional impact.
- Indirect questions may help: 'Did he talk before he walked?'; 'How does she compare with your other children?'; 'What was he doing on his first birthday?'.
- Developmental history is required in most children seen in community paediatric/neurodevelopmental clinics (see 📖 pp44–54).
- Any loss of previously acquired skill (see 📖 p253) must be established beyond doubt by asking for specific milestones, e.g. 'Baby who could stand and hold a spoon is not able to do now …'
- PCHR can supplement parental recall of developmental milestones.
- Important to emphasize positive aspects of development; to record what the child can do.

- Details of educational achievement/schooling can provide useful additional information about child's behaviour and intellectual ability (see 📖 p520).
- Elicit history of behavioural difficulties in different settings (see 📖 p340).
- Condition specific history should be taken according to presentation (e.g. in autism ask specific questions re: communication, social interaction difficulties, behaviours, etc. Also see particular points for condition-specific history in individual chapters).
- General system-specific enquiry:
  - Respiratory system (RS): cough, breathing difficulty, wheezing, choking (with feeding/saliva).
  - Gastrointestinal (GI): vomiting, reflux, diarrhoea, constipation.
  - Central nervous system (CNS): fits, funny turns, drop attacks, etc.
  - Other system-specific symptoms as indicated including diet (as well as any restrictions), sleep, etc.

Past history
- Pregnancy: antenatal monitoring and growth, folate supplementation, exposure to alcohol, smoking, recreational drugs, medications, intrauterine infections, bleeding, quality of fetal movements, etc.
- Birth: gestation, meconium staining of liquor, mode of delivery, Apgar scores, birth weight, difficulties in neonatal period, admission to neonatal unit, jaundice, condition at discharge, etc.
- Mode of feeding, age at weaning (any problems with solids or liquids).
- Hospitalization, operations, medications, infections, fractures, etc.

Developmental history
- Age at first smile, sitting, crawling, standing, walking, first independent step, first clear single words, two-word phrase ('ball gone' rather than 'all-gone').
- Toilet training, concerns about vision (see 📖 p271) or hearing (see 📖 p296), school performance compared to siblings (see 📖 p520).

Current development and functioning
- Current level of independent mobility (with or without mobility aids): rolling over, sitting, crawling, cruising, walking, jumping, hopping, climbing stairs, kicking a ball, riding a bicycle, tendency to fall, any concerns about gait, clumsiness.
- Hand preference, pincer, transfer across midline, use of cutlery, scribbling.
- Current method of communication: gestures, verbal, eye pointing, signing, eye contact while communicating, clarity of speech, sharing of interest, protodeclarative pointing, age appropriate pretend play, interest in other children, number of single words, joining words in phrases.
- Self-care: feeding, indication of toilet needs, brushing teeth, dressing/ undressing, continence.
- Emotional and behavioural: concerns about behaviour, temper tantrums, challenging, repetitive or stereotypic, response to change in routine, situational variation (e.g. worst in crowded situation/school), emotional responses to family/strangers.

- Learning: any concern about learning, school progress, any loss of skills/regression. School report may be helpful. Exceptional abilities, e.g. computing, puzzles, memory, music.
- Concerns about hearing, ear infections, if tested—test results. Concerns about vision, squint, nystagmus, results if tested.

Family history
- Consanguinity, parental age and occupation, previous miscarriages, unexplained death, family's understanding of child's difficulties, parental occupation (expectation from child), health, development, and learning ability of siblings and other relatives.
- Specific family history of problems with hearing, vision, speech, learning, epilepsy, fits or funny turns, muscle problems, physical disability, or mental health.
- Any family member attending special school?

Social history
- Home situation, housing, neglect (see 🕮 p449), abuse, being in public care, family support, allowances (see 🕮 p514).
- Schooling (see 🕮 p520 and p522).
- Grade, academic performance, extra support, friendship, bullying (see 🕮 p324), attendance, transport.

Immunisation
- Status vs UK vaccination schedule (see 🕮 p620).
- Indication for special vaccines, e.g. flu (congenital heart disease), hepatitis B, etc.

Current management
- Other professionals involved (e.g. child psychiatrist, speech and language therapist (SLT), etc.).
- Medications, allergies.

Things to be aware of
- Safeguarding issues.
- Inappropriate use of medical terminology by caregivers.
- Accepting diagnosis made previously without clear evidence.

Examination

Equipment
- Have the following available to you/carry:
  - Tools: stethoscope, ophthalmoscope, auriscope, tendon hammer, Wood's lamp, tape measure, sphygmomanometer, orchidometer, toniometer.
  - Preferred development testing set.
  - Growth charts including specific charts for individual conditions (DS, Williams syndrome).
  - Diagnostic checklists, e.g. Asperger syndrome (AS), developmental coordination disorder (DCD), ADHD, etc.
  - Standard Snellen test chart.
  - Paper and pencil to assess drawing skills.
  - Wooden cubes (1 inch/2.5cm), rattle, etc.
  - Finger puppets.

Equipment/resources
- You should have ready access to:
  - Variety of small toys.
  - Age-appropriate books.
  - Facilities for weight and height measurements.
  - Developmental screening tools: Denver Development Screening Test (DDST)/schedule of growing skills (SOGS).
  - Developmental test tools: Griffiths Mental Development Scales-Extended Revised (GMDS)-ER/Bayley.
  - Pro-formas/scales, e.g. Conner Parent Rating Scale/Teacher Rating Scale, strengths and difficulties questionnaire (SDQ), etc.
  - Computer with Internet facilities.

Clinical examination
- Is often dictated by presenting complaints, child's compliance, and available opportunities during consultation.
- Detailing systemic examination is outside the scope of this book. For some of the relevant observations that need to be made in a community paediatric clinic see Box 1.1.

Box 1.1 Things to look for

Posture and demeanour: abnormal posturing (spastic quadriplegia, hypotonia), tremors (Wilson's disease), seizure activity or unusual hand/body movements (epilepsy), hand flapping (autism), tortuous wringing of hands (Rett syndrome), excessive laughter (Angelman syndrome), etc.

Dysmorphic features (see 📖 p384): e.g. upward slanting eyes (DS), coarse features (mucopolysaccharidoses (MPS)), elfin facies with large mouth and upturned nose (Williams syndrome), elongated face (fragile X), micrognathia (Treacher Collins syndrome, Pierre Robin sequence).

Box 1.1 (Continued)

Neurocutaneous skin marks (see 📖 p250): e.g. noticed on Wood's lamp; hypopigmented macules (TS), multiple café au lait spots (Neurofibromatosis type 1 (NF1)), vascular malformation in trigeminal distribution (Sturge–Weber syndrome).

Other skin abnormalities (see 📖 p96): such as severe eczema (phenylketonuria (PKU)), thickened skin (MPS), aplasia (cutis aplasia congenita), nail abnormalities (clubbing).

Examine head (see 📖 p231): for scars, shunt, fontanelle, degree of head control.

Eyes (see 📖 p269): eye contact (pervasive developmental disorder (PDD), visual impairment), microphthalmia (congenital toxoplasmosis, trisomy 13–15), epicanthic folds, conjunctival telangiectasia (ataxia-telangiectasia), Brushfield spots (DS), corneal abnormalities (clouding in MPS), squint, ocular movements (limited abduction and retraction on adduction in Duane syndrome), nystagmus, fundoscopy (cherry spots in Tay–Sachs disease), lens dislocation (Marfan syndrome). Arrange formal vision test.

Ears (see 📖 p297): size; prominent ears in (fragile X), low set in CHARGE (choanae, heart, anal, growth, and ear anomalies), malformation (microtia in Goldenhar syndrome), hearing aids. Arrange formal hearing testing.

Oral examination: for dental health (see 📖 p165), tongue (fasciculations in spinal muscular atrophy (SMA)), drooling (see 📖 p92), palate (submucous cleft) tonsils (ask about snoring (see 📖 90) and sleep (see 📖 p168)).

Hands: single crease (DS), polydactyly (Laurence–Moon–Biedl syndrome), syndactyly (Apert syndrome), arm span if tall stature (Marfan syndrome), manoeuvres for hyperextensibility, the 'thumb sign'.

Feet (see 📖 p422): tight Achilles tendon (cerebral palsy (CP)), pes cavus (Friedreich's ataxia), rocker bottom feet (trisomy 18).

Note: spontaneous speech, general play and interaction, mobility and general coordination.

Special equipment: examine wheelchair, orthotics, specialized shoes for size and signs of wear and tear.

Growth parameters
• Weight: underweight (neglect, coeliac disease), overweight (Prader–Willi syndrome, hypothyroidism).
• Height: tall (Marfan syndrome), short (skeletal dysplasias, chromosomal disorder, Turner syndrome etc.).
• Head circumference: increased (hydrocephalus, familial macrocephaly, neurodegenerative conditions), small (Rett syndrome). Measure parental head circumference.

Neurological examination (see 📖 p228): depending upon age and abilities.

Box 1.1 (Continued)

Gait assessment (see 📖 p433): in older child—limp, Fog's manoeuvre for soft signs, calf hypertrophy, foot drop, etc.

Spine (see 📖 p416): check for scoliosis (idiopathic, CP) by asking to touch toes in standing position, kyphosis (MPS).

Gross motor skills: assess these. See 📖 p176.

Limb examination:
- Asymmetry, pressure points for soreness, calf hypertrophy.
- Tone: raised (CP, Gaucher disease) or reduced (DS).
- Reflexes: hyper-reflexia (CP), hyporeflexia (peripheral neuropathy).
- Power: weakness (neuromuscular conditions).
- Range of movements at various joints: hypermobility (Marfan syndrome, Ehler–Danlos syndrome) or contractures (CP, arthrogryposis).
- If possible ask to draw some basic shapes and write name (coordination, look for pencil grip).

Other systemic examination:
- Cardiovascular system: murmur (DS, Noonan syndrome), BP (medications effect, e.g. methylphenidate, NF1).
- Chest: Harrison sulcus (chronic respiratory difficulties).
- Abdomen: hepatosplenomegaly (storage disorders, inherited metabolic disorder (IMD)), genitals (undescended testes), inguinal/umbilical hernia, anorectal malformation, nappy rash (?neglect), hips examination (developmental dysplasia of the hip (DDH)).
- Musculoskeletal: spine (scoliosis/kyphosis), gait, hips (dislocation), ankles (Achilles tendon tightening)

Developmental assessment: see 📖 p36.

Child development

History of child development

- Charles Darwin, in 1877, published a detailed account of the development of one of his own 10 children, interest was aroused. He wrote 'My first child was born on 27th December 1839 and I at once commenced to make notes on the first dawn of the various experiences which he exhibited, for I felt convinced, even at this early period, that the most complex and fine shades of expression must have had a gradual and natural origin'.
- He described the cephalocaudal sequence of development, hand regard at 4 months, recognition of own name at 7 months, etc.
- 1912: Stern and Kuhlman suggested that a child's relative status could be indicated by a ratio between his mental age and his chronological age—the intelligence quotient.
- 1925: Arnold Gesell published 'norms' of development describing the development of infants and children from newborn to 5 years.
- 1933: Nancy Bayley established norms on a large number of children.
- 1954: Ruth Griffiths tested 571 children aged 14 days to 24 months, publishing *The Abilities of Babies*.
- 1967: Denver Developmental Screening Test (DDST) sample of >1000 children was published.
- 1970: Griffiths scales extended from birth to 96 months was published.

Principles of child development

- Development is a 'continuous' process from conception to maturity. It must not be thought of in terms of mere milestones.
- Development is a 'reflection' of the maturation and myelination of the nervous system.
- The 'sequence' of development is the same and relatively fixed for all, but the rate may vary, e.g. the child has to learn to sit before he can walk.
- Certain 'primitive' reflexes anticipate corresponding voluntary movement and must be lost before the voluntary movement develops, e.g. the grasp reflex has to disappear before the child can hold and manipulate the toy in his hand.
- The direction of development is 'cephalocaudal', i.e. head control has to come first before the child can sit or stand.
- Gross movements refine to finer ones. Generalized mass activity gives way to specific individual responses as the infant grows, e.g. a young baby shows generalized activity to pleasure by widening the eyes, increasing his breathing, kicking his legs, and moving arms vigorously.
- Attainment of skill is reached first. Then speed, strength, precision, balance, performance improves, e.g. a child learns to run at around 18 months of age but the speed, performance, balance, and skill of running continues to improve until adulthood is reached.
- No amount of practice can make a child learn the relevant skill until the nervous system has matured and myelinated, e.g. a child cannot sit

up at 3 months despite practice and opportunity. When the practice is denied the ability to perform the skill lies dormant, but is rapidly learnt as soon as an opportunity is given. External stimulation can hence influence the course of the child's development.

How common are developmental disabilities?
- In the UK it is reported that developmental disabilities affect ~12.5% of school children.
- In the US, developmental disabilities are reported to affect ~17% of children aged <18 years.
- The developmental disabilities include CP (see 📖 p67), learning disability (LD (see 📖 p117)), vision impairment (VI (see 📖 p275)), hearing impairment (HI (see 📖 p296)), ADHD (see 📖 p126), ASD (see 📖 p107), etc. These developmental disabilities result in substantial financial and social costs to the individual, their families, and to the wider society.

Factors that influence the course of child development
- Prenatal e.g. abruption, trauma, intrauterine growth retardation (IUGR), infections, etc.
- Perinatal, e.g. hypoxic-ischaemic encephalopathy, prolonged rupture of membranes leading to infection, etc.
- Postnatal, e.g. illness, infection, nutrition, trauma, etc.
- Genetic, e.g. parental intelligence, attitudes, health, etc.
- Environment, e.g. socioeconomic factors, cultural, health surveillance, etc.
- General, e.g. education, opportunities, intelligence, management of disability/inclusion, personality, gender, order of birth, etc.

Why is assessment of child development important?
- Parents/carers would like to know whether their child is developing normally especially if there have been problems in pregnancy or family.
- A family history of mental subnormality, epilepsy (see 📖 p240), cerebral palsy, sensory loss, etc. would understandably heighten parent/carer's anxiety.
- For obstetricians the developmental assessments provide information with regard to safety of special investigations and treatment they carry out, e.g. management in pregnancy, labour, *in vitro* fertilization (IVF), chorionic villus sampling, amniocentesis, management of medical illnesses, etc. For example, ORACLE II study showed that use of perinatal prophylactic antibiotics to reduce perinatal infections was leading to a higher incidence of CP.
- The knowledge of development is important to neonatologists to be able to assess the risks in the methods of management and treatment they offer in the intensive care unit (ICU), evaluate various interventions, provide counselling/decision-making in preterm resuscitation, e.g. the use of nitric oxide ventilation resulted in a fewer number of children with neurological deficits.
- Developmental assessments (see 📖 p36) will help surgeons in their decision before embarking on a risky procedure in a major congenital abnormality or epilepsy surgery.

- The knowledge of development assists paediatricians in identification of problems with hearing, vision, behaviour, dysmorphism, parenting (see 📖 p371), learning disorders, etc. An in-depth knowledge of child development will also help in providing medical opinion in adoption, fostering (see 📖 p480) and in medico-legal cases.
- Teachers would like to know the reason/s behind a child presenting with behavioural and educational difficulties (see 📖 p520) and knowledge of child development will help evaluate the cause/s behind such difficulties.

How to make up your mind regarding a given child's development

- Comment on his/her alertness, concentration, social interaction, interest and understanding of surroundings. These are all good markers of a child's cognition/developmental maturity.
- Ask yourself if the development is 'normal' or 'delayed' (see 📖 p36).
- If delayed, is it 'global delay' or delay in more 'specific areas'?
- What is the likely cause? Think of common things first.
- Carry out a quick developmental screen (see 📖 p42), even in the outpatient department (OPD), if possible.
- If you come across a very unusual, complex or confusing picture then consider:
  - Discussing with a colleague/senior
  - Arranging for in-depth developmental assessment
  - Investigating (including information from PCHR, HV, GP, nursery/school, etc.), or
  - Referring to an neurodevelopmental expert.

Working with child and family

Do what you can, with what you have, where you are.
Theodore Roosevelt, 1858–1919

Communication with children

Fundamental principles for communicating with young people

- Awareness of the cultural and social background of children and their families.
- Being non-judgemental, respectful, and fair.
- Acknowledging their rights to equality and diversity.
- Understanding that communication is a two-way process.
- Patient listening to encourage their feeling of participation, empowerment, and respect.
- Using clear common language without technical words or jargons.
- Realization of the importance (and effect) of non-verbal communication (facial expression, tone of voice, body language, etc.) on children.
- Offering information to children and young people (C&YP) in a way to match their level of understanding.
- Use of real-life situations to put information in the right perspective.
- Frequently checking their understanding through discussion, and summarizing key points at the end of the meeting.
- Offer to talk to young people, especially teenagers, separately from their parents and deciding together how to involve parents or carers in decision-making process.
- Asking open questions to widen the topic of discussion and encouraging expression of their feelings.
- Use of multisensory methods of communication such as drawing and models to get important and complicated information across.
- Presenting genuine choices and options in decision-making process.

Techniques of communicating with children
Verbal
- Use of 'I'/'me' instead of 'you'.
- Third-person technique, e.g. 'Sometimes when someone is hurt he is angry or sad. Do you sometimes feel like that?'.
- By being non-judgemental and legitimizing their feelings, e.g. 'It is sometimes OK to feel hurt'.
- Story telling—telling two stories with different outcomes.
- 'What if' question—by encouraging the child to use alternative options to deal with a different situation.
- 'What would you ask if you have three wishes?' may help in exteriorizing a child's feelings and help in establishing rapport.
- Using a rating scale, e.g. 'How will you rate tummy ache on a scale of 1 to 10?'.

Non-verbal
- Writing—feelings or thoughts, keeping a diary.
- Drawing.
- Play—spontaneous play with ordinary toys or directed play, e.g. to involve them in imaginative play.
- Use of models to explain complicated topics.

Communicating with children at different ages

Infants
- Mainly non-verbal, vocalization, cuddle, and careful handling.
- Beware of stranger anxiety.

Early childhood
- Focus on individual child.
- Personalize experience to them.
- May prefer to touch and feel examination equipments.
- Concrete thinking—avoid abstract concepts or language.

School-age children
- Want straight explanations and reasons for everything, but would be happy to accept if given in simple language.

Adolescents
- Respecting their views.
- Respect privacy and right to confidentiality (except if safeguarding or other serious issues involved).
- Undivided attention and good listening.
- Keeping open mind and calm.
- Avoid judging.

Barriers to effective communication

- Defending a situation or opinion.
- Stereotyped comments and clichés.
- Direct/close-ended questions from the start.
- Interfering and finishing other's sentences.
- Talking more than listening.
- Frequent change of topic/focus.

Clues/signs of poor communication
- Long periods of silence.
- Constant fidgeting.
- Tapping, playing with hair.
- Looking around, yawning.

Difficult communication

See 📖 Consultation in community p4.

Child- and family-centred care

- During the latter half of the 20th century there has been a growing understanding of the family's role in a child's life. It is recognized that *each family is unique and family members are the experts and best advocate of a child's needs.*
- Family-centred care puts children and their families at the heart of care provisions and is a significant shift from the traditional *biomedical model* of care which focuses on biological rather than social and emotional aspects to deal with the disease process.

Why is child- and family-centred care important?

- For family to accept child's condition.
- To manage child's condition on day-to-day basis.
- To meet child's normal developmental needs.
- To meet sibling's developmental needs.
- Coping with ongoing stress and periodic crises.
- To assist family members in managing their feelings.
- Educate and inform others about the child's condition.
- Establish a support system.

Key principles of child- and family-centred care

- Recognition that family occupies a central and constant position in a child's life.
- Acknowledging that family members are the experts about a child's condition and that they are the best advocates of a child's needs.
- Family–professional collaboration at all levels of healthcare, professional education, policy-making, and programme development to optimize care.
- Effective communication and negotiation of care.
- Recognizing and building on the strengths of each child and family, even in difficult and challenging situations.
- Empowering each child and family by free exchange of information backed by professional support to ensure their involvement in decision-making process.
- Recognition and respect for cultural, racial, and social diversity.
- To fit various support services around the child's and family's needs rather than to suit care provider's convenience.
- Encouraging networking and family-to-family support to facilitate learning from each other's experience.

Advantages of child-centred and family-focused care

- Greater patient, family, and professional satisfaction.
- Improved patient and family outcome.
- Decreased healthcare costs.
- More effective use of healthcare resources.

Example of child- and family-centred care

Harry is a 2-year-old boy seen in clinic for developmental delay. On assessment it became clear that he has autism with general delay in cognitive development. His parents are distraught with this news and would like to know about the best way forward.

They would also like to know:
- What they can do as a family to optimize his development?
- What and how to tell their family and friends?
- How can professionals help?

A family-centred approach will involve:
- Discussion with parents (and with extended family if needed) reflecting respect, involvement, and empowerment.
- Explaining autism with details on how it is affecting Harry rather than discussing about a 'typical case of autism'.
- Highlighting Harry's unique strengths and difficulties.
- Providing best available information (ASD support groups, benefits, etc.) for family to go through at their own pace.
- Honest opinion about prognosis, leaving room for hope in view of young age.
- Arranging appropriate referrals to SLT, occupational therapist (OT), early years special educational needs inclusion team (EYSENIT), and social services (SS) with clear information about who is going to be offering what.
- Clear overview of coordination and delivery of services.
- Discussions followed by written report/letter containing the details of assessment and plan.
- Clear plan for follow-up and information about contact prior to next meeting if needed.

Child development teams

In 1976, Donald Court's report commissioned by the British government drew particular attention to service provisions for children with disabilities and recommended creation of a district team which should include a number of professionals providing multidisciplinary support (see 🕮 Foreword).

Child development team (CDT)

- Is a secondary level service provision for children with neurodevelopmental disability, providing multidisciplinary assessment and support in a local health district.
- Provides a cohesive service ideally from a common location.
- Makes sure that service provisions are responsive to the individual needs of families and children.
- Usually serves preschool children.

Functions of a CDT

- Specific assessment and therapy.
- Information about specific conditions and about disabilities in general.
- Emotional support.
- Link with other families with similar conditions.
- Easy access to other agencies such as education.
- Prompt, efficient supply and repair of equipment.

Structure and composition of a CDT

- Can vary but usually include staff from healthcare, education, and social care (see Fig 2.1).
- It usually includes:
  - Community paediatrician
  - Clinical (or educational) psychologist
  - SLT
  - OT
  - Physiotherapist
  - Preschool teacher/portage worker/EYSENIT
  - SW
  - Specialist HV/key worker
  - Audiologist
  - Allied disciplines, e.g. orthoptist, child psychiatrist, dietician, dentist, play specialist, etc.

Assessment by a CDT

- Assessment may take place jointly at a central facility (child development centre (CDC)) but is more commonly performed at different times by individual team members.
- Some teams may also assess children at a variety of sites outside the CDC including local nurseries, educational units, and home.
- Team meetings and discussions form the core of the CDT to facilitate:
  - Coordination of appropriate service provisions and to avoid duplication (case management).
  - Discussing new referrals to plan and coordinate future assessments.
  - Reviewing policy and team organizations.
  - In-service training, audit, etc.

- Combined health, educational, and care needs of children attending special schools can be discussed in multidisciplinary school meetings.
- Information obtained during assessment process is shared with the parents and (other) professionals working with the child.
- A detailed written report is provided to parents at the end of assessment and shared with partner agencies with parental consent.

Advantages of a CDT
- Detailed multidisciplinary assessments identify needs enabling appropriate service provisions.
- Seamless communication between various professionals/disciplines.
- Avoidance of duplication of assessment with improved coordination.
- Team members learning from each other.

Disadvantages of a CDT
- Risk losing an overview of the child if not coordinated well.
- Lack of accountability and responsibility.
- Dual accountability of practitioners to the team and their line manager with potential for conflict.
- Excluding older children and those without multiple needs who may still benefit from CDT input.
- Risk of becoming CDT centred rather than family centred.

Changing face of a CDT
- Move from 'expert' model to 'empowerment' model.
- Parental expectation and better access to information.
- Changing role of therapists with more parental involvement and enablement in therapeutic interventions.

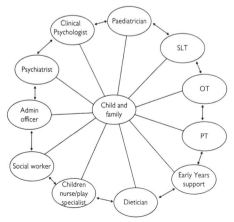

Fig. 2.1 Child development team.

Child development centres

Some CDTs operate from a base while others gather at different locations to meet.

Advantages of a CDC
- Better communication and coordination of services.
- Purpose built facilities and co-location of various support services.
- Recognizable point of contact for families and other professionals.
- Can be used for health promotion activities.
- Can be used as a base to provide various resources by other professionals and local community, e.g. DS support group meetings, parenting programmes, early bird courses, etc.

Disadvantages
- Risk of isolation from families and local services.

Children likely to benefit from CDT/CDC input
Those with:
- Learning disabilities (see 📖 p117).
- Gross motor impairment:
  - CP (see 📖 p67).
  - Neuromuscular disorders (see 📖 p257).
  - Chronic neurological conditions, e.g. post meningitis, brain malformations, survivors of severe head injury (see 📖 p267).
- Fine motor difficulties:
  - DCD/dyspraxia (see 📖 p136).
- Speech, language, and communication disorders:
  - Severe language disorder (see 📖 p200).
  - ASD (see 📖 p107).
- Visual impairment (see 📖 p275).
- Hearing impairment (see 📖 p296).

Multidisciplinary working

- Children with complex needs and their families require support from multiple agencies. Families can sometime get overwhelmed with multiplicity and duplication of input if these agencies work in isolation.
- Various professionals involved may represent public, private, or voluntary organizations. It is crucially important for various professionals, often working across different agencies, to work together in order to meet the family's needs in an effective and efficient manner (see 📖 p547).
- Multiagency support can be provided in the form of team around a child (TAC) model or by assembling multiagency teams or panels.

Advantages of multidisciplinary working

- Effective and efficient provision of services with improved quality of care.
- Better coordination with minimization of duplication of assessments and support, therefore increasing cost effectiveness.
- Beneficial for families by reducing the number of different agencies they have to deal with.
- Key worker or coordinator can provide easy point of access.
- Improving skills of professionals by working together and learning from each other, e.g. joint home visit by preschool teacher and various therapists.
- Increases patient and family's satisfaction.

Skills required for multidisciplinary team working

- Good communication skills.
- Willingness to work with others along with commitment to team process to help children and families.
- Ability to listen and see other's perspective.
- Have mutual respect and trust other team members.
- Understanding of partner agencies' working.

Key principles which underline successful multidisciplinary working

- General knowledge and understanding of the range of organizations and individuals working with children and young people.
- Knowledge and appreciation of common principles and procedures of joint working including those for consent, assessment, confidentiality, and information sharing.
- Clarity about individual roles along with respect and value for other's contribution.
- Effective communication with appropriate information sharing, avoiding jargon and abbreviations.
- Being proactive and assertive to be able to make significant contribution.
- Confidence to challenge situations by asking considered questions.
- Putting children and their families at the centre of decision-making process.
- Common language of terminology.

- Awareness of the partner agencies' policies and working practices.
- Co-location of services.
- Joint budgetary control if possible.

Potential disadvantages of multiagency working
- Lack of responsibility and accountability. This can be overcome by appointing a coordinator or key professional who can liaise with other professionals.
- Potential to confuse families and young people about whom to contact during times of specific needs.
- Time and resource intensive.

Barriers to effective multiagency working
- Poor communication and information sharing.
- Differences in organizational aims.
- Lack of support and commitment from senior management.
- Constant reorganization.
- Frequent staff turnover.
- Financial uncertainty.
- Different professional ideologies and agency cultures.

Example of a multidisciplinary team
See Fig. 2.2.

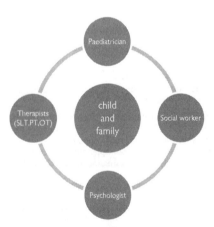

Fig. 2.2 Example of a multidisciplinary team.

Multidisciplinary team process
See Fig. 2.3.

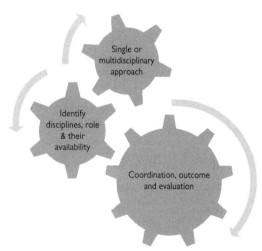

Fig. 2.3 Multidisciplinary team process.

Breaking bad news

Setting the scene

- Most senior person who knows the family best should give the news.
- Collect appropriate information, anticipate likely questions, and prepare answers.
- Make sure there is no interruption during consultation.
- Keep box of tissues, drinking water, etc. in the room.
- Sitting down, face-to-face conversation.
- Preferably with both parents present. Suggest inviting a relative or friend especially for single parents for support.

Consultation

- Introduce yourself if you are not already known, and address child by name.
- Establish what is already known to the family.
- Gently build up before delivering the bad news, e.g. 'As you are aware, Jack had a MRI scan of his brain. I am afraid it is not normal'.
- Avoid jargon and speak at a pace the family can understand.
- Be honest and straight to the point.
- Reassure them that everything that needs to be done is being done. Don't promise anything you are not sure you can deliver.
- Be sensitive to a parent's reaction.
- Provide plenty of time and opportunities for asking questions.
- Be willing to repeat information if necessary.
- Give clear plan of action and follow-up.
- Provide contact details to family for further questions if necessary.
- Offer to share information with the child or others involved in child's care.
- During a multidisciplinary assessment/briefing offer to speak to parents privately prior to joint meeting with other team members (see 📖 p23).

Follow-up

- Write to family to supplement verbal discussion.
- Offer a follow-up appointment to meet family.

Common scenarios—includes giving diagnosis of:

- CP (see 📖 p67).
- Autism (see 📖 p107).
- Developmental testing revealing global developmental delay (GDD) (see 📖 p117).
- Genetic investigations, e.g. *MECP2* mutation detection confirming Rett syndrome (see 📖 p405).
- Lab confirmation of an IMD (see 📖 p153) etc.

Effects of illness and disability on family

Causes of increased burden of illness and disability on families

- Better survival of extremely premature neonates and those born with birth defects.
- Early intervention with longer life span for some of the babies with treatments previously not offered, e.g. cardiac surgery for children with DS (see 📖 p387).
- Better awareness and early identification of conditions such as autism (see 📖 p107).
- More children with disabilities now living at home and attending mainstream schools.

Negative consequences of disability

A child's disability can affect the entire family's well-being by:
- Feelings of guilt, blame, and reduced self-esteem which may either lead to rejection or overprotection of the affected child.
- Limiting and interrupting family activities.
- Feeling of helplessness due to lack of information and awareness of service provisions.
- Consuming large majority of parental time, energy, and attention (see 📖 p371).
- Relative neglect of siblings and other family member's needs (see 📖 Care of siblings p32).
- Poor peer activities and cognitive development in siblings.
- Affecting family income due to parents taking time off or leaving jobs.
- It can be a source of parental emotional distress and mental health problems affecting relations and living arrangements (see 📖 p363)
- Social isolation from peers and neighbours due to perceived stigma attached to disability.

Positive effects of disability

Having a disabled child can be a unique family experience which may also:
- Enhance family cohesion and encourage links with community groups.
- Increase awareness of inner strength.

Minimizing the negative effects of disability

To achieve this, health professionals need to adopt a *family-centred approach* (see 📖 p18). Families caring for children with disabilities can be helped by:
- Addressing their (child and family's) complex medical, developmental, educational, social, emotional, recreational, and care needs.
- Informing families about the range of services required for a particular child (see 📖 p29).
- Arranging required services locally as far as possible.
- By understanding and supporting families through the grieving process (see 📖 p373).

Sources of support

- Acute and primary healthcare services to manage long-term conditions, e.g. children's community nurse (CCN (see 🕮 p545)), therapy services (see 🕮 Chapter 5), etc.
- Social services for financial support, respite, home adaptations (see 🕮 p514), etc.
- Education services for providing special education need provisions (see 🕮 p524).
- Voluntary organizations (see 🕮 p547).
- Parent support groups.

Further resources

Carers Trust: ☎ 0844 800 4361 🖰 http://www.carers.org
Sibs: ☎ 01535 645453 🖰 http://www.sibs.org.uk
Young Carer's Net c/o PRTC: 🖰 http://www.youngcarers.net

Providing information, support, and advice

There was no substitute for real people, written information is nice to have as a comfort factor, but you really get your information from people, talking face to face with them.

Parent with a child with learning disabilities

You could talk to her about anything, and she was really good. She knew people who could help you if you were stuck, or would say 'well, you could try this, or that, or something else'.

Parent of a child with learning disabilities

Living with a disabled child presents a number of challenges even for more resourceful and well-informed parents. It is a juggling act, balancing routine parenting tasks with treatment programmes and additional physical and emotional demands (see ☐ p27).

Adequate information is crucial:
- To understand the impact of disability on family life.
- To facilitate adjustment to disability.
- To empower parents—helps in coping and transitions.
- Non-directive information can be valuable during periods of crises.

Settings

Exchange of information can take place:
- In a multidisciplinary case conference.
- During home visit.
- At an outpatient/school clinic.
- During a hospital admission on the ward.
- Over the telephone or by email.
- In the form of a clinic letter.

Types of information

- New diagnosis: provide information about the condition, its complications, long-term outcome, etc.
- Information regarding various management options.
- About engaging other professionals for further assessment/support (see ☐ p23).
- About local and national support agencies, e.g. voluntary organizations and charities (Hemihelp for hemiplegia, Scope for CP (see ☐ p67), etc.).
- For support from statutory agencies (e.g. statutory assessment for special educational needs (SEN (see ☐ p524)), disability living allowance (DLA)).
- To inform about local parents support group, e.g. local DS groups for newly diagnosed child with DS (see ☐ p387).
- Internet-based resources, e.g. ERIC for incontinence (see ☐ p162).

Ways in which families receive information

- Personal communication with professionals:
  - Most frequent and highly valued mode of information.
  - Verbal information supported by written/printed material helps to reinforce the message delivered during consultation.
- Direct contact with other parents and voluntary organizations.

- Locally produced booklets (rather than general publications) are more relevant and better appreciated by families.

Advantages of appropriate and timely information

This enables parents to:
- Access suitable services and benefits.
- Enhance management of their child's condition and behaviour.
- Plan, prepare, and hence feel more in control.
- Link with support agencies to adjust emotionally to their child's disabilities and reduce feeling of isolation.

Type of support needed by families with complex needs children

Information

- About long-term outcome, treatment options, prognosis, and its impact on family life (see 🕮 p63).
- About condition-specific support groups via Contact a Family (CaF) directory (see 🕮 p579).
- Benefits, allowances, equipment, and details of local agencies (see 🕮 p514).

Education

- Acknowledgement and understanding of child's difficulties in educational setting while promoting inclusion. CCN (see 🕮 p545) and school nurses (see 🕮 p542) play a valuable role in support.
- Good ongoing liaison between parents, school, and health services.
- Identification and provision for special education needs—equipment, medications.
- Home teacher or home-school link worker for prolonged periods of absence secondary to illness (see 🕮 p534).
- Special school provisions and support from specialist advisory teachers if necessary, e.g. autism advisory teacher, specialist teacher for visual or hearing impaired.
- By providing transition programmes and specialized job training during teenage years (see 🕮 p171).

Financial support

- Allowances and benefits (see 🕮 Certification and Benefits p514).
- Home adaptation (see 🕮 p191).

Social and emotional support

- Directing parents and siblings to local support agencies and advocacy groups (see 🕮 p516) to share information and meet other families affected with similar condition (e.g. autism family support).
- Respite care including support for siblings and parents (see 🕮 Care of sibling p32).
- Support from extended family and friends.
- Psychological support from counsellors, family therapy (see 🕮 p373).
- Spiritual support from faith leaders.

Support for practical issues

- Good liaison between hospital and community teams for issues such as home oxygen, suction, specialized bed, mobilization devices, feeding pumps, etc.

- Training of parents and other carers for managing specialized procedures such as gastrostomy feeding, administering rescue medications such as buccal midazolam, managing Hickman line (see 📖 p18), etc.
- Details of continuing supplies such as oxygen, medications, and other consumables.
- Contact details of key worker, link professional, and other members of multiprofessional teams, arrangement of open access at local paediatric unit (see 📖 p20), etc.

Further resources

Contact a Family: ℅ http://www.cafamily.org.uk
National Parent Partnership Network: ℅ http://www.parentpartnership.org.uk
Parents for Inclusion: ℅ http://www.parentsforinclusion.org
Scope: ℅ http://www.scope.org.uk

Care of siblings

- Siblings share their culture, heritage, parents, and a whole host of environmental factors throughout their lives.
- Disability or a chronic illness in a child therefore is bound to have a significant and long-lasting impact on siblings.
- Siblings of children with disability react in different ways according to their age and understanding about their sibling's disability. Their resilience and adjustment to sibling disability is also influenced by factors affecting family and social environment.

Factors contributing to sibling adaptation to chronic illness or disability

- Socioeconomic status.
- Parental stress (see 📖 p371).
- Family cohesion (see 📖 p363).
- Consistent routines.

Emotions in siblings of disabled children

- Worry, fear, and anxiety.
- Embarrassment and shame.
- Jealousy, anger, resentment, and a sense of injustice.
- Isolation and loneliness, especially if sibling requires/receives significant amount of parental attention.
- A sense of loss and sadness.
- Increased levels of anxiety (see 📖 p354), depression (see 📖 p350), peer problems, and behavioural difficulties (see 📖 p340).

Positive attributes seen in siblings of a disabled child

- Often more caring, empathetic, and sensitive to others' needs.
- More responsible and tolerant behaviour with maturity and independence.

Signs of difficulty in coping with the situation

- Help should be sought if a sibling is:
  - Having difficulty with sleep (see 📖 p168) or appetite.
  - Avoiding the sibling.
  - Apathetic with low self-esteem.
  - Has behavioural difficulties (see 📖 p334).
- Siblings have specific needs that require attention at different stages of their lives.

Strategies which can help children cope with their sibling's disability

These include:
- Clear and factual information about child's disability to siblings (see 📖 p29).
- To acknowledge and appreciate sibling's emotions and feelings.
- Parents spending some quality time with siblings especially sharing activities which mean a lot to them.
- Appreciating and encouraging good qualities and behaviours in siblings (see 📖 p210).

- Providing siblings with their own personal space.
- Ask siblings if they would like to be involved in care-giving responsibilities appropriate to their abilities and respecting their wishes if they don't want to.
- Individual sibling support or combined family intervention programmes can be helpful in protecting their physical and emotional well-being (see 📖 p373).

Further resources

Carers Trust: 📞 0844 800 4361 🖰 http://www.carers.org
Sibs: 📞 01535 645453 🖰 http://www.sibs.org.uk
Young Carer's Net c/o PRTC: 🖰 http://www.youngcarers.net

Development

A stitch in time saves nine.

English proverb

Developmental assessment

A hundred years from now it will not matter what my bank account was, the sort of house I lived in or the kind of car I drove…but the world may be different because I was important in the life of a child.

Forest E. Witcraft

Identifying developmental delay

- Developmental delay can be picked up in two ways:
- Developmental screening.
- Developmental assessment.

Developmental screening

- Screening tests are used to identify children whose development is unknown or when there is a suspicion of developmental delay. Screening tests ask the question 'Is this normal? Yes/No'.
- Screening tests produce two outcomes:
  - 'Pass' (development is within normal limits).
  - 'Fail' (there is likely to be developmental delay).
- Screening tests carry a risk of false positives/negatives, either over- or underidentifying children with developmental delay.
- Screening tests can take the form of either:
- A questionnaire handed out to the parent/carer, or
- A checklist, i.e. ticking the milestones achieved by the child.
- Screening tests are carried out by HVs (see 🕮 p540), GPs, EYSENIT (see 🕮 p544), and professionals in primary care.
- The following tests are widely used:
  - The 'Ten Questions' test (widely used in developing countries).
  - 'Schedule of Growing Skills' (widely used in UK).
  - 'Denver Developmental Screening Test' (widely used outside the UK).

Developmental assessment

- Developmental assessments are used to answer the question 'At what level (i.e. mental age/developmental age) is this child functioning and why?'.
- Assessment is an in-depth evaluation of a child's abilities and is carried out by trained professionals such as developmental paediatricians, educational psychologists (see 🕮 p531), neuropsychologists (see 🕮 p212), neurologists, etc.
- Developmental assessment is usually part of a process of establishing developmental diagnosis.
- Developmental assessment gives a detailed understanding of a child's strengths, weaknesses, and attainment levels by providing developmental results in the following forms:
  - Percentiles.
  - Quotients.
  - Standard deviation (sd) or 'z' scores.
  - Age equivalent scores etc.
- The following tests are more widely used for developmental assessment by paediatricians, psychologists, and therapists:
  - Griffiths Mental Developmental Scales-Extended Revised (GMDS-ER).
  - Bayley Scales of Infant and Toddler Development-III.

Establishing developmental diagnosis

- ❶ In developmental assessment there is no place for 'spot' diagnoses.
- Diagnosis consists of not only observing what a child does but how he does it, the degree of maturity he shows.
- Developmental diagnosis should never be made on clinical impression alone, but should be based on:
  - History.
  - Examination.
  - Developmental assessment.
  - Clinical observations.
  - Special investigations, where relevant.
  - 'Interpretation' of all the above.

How does developmental assessment help us?

- Certain developmental profiles (see below) are suggestive of specific developmental disorders/diagnoses and hence help in formulating a diagnosis of developmental disorder/disability.
- Developmental profiles help our understanding of the child by providing the developmental age/mental age, strengths, and weaknesses.
- Guide our decision to undertake further investigations for delay/ disorder, e.g. if the results show a severe delay/deviation, you are more likely to consider investigations (see 📖 p123) vs if the results were to reveal mild delay.
- Results of assessments help in making appropriate referrals for therapeutic interventions, e.g. PT (see 📖 p176), OT (see 📖 p188), SLT (see 📖 p200), audiologists, psychologists, etc.
- Lead us in our referrals to educational/early intervention programmes (📖 p59).
- Help in assessing the impact of the interventions, programmes, and therapies offered to the child.
- Direct our decisions about educational placement/options (see 📖 p533 and p534) to be offered to the child.

Developmental profiles

Relative discrepancies in the percentile score from a mean of the 50th percentile by more than 2 sd or by comparison between the domains or over several assessments give valuable indication of the child's strengths, weaknesses, and rate of progress.

The following *developmental disorders* are more likely to produce *typical developmental profiles* on developmental testing, if there are no added comorbidities:

- Autism (see 📖 p107): very low scores in language (Lang) and social (PS) scales. Low scores in eye–hand coordination (EHC) and patchy abilities in practical reasoning (PR).
- Asperger syndrome (see 📖 p329): low in PS, average in Lang. Low in performance (Perf), EHC, and Loco if they are also dyspraxic.
- General learning disability (see 📖 p117): low scores (the degree depends on the severity of LD) across all skill areas, i.e. locomotor (Loco), PS, Lang, EHC, Perf, PR.
- Hearing impairment (see 📖 p296): low scores on Lang, PR, and PS subscales in items which are language dependent.

- Vision impairment (see 📖 p275): very low scores in EHC and Perf which are more vision dependent. Low scores in PS, Lang, and even PR, if autistic features.
- Developmental coordination disorder (see 📖 p136): low scores (depends on the severity of the disorder) in EHC, Perf, and Loco.
- Specific learning disability (see 📖 p145), e.g. dyspraxia: Lang good, low on EHC, Perf, and PR.
- Physical disability (see 📖 p67) e.g. CP, hypotonia: low in Loco, EHC, and Perf. Lang, PS, and PR are not affected to similar extent.

Cautions when using developmental tests

- Compare one's findings with the history given before reporting the results of developmental assessments.
- Shyness and failure to cooperate should not lead to hasty conclusions. In doubtful cases with unusual features, it is better to repeat the test after an interval.
- Important aspects such as the alertness, the rapidity with which tests are performed, the degree of the understanding displayed by the child, the interest shown in their surroundings, his/her personality are usually not recorded quantitatively by many developmental tests.
- Don't make 'predictions'! Mental subnormality can never be diagnosed on account of delay in any one skill such as sphincter control, locomotion, or speech. It can largely be eliminated by the normal or early development of speech. There are many variables, hence one cannot predict the effect that opportunity, education, personality, motivation, illness, injury, and care received will have on the development of the child.
- 'Milestones' are just milestones! It is wrong to say that a child should pass a certain milestone at a certain age. All one can say is that the further away from average he is in anything, the less likely he is to be normal.
- The maturity and quality of speech has the highest correlation of all aspects of behaviour with the child's later intelligence. Gross motor development with the age of sitting and walking has the lowest correlation with subsequent intelligence.

❶ Failure to present the tests correctly can affect the performance of the child and lead to fallacious results.

Principles of neurodevelopmental testing

Aims

- Ask yourself what are you really testing and why? Is the testing to screen the child's development so far or is it to assess and quantify the exact degree of developmental delay?
- This will help you to choose an appropriate developmental test, i.e. screening test or a detailed/diagnostic test to address the given question.

General advice on testing

- Speak slowly and clearly.
- Engage the child's cooperation.
- Do the test only. Do not engage in prolonged general discussion or chatting during the test.
- Attract the child's attention before asking a question.
- The test items are not toys. Put away each piece of equipment after testing, having only one item before the child at a time. Put the equipment, e.g. picture cards, in the correct order after finishing. (If you lose one test item, e.g. a piece of a form board, then a whole sequence of test items across a wide range of ages may be inaccessible!)
- Hygiene: clean the soiled test items with warm water and soap/ antiseptic solution. Follow local infection control guidance.
- Safety: watch children so that they do not put small beads in their mouth etc. Be careful on stairs. Children need to be supervised at all times.

Testing environment

- Most developmental tests can be administered in a variety of settings, e.g. clinic, home, school, nursery, etc.
- Testing room/adjoining corridor should be large enough to administer locomotor scales.
- The room should have adequate lighting, heating, and ventilation.
- There should not be any distractions, e.g. posters, on the walls or non-test items within view of the child during the test itself.
- Seating: there should be a table and chair of suitable height, i.e. the child's feet should be on the floor and the child is able to place elbows at right-angles and hands on the table surface.
- Additional equipment: paper, pencils, crayons, story books for different ages, and access to stairs may be needed in addition to the test items/ equipment.

Method of administration

Success comes when preparation meets opportunity.

                                                              Henry Hartman

- Follow the standardized procedure as mentioned in the administration manual/section.

- Practise the presentation of items in the way that was used to standardize the test. If the instructions are not followed exactly then the results of the developmental assessment would be unreliable and not comparable to the standardization norms in norm-referenced tests.
- Save time by administering all tests using the same equipment consecutively.
- Test sequence: generally use non-verbal items, e.g. form boards, before verbal items, e.g. comprehension questions. Also leave the locomotor scales to last as the child may not re-engage easily once he/she gets off the chair.
- Time taken to administer the test varies according to the skill of the examiner in selecting correct age range of items, ability to move efficiently between different scales to reach a basal/ceiling score, the child's concentration, cooperation, and ability.
- Do not hurry with the test.
▶ Refer to 'administration' instructions on regular basis.

Scoring

- Score each item marking '√' for 'pass' and more discrete '–' for 'fail'.
- Know the principles of scoring. Get the baseline and 'ceiling' for each scale before moving to the next scale/domain wherever possible.
- Be careful in transferring and calculating the scores. Inaccuracy unsurprisingly leads to false interpretation and a wasted opportunity to help the child.
❶ Re-check if scores are contradictory to the clinical picture.
- Add the scores correctly for the test used to get 'RAW scores' for each scale.
- Obtain relevant standard scores, e.g. 'percentiles', 'z-scores', 'age equivalent/mental/developmental age', etc.
- The same record book may be used for reassessment of the same child at a later date, using a different coloured pen, to demonstrate new skills or regression.

Interpretation

All human knowledge takes the form of interpretation. All meanings, we know, depend on the key of interpretation.

George Elliot

❶ Do not interpret the results in isolation.
- Take all the history, parental/school concerns, your general observations, the child's interaction and behaviour into consideration before you draw conclusions. There is more to developmental testing than meets the eye. You could gain a great deal of information from testing situation from:
  • A=Attention, alertness.
  • B=Behaviours and mannerisms.
  • C=Cooperation/refusal, Concentration.
  • D=Dysmorphism, Disabilities.
  • E=Eye contact, Exploratory behaviour.

- F=Family interaction with primary carer.
- G=General aspects, e.g. spontaneous speech, articulation, etc.
- Relative discrepancies in the percentile score from a mean of the 50th percentile by >1 sd or by comparison between the subscales gives an indication of the *child's strengths, weaknesses, and profile*.
- Interpretation of the results obtained using item analysis of each scale - the *'construct model'* of the test, e.g. in GMDS-ER test:
  - *Practical reasoning* subscale would give information about moral/ social/everyday reasoning, sequential reasoning, analogical reasoning, concept formation, general cognitive functioning (memory, attention, learned knowledge).
  - *Locomotor subscale* would give information on power, strength, agility, depth perception, gross visuomotor coordination, balance, etc.
- Each developmental disorder can create a specific profile or signature on developmental assessment (see 📖 pp37–8).

Conclusions

In addition to the uses of developmental screening (see 📖 p37), detailed neurodevelopmental assessments help us by:

- Providing corroborative evidence for 'developmental diagnosis'.
- Identifying comorbidities/hidden disabilities, e.g. a child assessed for language delay could also show moderate/severe coordination difficulties.
- Giving an opportunity to identify additional features, e.g. sensory processing disorder, hypermobility, neurocutaneous markers, asymmetric weakness, hemihypertrophy, dysmorphic features, involuntary movements, etc.
- Alerting us to the need for further investigation of the child's circumstances when results are 'odd' or inconsistent, i.e. when profile/ scores contradict the history or clinical picture.

Tips for 'real-world' developmental assessments

Starting points

- Having some information/knowledge about age-appropriate and current TV programmes, fads, toys, computer games, music, books, etc. will help you engage the child and provide conversational content.
- Be prepared to talk about school likes/dislikes, friendships, 'sleep overs', whether they are invited to play or parties, etc.
- Humour can be helpful.
- Consider having age-appropriate toy selection, drawing materials, puzzles, blocks, toy animals, etc. available to occupy child whilst consulting parent/carer so as only to use test equipment for assessment.
- Personally collect the child and parent from the waiting area. Watch the gait, disposition, parent–child interaction, etc.
- Warm up! Begin by introducing yourself to parent/carer, listen to their concerns/questions, while the child warms up to the new environment.
- Sighting shot! Place a box of 10 bricks on the table. While introductions are going on, the child might start exploring, manipulating, building with the bricks. You'll get an idea of where the child's development is and help you decide which tests items you need to administer further.

Involving the child

- Introduce yourself to the child: Say 'We are going to play some games, which you will enjoy. You will find some games easy and some difficult. Just do your best'.
- Establish rapport and maintain a play-like rapport. Smile. Compliment the child. Be opportunistic.
- Mind your language! Don't give a choice to the child by saying 'Would you like to…' or 'Can you do this for me?'. Instead say 'Now it's your turn to do this and this'.
- Encourage. Praise the efforts of the child by saying 'keep going', 'good try', 'great effort', etc. But do not say whether their answer is right or wrong, as this could influence their score on a subsequent item.
- Sustain the child's attention by knowing your presentation well. Direct them to the equipment or test items you want them to play with. An appropriate testing environment (p39) will help.
- If the child loses concentration or appears tired then move on to different scales or test items or give them a short break/food/drink accordingly. Do not show your dissatisfaction with the child's response.
- Administer tests or items that utilize his/her curiosity or interest of the moment.
- Observe, observe, observe! OWL approach = Observe, Wait, Listen. Observe for any unusual behaviours, mannerisms, carer–child interaction, engaged–withdrawn, impulsivity, overactivity, social interaction/disinhibition, etc. Listen for any spontaneous speech.

❶ Beware of the parent talking 'over' or for the child.

Involving parents/carers
- Always begin by asking parents what their 'concerns' are (see below
  📖 p43).
- Parents should then sit out of the child's view.
- Involve them only where necessary, i.e. on the staircase/steps etc.
- If the child refuses to attempt a number of items repeatedly, then
  ask the parent/carer to administer those items according to your
  instructions.

Simple tests
- Goodenough–Harris 'Draw a man test' (general mental level 3–15
  years, standardized in the 1980s).
- Verbal fluency, e.g. test by number of different types of 'food' child
  could say in 60 seconds; mean:
  - 6 years = 10 (sd 3).
  - 8 years = 11 (sd 3).
  - 10 years = 14 (sd 2).
  - 12 years+ (approximate adult levels) = 18 (sd 4).
- Describe a picture (note: naming, narrative, perception, articulation).
- Three-part instruction (most can manage by 4 years).
- Literacy/numeracy: check reading, reading comprehension, spelling,
  times tables, addition/subtraction, and writing. Levels of expected
  attainment strongly dependent upon age and quality of education.
- Copying shapes, e.g. Aston Index Test.
- Read analogue clock face, left–right, and other person left–right
  orientation.
- General screening questionnaires, e.g. 'Strengths and Difficulties'.
- Develop selection of simple tests that can be applied across age bands
  (i.e. describe a picture), and stick with it; if given to enough children in
  a consistent fashion you will in time develop a sense of what a broadly
  'average' performance is for a given age.

Useful general questions
- How much do you think the child is behind other children in
  development?
- What do you think is the child's biggest problem?
- Have I seen a fair picture of what the child can do?
- How does he/she spend her time/interests/concentration?
- Does the child pretend or show imagination/humour? Could you give
  an example?

Gross motor milestones

Assessment of a child's gross motor skills gives us information about his/her gross body coordination, gross visual-motor coordination, strength, agility, flexibility, and balance (Table 3.1).

Table 3.1 Gross motor milestones. These milestones should only be used as guide to average development. There can be wide variation within normal development. These milestones do not replace the role of detailed 'neurodevelopmental testing' which should be undertaken if there are concerns regarding a child's development or behaviour.

3 months	Supine: turns head side to side. Brings hands to midline. Prone: forearm prop, face vertical. Pull to sit: minimal head lag.
6 months	Rolls prone to supine. Prone: pushes up on extended arms. Sitting (5–9 months).
9 months	Rolls supine to prone. Crawls on hands and knees. Pull to stand at support.
1 year	Cruises at support. Walk (average 13 months). Stairs: crawls up.
2 years	Run: start, stop. Kick: walks into ball. Stairs: walks up and down, 2 feet to a step. Jump. Climb up onto chair. Throw: ball over arm.
3 years	Kick: with force. Run: turn around obstacles. Pedal tricycle. Stairs: walks up with alternating feet, down 2 feet to a step. Stand on 1 leg: momentarily. Stand and walk on tiptoe. Catch: large ball on extended arms.
4 years	Stairs: Walk or run up and down with alternating feet. Stand on 1 leg: 3–5 seconds. Hop. Throw and catch: large ball, bounced ball to/from another person. Start using bat.

Table 3.1 (Continued)

5 years	Stand on 1 leg: 8–10 seconds. Heel–toe walk along line. Throw and catch—large ball: throw, catch, and bounce to self.
6 years	Stand on 1 leg: 15–20 seconds. Ride bicycle. Throw and catch—tennis ball: throw, catch, and bounce to self.
7 years	Stand on one leg: 20–25 seconds. Throw and catch: 1 hand.
8 years	Stand on 1 leg: 25–30 seconds.

Fine motor milestones

- Fine motor skills are patterns which include reach, grasp, carry, and voluntary release, as well as more complex skils of in-hand manipulation, form perception, and bilateral coordination.
- The development of fine motor skills depends on adequate postural functions and sufficient visual-perceptual and cognitive development.
- There is a wide variation within/to normal range of fine motor skills acquisition.
  (Table 3.2).

Table 3.2 Fine motor milestones. These milestones should only be used as guide to average development. These milestones do not replace the role of detailed 'neurodevelopmental testing' which should be undertaken if there are concerns regarding a child's development or behaviour.

0–3 months	Focuses eyes, follows faces/objects moved from side towards midline.
	Beginning to open hands occasionally.
	Extensor movements of limbs cause fingers and toes to fan out.
3–6 months	More visually alert, regard for own hands when lying supine.
	Brings hands into midline over chest or chin.
	Clasps and unclasps hands, presses palms together.
	Holds rattle for few moments, can visually regard rattle at same time as holding/moving it.
6–9 months	Eyes move in unison to follows activities across room.
	Purposeful alertness.
	Grasp toys/objects within 15–30cm using palmar grasp, passes toy from one hand to another.
9–12 months	Manipulates toy by passing from hand to hand and turning over.
	Points with index finger at distant objects.
	Picks small objects up between index and thumb (inferior pincer grasp).
	Releases toy by dropping—not yet placing down voluntarily.
12–18 months	Picks up small object between tip of index finger and thumb (pincer grasp).
	Uses both hands freely but hand preference emerging .
	Holds 1 cube in each hand with tripod grasp. Bangs cubes together. Build tower of 2 cubes after demonstration.
18–24 months	Spontaneous and fro scribble with either hand holding crayon/pencil in a fisted grasp, shoulder stabilized while arm moves as a unit.
	Builds tower of 2–3 cubes.
	Points with index finger to emphasize interest or demand objects out of reach, turns pages of book several pages at a time.
	Hand preference establishing.

Table 3.2 (Continued)

24–36 months	Builds tower of 6–10 cubes.
	Spontaneous circular scribble, holding pencil proximally with all fingers and thumb pointing downwards towards tip of pencil (digital pronate grasp), elbow stabilized while forearm moves as a unit, imitates vertical line, horizontal line, copies circle.
	Picks up tiny objects accurately and quickly and places down neatly with increasing skill.
	Turns pages of book singly, threads large wooden beads on a shoelace, cuts with toy scissors.
3–4 years	Builds a bridge of 3 cubes from a model using 2 hands. Builds tower of 10 or more cubes. Builds 3 steps with 6 cubes after demonstration.
	Holds pencil in preferred hand, grasped proximally between first 2 fingers and thumb (static tripod grasp), wrist joint stabilized while hand moves as a unit. Copies a cross (+) and draws a person with head and 3–4 body parts.
4–5 years	Builds 3 steps with 6 cubes from a model; sometimes 4 steps from 10 cubes.
	Holds pencil distally between first 2 fingers and thumb with precise opposition of pads of thumb, index, and middle fingers (dynamic tripod grasp) with metacarpophalangeal joints stabilized during proximal interphalangeal movements. Draws person with head, trunk, and legs, usually arms and fingers.
	Imitates thumb touching each finger with either hand.
5–6 years	Dynamic tripod grasp. Copies square, then a triangle, copies several letters and writes a few letters spontaneously, draws a person with head, trunk, legs, arms, and features.
	Picks up and replaces tiny objects carefully.
6–8 years	Copies a diamond and other more complex and unfamiliar shapes.
	Uses dominant hand while stabilizing with non-dominant hand. Posts coins into a slot quickly and accurately.
	Threads beads onto a string quickly and accurately using in-hand manipulation to turn beads in fingertips.

Development of vision/visual milestones

- The first few years of life are crucial for visual development.
- Adequate stimulation of both eyes in the first 6–8 years of life is essential to achieve normal visual acuity as adults.
- Visual deprivation of one or both eyes from any reversible cause can result in amblyopia (lazy eye).

The various stages of visual development are listed in Table 3.3.

Table 3.3 Stages of visual development

0–3 months	Briefly holds gaze. Takes interest (stares) in surroundings, Blinks at bright lights. Tracks vertically and horizontally. Makes eye contact at 6–8 weeks, fixes on mother's face.
3–6 months	Follows adults or moving objects with eyes across. midline. Observes own hands face. Displays interest in human faces. Briefly fixes and reaches for small objects.
7–12 months	Recognizes objects at home, tracks across the room. Interested in pictures, inspects toys, enjoys hide-and-seek (recognizes partially hidden objects). Responds to smiles and voices, develops stranger anxiety.
1–1½ years	Enjoys picture books and points to pictures. Holds objects close to eyes to inspect.
2–3 years	Recognizes faces in photographs. Begins to inspect objects without touching them. Likes to watch moving objects, such as wheels on toy vehicle. Watches and imitates other children. 'Reads' pictures in books.
3–4 years	Copies patterns. Recognition of colours. Can close eyes on request and may be able to wink.
4–5 years	Draws recognizable person and house and names pictures. Uses eyes and hands together with increasing skill. Moves and rolls eyes expressively. Can place small objects into small openings. Demonstrates visual interest in new objects.

Personal–social milestones

Personal–social skill can gives us an insight into child's communicative intent, interpersonal skills, concept of self, self-care skills and domestic skills (Table 3.4).

Table 3.4 Personal–social milestones. These milestones should only be used as guide to average development. These milestones do not replace the role of detailed 'neurodevelopmental testing' which should be undertaken if there are concerns regarding a child's development or behaviour.

0–3 months	Recognize mother. Social smile. Follows a moving person at close distance. Brings hand to mouth.
3–6 months	Spontaneous smile. Enjoy 'to and fro' communication with sounds. Recognizes primary caregivers. Greets with squeals and vocalizations. Holds bottle briefly.
6–9 months	Joint attention, i.e. looks at an object with parent. Gaze monitoring, i.e. follows adult's gaze with own. Separation anxiety emerging. Vocalizes to seek attention. Holds own bottle. Finger feeds. Can pull hat off.
9–12 months	'Protoimperative pointing' established, i.e. pointing to ask for an object. Separation anxiety established. Put arms up to be picked up. Recognizes/responds own name. Recognizes self in a mirror. Plays 'peek-a-boo'. Gives affection. Can wave 'bye-bye'. Interested in watching other children. Drinks from an open cup held to lips.
12–18 months	'Solitary play', i.e. play away from caregiver for a short while. 'Functional play' established, i.e. child's manipulations become object specific (vs indiscriminate banging). 'Protodeclarative pointing', i.e. use index finger to indicate an object of interest to others. Enjoys sharing a book with parent/carer. Responds to simple commands, e.g. 'Give me the spoon'. Uses spoon with some spilling. Picks up and drinks from a lidded cup. Remove sock/shoe or a garment.

Table 3.4 (Continued)

18–24 months	'Pretend play' established, e.g. 'pat-a-cake'.
	'Symbolic play' emerging.
	Possessive of own toys. Can't share. Parallel play.
	Helps put toys away on request.
	Imitates household chores.
	Indicates toilet needs.
	Helps with dressing, i.e. put arms and legs through.
	Uses spoon well.
	Drinks from an open cup, if held.
	Sucks through a straw.
24–30 months	Beginning to share and joins others briefly in play.
	Symbolic play established, e.g. rides a broomstick for a horse.
	Knows gender.
	Participates in simple group activities.
	Cooperative play emerging.
	Uses fork and spoon well.
	Washes hands and dries them.
	Pulls off a T-shirt.
30–36 months	Cooperative play emerging, i.e. taking turns.
	Starts to share.
	Knows own age.
	Toilet trained.
	Wears dress, but needs help with buttons and zips.
	Can finish a meal unaided if food is cut 'bite-sized'.
	Brush teeth with assistance.
3–4 years	'Imaginative play', i.e. child's imagination doing the work vs design and function of the toy, e.g. play with dolls.
	Can share without prompts.
	Independent with toilets.
	Can wash hands and face.
	Can unbutton and then learns to button up.
	Puts shoes on without laces.
4–5 years	Group play, i.e. joins in play with other children.
	Can give family name.
	Can brush teeth without assistance.
	Can put on an overcoat or cardigan.
	Can fasten buckle of a shoe.
5–6 years	Has a special playmate. Chooses own friends.
	Apologizes for mistakes.
	Can choose own clothes, i.e. for summer/winter etc.
	Can take part in competitive games.
	Knows address.
	Can spread with knife.
	Can wash hands and face, and dry them with no help.

Table 3.4 (Continued)

6–7 years	Knows birthday—date, month, and year.
	Knows 'full' address.
	Can play board games with rules.
	Can distinguish fantasy from reality.
	Can dress and undress completely.
	Can lay a table with some supervision.
7–8 years	Learns from mistakes.
	Can do homework on own.
	Helps others/younger children.
	Can delay gratification and awaits his/her own turn.
	Can shampoo hair, have bath or shower on own.
	Can lay a table completely without supervision.
	Can tie shoelaces.

Speech and language milestones

Assessment of SAL skills gives us information about a child's receptive language, expressive language, linguistic and applied knowledge, verbal reasoning, auditory memory, and conceptualization (Table 3.5).

Table 3.5 Speech and language milestones. These milestones should only be used as guide to average development. These milestones do not replace the role of detailed 'neurodevelopmental testing' which should be undertaken if there are concerns regarding a child's development or behaviour.

0–3 months	Crying.
3–6 months	Cooing and gurgling.
6–9 months	Double syllable babble. Reaches up to be picked up and to request.
9–12 months	Waves and claps. Babble conversations. Jargon-like babble. Responds to 'no' and 'name'. Context dependent comprehension.
12–18 months	Increasing comprehension of everyday words. First early words emerge—up to 20.
18–24 months	Points to show/request. Comprehension of many single words—nouns and verbs. Words increase up to 50.
2 years	50 words some 2-word phrases. Words usually contain /m p b t d n/ sounds. Often word endings are omitted.
2.6 years	3–4 word sentences. Understood by familiar adults, lots of sound simplifications, especially with 'f' 's' 'sh' 'ch' sounds.
3 years	Sentences of 5–6 words, use of some pronouns (me, he, she). Understands basic concepts of big/little, on/under. Understood most of time by strangers. Begins to ask 'why' questions. Can tell a story. Has a vocabulary of nearly 1000 words. Beginning to understand 'yesterday/tomorrow'.
4 years	Sentences fluent, able to converse and explain at simple level. Can talk about things they have done and will do. Can tell stories in their play. Can still make errors especially with past tense, e.g. falled.

Table 3.5 (Continued)

	Understands more 'time' words (morning, afternoon).
	Speech intelligible but may be errors with consonant blends (sp bl gr) and sh/ch.
5 years	Full adult grammar.
	Good reciprocal conversation and clear speech with only minor errors not affecting intelligibility.
6 years	Errors can still be evident with 'th', 'r', 's' or 'z'.
	Uses preposition 'above'.
	Begins to master exceptions to grammatical rules.
	Understands passive tense.
	Can give directions.
	Asks/answers factual and inferential questions.
	Answers complex how, who, why, when questions.
	Starts and takes turns in conversations.
7 years	Can listen for sustained periods of time.
	Follows complex directions/series of instructions without need for repetition.
	Uses language to problem solve and talk about feelings.
	Rephrases statements if not understood.
	Asks for clarification if doesn't understand.
8 years	Begins to understand and use idioms.
	Uses clear and subject related vocabulary.
	Explains what has been learned.
	Gives synonyms and categories in word definitions.
	Begins to understand jokes and riddles based on sound similarities.

Cognition milestones

- Assessment of a child's 'cognition' involves looking into the child's thinking, understanding of concepts, problem-solving, (moral/everyday/social) reasoning, and remembering (memory and learnt knowledge) skills (Table 3.6).
- The way the child thinks in each stage is different. The process of development is marked by a gradual decrease in egocentrism (being able to see only one aspect of a situation). The child constructs knowledge through actions then later mental actions (operations).
- Biological adaptation: cognition is a form of adaptation to the environment through two complementary processes:
  - Assimilation (incorporating new knowledge into existing) and
  - Accommodation (changing cognitive structures).
- Broadly, stages of cognitive development are as follows:
  - Object permanence.
  - Capacity for representation.
  - Symbolic language (signs/numbers/letters).
  - Decrease in egocentricity.
  - Formal operations (12 years onwards): ability to think about thinking—metacognitive activity.

Table 3.6 Cognition milestones. These milestones should only be used as guide to average development. These milestones do not replace the role of detailed 'neurodevelopmental testing' which should be undertaken if there are concerns regarding a child's development or behaviour.

0–3 months	Recognizes mother. Grasps rattle when given. Looks at a toy on the table. Visually explores environment.
3–6 months	Shows interest in toy. Grasps a toy. Shakes rattle. Passes toy from hand to hand.
6–9 months	Finds toy hidden under a cup. Manipulates 2 objects or bricks at once. Tears/crumples a tissue paper. Interested in a toy car. Casting, i.e. throws objects to the floor.
9–12 months	Holds pencil and makes random marks on paper. Plays with a brick box, takes lid off/bricks out. Unwraps toy under a cloth. Interested in pictures in a book. Can complete single-piece form board. Responds to simple commands, e.g. 'Give me the fork'.

Table 3.6 (Continued)

12–18 months	Knows function of objects, e.g. comb for hair, spoon to eat, etc.
	Can replace bricks back into the box and put lid on.
	Can complete 2-circle form board.
	Can pull cloth or a string to get a toy.
	Enjoys looking through a book.
18–24 months	Can complete a 3-shape form board.
	Can complete a shape form board rotated.
	Can draw horizontal and vertical stroke with pencil.
	Can open a screw toy.
	Can make a tower of 5–7 bricks.
24–30 months	Matches objects to appropriate pictures.
	Matches colours and shapes.
	Can repeat single digits on request.
	Can compare sizes, i.e. big and small.
	Points to pictures in a book.
30–36 months	Can count up to 4 correctly.
	Can compare 2 lines for length.
	Can compare 2 brick towers for height.
	Can talk about what he/she did.
36–48 months	Can draw a 3–4-part person.
	Can follow a 3-step command.
	Can count up to 10 correctly.
	Moral reasoning e.g. 'Is it right or wrong to hit someone?' answers correctly.
	Uses 'why' and 'how' questions.
	Matches some colours.
4–5 years	Can draw a 7–8-part person.
	Can count correctly up to 15.
	Social reasoning emerging, e.g. 'Which costs more money, a watch or a drink?' answers correctly.
	Knows 4–6 colours.
	Knows 1 or 2 parts of his/her address.
	Understand functional concepts, e.g. use of appliances.
	Understands concept of time, i.e. past/present.
5–6 years	Can draw a 10–12-part person.
	Can count backwards from 10.
	Count up to 30.
	Knows 10 colours.

Table 3.6 (Continued)

	Knows most sounds/letters.
	Can explain about an incident at school.
	Knows number of fingers on both hands put together.
	Can name some days of the week.
	Understands seasons.
6–7 years	Can do single digit addition and subtraction.
	Begins to spell out words/read few sentences.
	Begins to read words.
	Can count backwards from 15.
	Can name all the days of the week in correct order.
	Knows 'directions' and 'sides of a body', e.g. left hand/ right leg.
7–8 years	Can count backwards from 30.
	Can read sentences (without unusual words) more fluently.
	Can repeat 5 digits, e.g. 4–7–1–9–6 forward on request.
	Can repeat 3 digits backwards, e.g. 5–2–9, answer 9–2–5.
	Can arrange 4–5 pictures in correct sequence and tell a story.
	Can draw a person or house with use of creativity and imagination.

Warning signs: 'red flags' in child development

See Table 3.7.

Table 3.7 'Red flags' in child development. More than 1 feature in any aspect of child development should raise concern.

Gross motor development	Has a floppy or limp body posture compared to other children of the same age.
	Has stiffness in arms and/or legs and paucity of movements.
	Uses 1 side of body in preference to the other, before 1 year of age.
	Is very clumsy or poorly coordinated when compared with other children of the same age, e.g. gait is wide or dyskinetic.
	Difficulties in keeping balance while sitting, walking, playing, or frequent falling.
Fine motor and vision development	Turns, tilts or holds head in unusual position when trying to look at or follow an object.
	Seems to have difficulty finding or picking up small objects dropped on the floor (after the age of 12 months) or lacking pincer grip. Has tremor.
	Rubs eyes frequently.
	Eyes appear to be crossed or turned in/out.
	Closes 1 eye when trying to look at distant objects.
	Brings objects too close to eyes to see 1 or both eyes/pupils appear abnormal in size.
	Difficulty in manipulating small objects after 3 years of age.
Hearing and language development	Doesn't startle to loud noises or resists them with hands over ears.
	Ears appear small or deformed.
	Talks in a very loud or very soft voice.
	Seems to have difficulty responding when called from across the room.
	Does not make sounds in response to others after 12 months.
	Turns body so that the same ear is always turned toward sound.
	Has difficulty understanding simple sentences after once he/she has turned 3 years of age.
	Fails to develop sounds or words that would be appropriate at his/her age.
	Dribbles excessively. Cannot chew or chokes on food or drink.

Table 3.7 (Continued)

Social interaction and communication development	Avoids or rarely makes appropriate eye contact with others.
	Lack of reciprocal or social smile.
	Inability to communicate using non-verbal behaviours, e.g. lack of finger pointing, facial expressions, body language, gestures, eye-pointing, waving bye-bye, etc.
	Poor attention, impulsivity or inability to stay focused on an activity.
	Focuses on unusual objects for long periods of time or observes them from unusual angles; enjoys this more than interacting with other children/adults. Does not seek love and approval from a caregiver or parent.
	Lack of sharing interest or enjoyment with others, prefers to play alone. Withdraws, 'in a world of his own'.
	Does not respond to his/her name being called. Lack of social anticipation.
	Gets unusually frustrated when trying to do simple tasks that most children of the same age can do. Difficulty in seeing a coherent whole, rather notices small fragmentary features in a picture or puzzle.
	Dislikes hugs, kisses, cuddles, and close physical contact. Misjudges personal space.
	Unusual prosody (little variation in tone, intonation or pitch, rhythm, voice quality).
Behaviour/personality development	Unusual motor mannerisms, e.g. hand flapping, twisting, spinning, stares into space, rocking body, tip-toeing, etc.
	Restricted and repetitive range of interests and activities e.g. playing with a single toy or part of a toy.
	Difficulty to cope with change or abnormal reaction to change in routine, especially if a minor change.
	Shows aggressive behaviors, hyperactive, uncooperative, or oppositional.
	Displays temper tantrums or violent behaviours on a daily basis.
	The child shows unusual attachments to toys, objects, or parts of objects and does not play with the toys in a way they are intended or designed.
	Child spends a lot of time lining things up or putting things in a particular order.

Early Intervention

Early intervention maximizes the opportunity for the child to achieve his/her potential. Subsequent to the developmental diagnosis, a paediatrician can refer a child to a variety of different resources with the following aims:
- Involve appropriate therapy services specifically tailored to meet the needs of the child.
- Provide information, support, and advice to families to enhance the child's development.

The resources/services can include any number of the following:
- Physiotherapy (see 📖 p176).
- Postural management services (see 📖 p183).
- Occupational therapy (see 📖 p188).
- Speech and language therapy (see 📖 p200).
- Psychology.
- Counselling services (see 📖 p373).
- SEN programmes (see 📖 p524).
- Audiology (see 📖 p296).
- Ophthalmology and orthoptics (see 📖 p271).
- Assistive technology (see 📖 p186 and p225) (wheelchair, keyboard, etc.).
- Community nursing (see 📖 p545).
- Dietician and nutritionists (see 📖 p87).
- Respite services.
- Social services for benefits, allowances, housing adaptations (see 📖 p514).
- Orthopaedic services (gait analysis, spasticity/dystonia treatment/botulinum toxin, etc. (see Chapter 11 📖 p410)).
- Dentist (see 📖 p165).

Why is an Early Intervention Programme important?

Early intervention is important for various reasons:
- Early enablement has better results/outcome when compared to later intervention.
- Sometimes a delay in one area (e.g. vision) can affect other developmental areas (e.g. gross and fine motor coordination, social interactions, etc.).
- Late/inadequate intervention can result in poor self-esteem, avoidance of learning opportunities, educational difficulties, difficulties with integration into mainstream school/society, etc. Early intervention could aid the development of good self-esteem.

Early Support Programme

- The Early Support Programme is a UK government funded programme for the families and carers of disabled children under 5 years of age.
- The programme allows families to coordinate the support they receive from health, education, and social care professionals and organizations via a 'key worker' (see 📖 p23).
- The key worker could be someone who already works with the child, such as a HV (see 📖 p540), EYSENIT (see 📖 p544), or SW (see 📖 p546).
- The programme offers *training courses* for parents and families.
- Through the programme families receive a *'family pack'*. This pack contains or could be a resource to carry:
  • Information on child's disability, medical history, dietary needs, etc.
  • Record of the child's progress.
  • Copies of any letters or details of any assessments the child has had.
  • Record of professional contacts, important numbers, referrals, etc.
  • Section to write notes about what happened at each meeting.
  • Booklets explaining childcare, financial help, e.g. DLA, education/ health/social services, useful contacts and organizations.
- Moreover there are *downloadable packs/journals* on the following conditions (see weblink under Further resources):
  • ASDs (see 📖 p107).
  • CP (see 📖 p67).
  • Deafness (see 📖 p296).
  • DS (see 📖 p387).
  • If your child has a rare condition.
  • Learning disabilities (see 📖 p117).
  • Multisensory impairment (see 📖 p278).
  • Speech and language difficulties (see 📖 p200).
  • Visual impairment (see 📖 p275).
  • When your child has no diagnosis.
- The Early Support pack:
  • Focuses on what a child can do.
  • Facilitates interagency coordination of services.
  • Provides better assessments of families and children.
  • Improves communication between families and services.

Further resources

Directgov—Caring for a disabled child: ℘ http://www.direct.gov.uk/en/ CaringForSomeone/CaringForADisabledChild/index.htm
NHS Choices: ℘ http://www.nhs.uk

Neurodevelopmental disorders

It is the rough road that leads to the height of greatness.

Seneca, 5 BC–65 AD

Introduction to neurodisability

Neurodevelopmental disorders are conditions involving the developing nervous system that have or are likely to have an impact on the future course of the child's development.

The field of neurodisability has made massive progress in the last two decades. This progress is due to many factors.

Firstly, there has been a change in the attitude and approaches to child hood disability. In the past the 'medical model' to disability was predominant and the 'focus' was to treat the diseases. Now these disorders are addressed by multidisciplinary and multiprofessional teams. Hence children and families have access to a much broader range of interventions in all dimensions of health, i.e. holistic care.

Secondly, services are increasingly becoming 'child and family centred'. Families of children with disability are being encouraged to participate actively in their child's enablement plan. Professionals now talk in terms of 'development goals' rather than medical goals. The physical, social, psychological, educational, emotional, and financial needs of the entire family are discussed and appropriate information, support, and advice is provided.

Moreover, changes in legislation such as the Disability Discrimination Act and the 'Every Disabled Child Matters' campaign have played a part by increasing awareness and accessibility for these children.

Furthermore, advances in neurosciences have shown us that the brain is 'plastic' and that the activity can influence the organization of the brain. The studies in adults have demonstrated brain plasticity and provided us with evidence for efficacy of CIMT (constraint-induced movement therapy), treadmill training, robotic training, neuromuscular stimulation, training in virtual environments, etc.

Adoption of evidence-based medicine in childhood disability is gradually changing the repertoire of interventions offered to children. Many therapists and professionals are gaining postgraduate degrees or diplomas in childhood disability and all of this is driving up the quality of care provided.

Guidance from institutes such as the National Institute for Health and Clinical Excellence (NICE) on conditions like epilepsy, ADHD, and ASD are influencing the availability of resources to manage these conditions. Audits and continuing professional development are improving the overall standard of care for children with neurodevelopmental disorders.

In addition to this, the spectacular advances in neurosciences have furthered our knowledge and understanding of these conditions. Risk genes for complex neurodevelopmental disorders are being identified. Advances in pharmacokinetics has lead to increased availability of medications for treating seizures, hyperactivity, spasticity, sleep disorders, depression, movement disorders, etc.

Spectacular technological advances have helped in developments of 'intelligent aids'. Assistive devices are helping to overcome functional impairments and enable these children to participate in daily activities, e.g. accessing computers, communication, independent feeding, living skills, mobility, postural stability, nutrition, etc.

ICF-CY and application of ICF model to children with disability

What is ICF-CY?

- ICF-CY stands for 'International Classification of Functioning, Disability and Health for Children and Youth'. It has been derived from the World Health Organization's (WHO) International Classification of Functioning, Disability and Health (ICF).
- ICF is a framework designed to record the characteristics of the developing child and the influence 'environment' and 'personal' factors have on the child's activities, participation, and engagement in life.

Components of ICF-CY framework

Body structure

Describes the various structures and systems of body with different codes for each, e.g. CNS (spastic quadriplegia), GI (unsafe swallow), eyes (microphthalmia), inner ear (damaged hair cells in cochlea), etc.

Body functions

Includes physiological and psychological functions, e.g. movements, speech, hearing, vision, attention, impulsivity, etc.

Activity (functional)

- Strengths: are activities of daily living (ADL) that child can do, e.g. feeding, dressing, walking, toileting, bathing, preparing meals, listening to music, playing games, watching TV, typing on keyboard, reading a book, communicating with a friend on Skype/text/email, etc.
- Weaknesses: e.g. inability to walk more than 30m, difficulty in writing with pen/pencil, poor articulation of speech, impulsive, attention span of 10–15min, poor verbal communication, difficulty in comprehending hence information has to be repeated and given in smaller chunks.

Participation

- *Facilitators:* includes examples of child's engagement and involvement in the local community, e.g. going to local church with family, visiting library with a family friend, going to shopping with neighbours, going to watch a play or film with grandparents, helping in the local community shop, etc.
- *Barriers:* includes, e.g. missing a film because of a seizure, local library prevents admission because of vocal tics, library does not lend audio books for more than a week and has penalties for being late, no access to after-care clubs as lack of trained supervisors to administer antiepileptic drugs, father works unpredictable shifts hence cannot do sleepovers at grandparents' house, etc.

Environmental factors

- Facilitators: e.g. low floor bus, access via ramp in a shop, audio books on loan at the library, induction loop at the theatre, DLA and mobility allowance by government, respite care/help at home service from social care, downstairs toilet and walk-in shower funded by local council, etc.

- Barriers: e.g. no public transport to go to library/shopping, lack of carer's allowance and respite care, lack of wheelchair repairs means no attendance/visits to day care centre, lack of adequate supervisors at the local pool leads to cancellation of swimming lessons etc.

Personal factors
- *Facilitators:* e.g. friendly, greets everyone, smiling, curious, willing to join others in play, loves music, loves outdoors, willing to try new foods/tastes etc.
- *Barriers:* e.g. drooling, tics, muscle spasms on loud noises, prefers sameness in routine, difficulty in understanding social cues, interrupts/intrudes in other's conversation/play, phobia about balloons/hairdryers/unexpected sounds, etc.

Advantages of ICF-CY

ICF-CY is a:
- Biopsychosocial framework (social model of disability) that enables physicians/services to see how a child might be disabled further by factors outside his/her control, i.e. environmental and social factors.
- Holistic tool that can easily be applied in a variety of scenarios to evaluate participation in everyday life. By doing so, it enables development of interventions to enable the child to function in family, school, and society.
- Common language that can unify medical, educational, and social services for children. It helps services identify where care, assistance, and changes are most needed.
- Tool that assists clinicians, researchers, commissioners, policy-makers, parents, and carers to document the factors of importance in promoting health, development, and engagement of the child in an array of everyday activities/life.
- Universal tool that can facilitate the documentation and measurement of health and disability in C&YP populations across localities, regions, nations, and over time.
- An evidence-based international WHO standard that can be used to advocate the universal needs and rights of children.

Example of using ICF-CY in clinical practice (Table 4.1)

Table 4.1 Application of ICF model to a 14-year-old girl with Down syndrome

Body structure	Trisomy 21/Down syndrome. Atrioventricular septal defect. Eye refractive error (hypermetropia). Past Hx of otitis media with effusion (had grommets, resolved).
Body function	Global hypotonia. Wears glasses for long sightedness. Short stature with short hands and feet. Unclear speech.

(Continued)

Table 4.1 (Continued)

Activity: strengths	Good at reading. Interested in reading story books. Can communicate her needs in short sentences Obliging and easy-going nature. Learns piano. Loves music. Independent with dressing, toileting, and self-care. Prefers indoor play with dolls, art and craft, painting.
Activity: weaknesses	Speech difficult to understand. Bored of being asked to repeat. Does not like physical activity, i.e. walking or outdoor play. Can miss out on fast moving situations with group of peers. Difficulty in writing. Written work slow, immature, and effortful. Coordination difficulties—takes twice as long to finish a meal, dress/undress. Delayed cognitive/ academic skills. Reading skills ~8-year-old child.
Participation: facilitators	Has Statement for SEN in a mainstream secondary school. Has 25hr/week of 1:1 help with TA in classroom and with SENCO at resource centre. TA/ teacher takes her to playground or outdoor activity for 30min/week. Has access to keyboard/laptop and a scribe when required. SLT provides exercises to address lisp/articulation difficulties 2–3 times/year. Teachers share her painting and art work with the class.
Participation: barriers	Misses school because of appointments with cardiologist, paediatrician, hearing, vision, dental, SLT, OT, psychologist, GP (minor ailments), etc. Annual individual educational plan review consumes lot of time and energy from parents. Frequent SLT changes. Parents constantly pleading for more SLT. Thumb sucking and drooling when concentrating on a task. Needs reminding.
Environmental: facilitators	Easy access to advice from paediatrician (email/ telephone). Teaching assistants (TAs) and teachers keen to learn more about DS and SLT exercises. In receipt of DLA and other benefits. Free glasses/ eye checks, dental checks/treatment. Local DS support group have hired a private SLT on annual basis. Parents attend annual DS conference, read newsletters, and work with professionals.
Environmental: barriers	On waiting list for OT and SLT. Frequent changes in primary care providers. School finding it difficult to accommodate for future years. May need to move the child to a special school. Father has to work away from home frequently hence miss out on weekend activities. Mother works in private sector. Cannot take time off at short notice. Lack of respite care means other 10-year-old child does not get special/ one-to-one time with parents.

Outcome

In addition to the listed advantages, ICF-CY can act as a good outcome monitoring and evaluation tool for the assessment of treatment/management offered to the child.

Cerebral palsy

Definition
- Cerebral palsy (CP) has been defined as: 'A group of disorders of the development of movement and posture causing activity limitations that are attributed to non-progressive disturbances that occurred in the developing fetal or infant brain. The motor disorders of cerebral palsy are often accompanied by disturbances of sensation, cognition, communication, perception, and/or behaviour and/or a seizure disorder.'[1]
- CP is an umbrella term for a group of disorders that are heterogeneous in aetiology, pathogenesis, and clinical manifestations.
- The CNS lesion or dysfunction may have occurred pre-, peri-, or postnatally.
- CP is not a result of a progressive or degenerative brain disorder. CP is static encephalopathy but the motor impairment and functional consequences may vary over time.

Epidemiology
- Globally prevalent. Pan-racial.
- Approximately 2–3 per 1000 live-births. Probably higher in developing countries.
- Slightly more common in boys than girls, 1.33:1. Lower socioeconomic class is another risk factor.
- Multiple gestation has 4 times higher rate of CP than singletons (7–12 per 1000)
- 10–15% of very low birth weight babies develop spastic CP.
- CP increases with decreasing gestation. 20% of infants born <28 weeks' gestation vs 4% born at 32 weeks
- CP increases with decreasing birth weight, e.g. babies between 32–42 weeks gestational age (GA) with birth weight <10th centile are 4–6 times more likely to have CP vs babies whose birth weight is in the reference range, i.e. 25th–75th centiles.

Aetiology
- A variety of causes/risk factors contribute to CP. These can be grouped according to the timing of insult (see Table 4.2).
- Majority of causes that lead to CP commence antenatally. ~80% of cases of CP are congenital. ~10–20% are acquired (vascular, traumatic, inflammatory, etc.).
- CP can be caused by multiple factors, i.e. the confluence of prenatal (extremely low birth weight, prematurity) and postnatal (chronic lung disease (CLD), intracranial haemorrhage (ICH)) factors *or* genetic and environmental aetiologies.

1. Bax M et al. Proposed definition and classification of cerebral palsy, April 2005. *Dev Med Child Neurol* 2005; **47**(8):571–6.

Table 4.2 Causes/risk factors contributing to CP

Prenatal	Perinatal	Postnatal/acquired
Prematurity. Low birth weight/growth retardation. Hx of infertility or IVF. Multiple gestations/births. Maternal age (<20 or >35 years). Hx of CP in previous births. Maternal conditions, e.g. thyroid, diabetes, chorioamnionitis, etc. TORCH infections (toxoplasmosis, other infections, rubella, cytomegalovirus, herpes). Thrombotic disorders, e.g. factor V Leiden mutations. Pre-eclampsia. Placental abruption. Teratogens, e.g. cocaine, alcohol, indomethacin, mercury, etc. Genetic disorders. Congenital brain malformations. Male gender	Birth asphyxia/ hypoxic ischaemic encephalopathy (HIE). PROM (prolonged rupture of membranes). Neonatal encephalopathy. Intracranial infections. Ischaemic stroke. Non-vertex presentation. Prolonged/ obstructed labour. Instrumental delivery. Birth trauma. Rupture of uterus. Hyperbilirubinaemia.	Intracranial infections. ICH. Respiratory distress syndrome (RDS)/ CLD. Traumatic brain injury (TBI), e.g. accidents, child abuse, falls etc. Prolonged mechanical ventilation/ hypocarbia. Postnatal steroids. Pneumothorax. Anoxic insult. Neonatal sepsis. Blood disorders e.g. sickle cell disease. Genetic disorders.

Pathophysiology

- A key concept in causation of CP is *'selective vulnerability'*, i.e. specific regions and cells in the brain are susceptible to insults during specific times in brain development, e.g. injury at:
  - <20th week of gestation can lead to neuronal migration deficit.
  - 26th–34th week leads to periventricular leucomalacia (PVL).
  - 34th–40th week cause focal/multifocal cerebral injury.
- Stages in human brain development:
  - Primary neurulation (3rd–4th week of gestation).
  - Prosencephalic development (2nd–3rd month).
  - Neuronal proliferation (3rd–4th month).
  - Neuronal migration (3rd–5th month).
  - Organization (5th month–beyond infancy).
  - Myelination (birth–6 years).
- There is likely to be a role for inflammatory mediators either causing brain damage or affecting brain development at critical/vulnerable periods.
- There are different risk factors for CP in preterm infants (e.g. ICH) and term (e.g. obstructed labour) infants.

- CP can vary according to the:
  - Timing of insult.
  - Type of insult.
  - Any exacerbating/remediating factors.
- Risk factors for stroke are multiple and include sepsis, peripartum asphyxia, polycythaemia, alloimmune thrombocytopenia, and less common genetic causes such as fibromuscular dysplasia, homocystinuria, factor V, protein C or protein S deficiencies.
- Intrapartum asphyxia or HIE accounts for a minority of cases of CP (~10–30%).

Criteria for defining an acute intrapartum hypoxic event

International Consensus Statement

Essential criteria:
- Evidence of metabolic acidosis in intrapartum fetal, umbilical arterial cord, or early neonatal blood samples (pH <7 and base deficit >12mmol/L).
- Early onset of severe or moderate neonatal encephalopathy in infants of >34 weeks' gestation.
- CP of the spastic quadriplegic or dystonic/dyskinetic type.
- Absence of other identifiable aetiologies.

Criteria that together suggest an intrapartum timing but by themselves are non-specific:
- A sentinel (signal) hypoxic event occurring immediately before or during labour.
- A sudden, rapid and sustained deterioration of fetal heart rate pattern usually after the hypoxic sentinel event where the pattern was usually normal.
- Apgar scores of 0–6 for >5min.
- Early evidence of multisystem involvement.
- Early imaging evidence of acute cerebral abnormality.

The term fetal distress has been replaced by the term 'non-reassuring fetal status'. >75% of cases of neonatal encephalopathy have no clinical signs of intrapartum asphyxia.

Factors that suggest a cause of CP other than acute intrapartum hypoxia

- Umbilical arterial base deficit <12mmol/L or pH >7.
- Infants with major or multiple congenital or metabolic abnormalities.
- Early CNS or systemic infection.
- Early imaging evidence of long-standing neurological abnormalities, e.g., ventriculomegaly, porencephaly.
- Infants with signs of IUGR.
- Reduced fetal heart variability from the onset of labour.
- Microcephaly at birth (occipitofrontal circumference (OFC) < 3rd centile).

- Major antenatal placental abruption.
- Extensive chorioamnionitis.
- Congenital coagulation disorders in the child.
- Presence of other major antenatal risk factors for CP, e.g. preterm birth at <34 weeks, multiple pregnancy, or autoimmune disease.
- Presence of major postnatal risk factors for CP, e.g. postnatal encephalitis, prolonged hypotension, or hypoxia due to severe respiratory disease.
- A sibling with CP, especially of the same type.

- In a child with motor impairment and abnormal tone the following features might point to an underlying IMD (see 🕮 p153):
  - Unexplained hypoglycaemia.
  - Recurrent vomiting.
  - Worsening seizures.
  - Hx of infant deaths in the family.

Clinical presentation

- As a rule of thumb, the more severe the CP, the earlier the presentation.
- Hence, severe CP could present soon after birth and mild cases could present even after 2–3 years.
- These are some of the common ways in which a case of CP might present to physicians:
  - Delayed motor milestones, e.g. sitting, crawling, walking.
  - Abnormal tone—floppy or stiff infant.
  - Abnormal posture, e.g. favouring one side of the body.
  - Abnormal movements.
  - Persistence of primitive reflexes.
  - Feeding and swallowing difficulties.
  - Speech impairment.
  - Voluntary movements are limited, stereotypical.
  - Discrete movements require marked effort, concentration, and often fail.
- Neurological findings often correlate with aetiological risk factors as well as location and extent of brain injury.
- A number of preterm babies can demonstrate transient abnormalities in tone and reflexes that interfere with acquisition of motor skills. Many of these transient manifestations of CP resolve at follow up by 1 or 2 years of age. In such a scenario:
  - All the necessary interventions/therapy should be put in place.
  - Parents should be informed about the fact that CP is a possibility.
  - All such patients should be followed-up.

Classifications
- CP can also be classified according to the functional limitations, i.e. mild, moderate, severe.
- Gross Motor Function Classification System (GMFCS, Box 4.1) is a functionally based system that has been documented to be stable over

time. Hence, GMFCS is increasingly used for research studies and to answer questions about prognosis such as ambulation and survival.

Box 4.1 GMFCS has five levels

- *Level 1:* walks without restrictions; limitations in more advanced GM skills.
- *Level 2:* walks without assistive devices; limitations walking outdoors.
- *Level 3:* walks with assistive devices; limitations walking outdoors.
- *Level 4:* self-mobility with limitations; children are transported or use power mobility outdoors and in the community.
- *Level 5:* self-mobility is severely limited even with the use of assistive technology.

- CP can further be classified according to the child's abilities and limitations as proposed by ICF (℅ http://www.who.int/classification/icf/en) (📖 p63).
- CP can also be classified according to resting tone and limbs involved (topography). See Table 4.3.
  - Many children manifest 'mixed' forms with varying degrees of spasticity and dyskinetic findings.
  - CP is not characterized by muscle weakness.
  - These phenotypes can be used to plan medical and rehabilitative management.

Table 4.3 Topography of CP

	Spastic	Ataxic/ hypotonic	Dystonic/ dyskinetic
Prevalence	Majority of cases. ~80%	Probably <5%	~10–15%
Aetiology	Term and preterm infants, PVL (spastic diplegia). Stroke, unilateral schizencephaly (hemiplegia). CNS infection, ICH, cerebral dysgenesis, periventricular white matter injury (PWMI) (quadriplegia).	Mostly genetic. 50% of cases are AR inheritance. Congenital cerebellar malformations. Mitochondrial disorders.	Typically affects term infants. Most result from severe acute perinatal asphyxia.

(Continued)

Table 4.3 (Continued)

Distribution /type	Unilateral: Monoplegia (rare) Hemiplegia (20–30%). Bilateral: Diplegia (30–40%) Quadriplegia (10–15%).	Involves the whole body.	Upper >lower extremity. Could be predominantly 'athetoid' or 'dystonic'.
Clinical features	↑ tone ↑ reflexes (hyper) Clonus. Extensor plantar response. Abnormal posture. ↓ range of movements likely.	↓ muscle tone. Incoordination. Movements have impaired accuracy and abnormal force. Speech slow, jerky, and explosive. Dysdiado-chokinesia	Varying muscle tone. Reflexes normal or ↓. Involuntary movements like athetosis, chorea, dystonia. Motor speech impairment.
Cognitive impairment	Intact or mild (hemiplegia). Mild to moderate (diplegia). Moderate to severe (quadriplegia).	Variable.	Intact to moderate.
Common associated disorders	Epilepsy. Orthopaedic deformities. Strabismus.	Undiagnosed genetic/ metabolic disorders.	Orthopaedic deformities. Genetic-metabolic disorders.

Associated disorders

Intellectual disability (mental retardation)
(See 📖 p117)
- ~50% have LD.
- Many others even with cognitive abilities in the broad normal range are likely to have specific learning disabilities (SpLD) (📖 p145), attention deficit disorder (ADD) (📖 p126), etc.
- Quadriplegic CP are likely to have severe LD and hemiplegics more likely to have mild LD or no LD.
- Augmentative communication aids (📖 p208) and assistive technologies (📖 p225) can enable pupils to perform to the best of their cognitive abilities.

Epilepsy (see 📖 p240)
- ~30–45% of children with CP.
- Seizures could be of any type and present at all ages.

- Monitor side effects more carefully as children with CP cannot communicate. AEDs can further impact on their cognition and behaviour.

Psychiatric disorders
(See 📖 Chapter 9)
- E.g. emotional behavioural disorders, obsessive–compulsive disorder (OCD), low self-esteem, depression are common.
- Children with, e.g. hemiplegia, can have the following difficulties:
  - Cognitive (performance IQ is lower than verbal IQ, visuospatial difficulties, specific learning difficulties).
  - Emotional and behavioural problems (irritability, anxiety, inattention, hyperactivity, shyness, specific phobias, etc.).
  - Relationship problems (peer relationships, prejudice).

Vision (see 📖 Chapter 7)
- ~50–80% have problems with vision (📖 p269).
- They include refractive errors, strabismus, visual field defects, ambylopia, dyskinetic eye movements, cortical vision impairment.

Hearing impairment (see 📖 Chapter 8)
- ~10–20% could have hearing impairment (📖 p295).
- Causes include middle ear dysfunction, ear infections, SNHL in kernicterus.

Speech impairment (see 📖 pp200–9)
- ~40% could have some speech impairment.
- Disorders include dysarthria, aphasia etc.

Gastrointestinal disorders
- Children with CP have feeding difficulties (📖 p82) due to poor oropharyngeal control, gastro-oesophageal reflux (GOR), poor oesophageal motility, postural control, involuntary reflexes/spasms, etc.
- There is a high risk of aspiration (📖 p91), undernutrition (📖 p86), oesophagitis, bleeding, pain, chest infections, progressive lung disease, etc.

Respiratory disorders
(See 📖 p90)
- E.g. repeated aspirations, reduced clearance of secretions, impaired cough, oropharyngeal incoordination lead to frequent pneumonia and chronic pulmonary disease.
- Chest deformity, obesity, and scoliosis further contribute to restrictive breathing.
- Acute airway obstruction can result with sedation.
- Obstructive sleep apnoea (OSA) (see 📖 p90) can present as snoring and disturbed sleep. Polysomnography (PSG) should be requested to confirm.

Nutrition and growth
(See 📖 p86)
- Children with CP are more likely to be underweight because of the previously mentioned GI disorders.

- Accurate measurements of height and weight are difficult.
- Short stature is likely secondary to chronic undernutrition and contractures.
- Involve a dietician who could give advice on caloric dense supplements, nutritionally complete drinks, etc.
- In a small proportion of patients excess weight can become an added secondary disability, posing challenges for ambulation and care giving.

Urinary problems
- E.g. frequency, urgency, stress incontinence, voiding difficulties, leakage are likely to be more common in children with severe CP (see ☐ p162).
- Factors contributing to this are low expectation of care givers, low cognition, poor communication, impaired mobility, etc.

Orthopaedic disorders
(See ☐ Chapter 11)
- Orthopaedicians can monitor musculoskeletal disorders of CP such as hip dislocations, contractures, scoliosis, etc. Hip dislocations and scoliosis are common complications.
- Treating these deformities can improve the quality of life and care giving.
- They are also best placed to monitor bone mineral density (BMD) (see ☐ p99).
- Impaired mobility/weight bearing, inadequate sun exposure, inadequate diet can result in frequent fractures secondary to osteopenia.

Diagnosis

Diagnostic evaluation should comprise of:
- *Comprehensive history.* Maternal Hx of reduced fetal movements is an important sign of prenatal CP.
- *Physical examination* should include *full neurological assessment* including observing primitive reflexes and abnormal movements. Hypotonia in young children can be confused with generalized weakness. Neurological findings can be correlated with specific cerebral lesions on neuroradiological examination.
- Despite technological advances the diagnosis of CP is based upon clinical assessment.
- Repeat examinations over a period of time may be necessary to confirm the type of CP.
- Diagnosis depends on a combination of findings including:
  - Abnormal neurobehaviour (difficult to handle, settle, or cuddle, sleeping difficulty).
  - Abnormal neurology (poor head control, delayed postural reactions, persistence of primitive reflexes, abnormal tone/deep tendon reflexes, etc.).
  - Evaluation of 'motor milestones' on a *developmental test*, e.g. GMDS-ER could reveal motor quotient of <50%. Delays in 3 or more milestones is very significant.

- CP is a static encephalopathy. Nevertheless, clinical signs evolve as the CNS matures. Hence spasticity may appear at 6 months, dyskinetic patterns not until 18 months and ataxia >2 years.
- Since signs of CP may be present in other conditions, follow-up neurological examinations and developmental assessments would be required to rule out other causes of DD and confirm CP. Therefore diagnosis may not be made until after 3 years of age.
- Accurate diagnosis enables planning therapy and treatment. It aids in giving prognosis and helps in recurrence risk counselling.
- Diagnostic evaluation and rehabilitative planning should involve *a multidisciplinary assessment* involving PT, OT, SLT, psychologist, audiologist, orthoptist, and, where required, a neurologist.

Differential diagnosis

- CP is a diagnosis of exclusion.
- It could be misdiagnosed because signs of CP, e.g. hypotonia, spasticity, dystonia, chorea, etc., may be present in other conditions (see Table 4.4).
- Hx of regression, decompensation during periods of illness/fasting, family Hx (FHx) of neurological disorder, presence of ataxia or weakness should raise the possibility of a metabolic or degenerative disorder.

Table 4.4 Differential diagnosis[a]

	Tests
With apparent or real muscle weakness	
Duchenne/Becker muscular dystrophy	CK in all, muscle biopsy to confirm
Infantile neuroaxonal dystrophy	CK in all, muscle biopsy to confirm
Mitochondrial cytopathy	CK in all, muscle biopsy to confirm
With predominant diplegia/tetraplegia	
Adrenoleucodystrophy	Abnormal MRI, ↑ VLCFA in blood
Arginase deficiency	Raised arginine levels in plasma AA
Hereditary progressive spastic paraplegia	X-linked AD or AR
Holocarboxylase synthetase deficiency	↑ lactate, 3-methylcrotonglycine
Metachromatic leucodystrophy	↑ urinary sulphitide ↓ lysosomal enzyme arylsulphatase A
With significant dystonia/involuntary movements	
Dopa responsive dystonia	Trial dose of levodopa

(Continued)

Table 4.4 (Cont.)

	Tests
Glutaric aciduria type 1	Urine organic acid analysis
Juvenile neuronal ceroid lipofuscinosis	Inclusion bodies in fibroblasts
Lesch–Nyhan syndrome	Deficiency of hypoxanthine guanine phosphoribosyl transferase, ↑ uric acid in urine
Mitochondrial cytopathies	
Rett syndrome	DNA analysis
With bulbar and oromotor dysfunction	
Bilateral perisylvian syndrome (opercular syndrome)	MRI scan
With significant ataxia	
Angelman syndrome	Typical EEG changes
Gangliosidosis	↓ B-galactosidase in leucocytes, cherry red macula
Niemann–Pick	Sea blue histiocytes in bone marrow, filipin test for cholesterol
Pontocerebellar atrophy/hypoplasia	MRI, EMG, sialotransferrins
Posterior fossa tumour	MRI brain including cerebellum
X-linked spinocerebellar ataxia	MRI brain including cerebellum

[a]Data from Gupta R, Appleton RE. Cerebral palsy: not always what it seems. *Arch Dis Child* 2001; **85**:356.

Investigations

Neuroimaging
- MRI is preferred because it can give clues to the cause of CP and timing of the insult. MRI identifies abnormalities in 80–90% of CP cases. Yield is higher in spastic and low in hypotonic types of CP.
- MRI can accurately identify and delineate neuronal migration disorders such as lissencephaly, double cortex syndrome, heterotopias, polymicrogyria, cortical heterotopias, schizencephaly, etc. It can identify other brain abnormalities associated with CP such as PWMI, PVL, cystic encephalomalacia, holoprosencephaly, posterior fossa malformations, agenesis of corpus callosum, congenital hydrocephalus to selective insults in the putamen, thalamus, basal ganglia, etc.

- Neuroradiological findings can help focus the diagnostic search. MRI at presentation can quickly reduce the list of possible causes/differential diagnosis.

Genetic testing (see 📖 p383)
- Seek genetic consultation if:
  - Clinical examination reveals dystonia, chorea, or ataxia (basal ganglia or cerebellar involvement) suggestive of a genetic disorder.
  - MRI reveals neuronal migration disorders such as lissencephaly and cortical band heterotopias.
- Request karyotyping or where available currently preferred comparative genomic hybridization (CGH) analysis in cases with severe microcephaly and dysmorphic features.

Metabolic work-up
(see 📖 p155)
Consider this when there is hypotonia, seizures, focal dystonias, encephalopathy, acidosis, hypoglycaemia, regression, worsening during illness or fasting, positive FHx, etc.

Coagulation screen
- Consider this in all cases of hemiplegic CP.
- Tests should include factor V Leiden, protein C, protein S deficiency, and lipoprotein A levels.

Electroencephalography
EEG is requested only if seizures are suspected in a child with CP. 40–50% of CP children have seizures.

X-ray/radiograph
- Clinical examination of hip state is insufficient. All children with bilateral CP require a radiograph which could be delayed until 30 months of age provided there is no earlier clinical sign of a hip problem.
- Radiograph of a spine where required.

Multidisciplinary management
▶Children should be referred to early intervention services even when CP has been suspected and motor delay has been recognized. 'Act early.' Don't wait until diagnosis is confirmed.
- Many CP cases could be mixed, but treatment is often directed towards the predominant neurological abnormality.
- Interventions should be aimed at improving the quality of life, enabling participation and helping the ADL.
- Multidisciplinary team should address the child's medical, psychological, social, emotional, educational, nutritional, and therapeutic needs.
- The management should be 'individualized', 'child-centred' and involve family, carers and teachers in the rehabilitation of the child. Such collaborative approach will help foresee barriers to management plan and maximizes adherence.

Medical interventions
- Botulinum toxin-A: has become a standard treatment for hypertonus in individual muscles in CP and is an alternative to global therapy such

as with oral antispasticity medications/intrathecal baclofen (see 📖 p431).
- Oral antispasticity medications: benzodiazepines (diazepam), oral baclofen, dantrolene, and tizanidine have been used to treat spasticity. Though they all reduce spasticity and improve the range of movement (ROM), side effects are common and hence long-term usage is limited.
- Antiepileptic medications: see 📖 p625.
- Anticholinergic medications: trihexyphenidyl, an anticholinergic agent reduces the severity of akinesia, rigidity, tremor, and secondary symptoms such as drooling.
- Dopaminergic medications: levodopa/carbidopa (Sinemet®) block cholinergic nerve impulses that affect the muscles in the arms, legs, and other parts of the body and help regulate extrapyramidal symptoms.
- Medications for bone health: address osteopenia by ensuring adequate intake of calcium, phosphorus, and vitamin D. Consider bisphosphonates where required, especially in children with repeated fractures (📖 p99).
- Antireflux medications: see 📖 p85.

Neurosurgical interventions
For intrathecal baclofen, selective dorsal rhizotomy, etc. please see 📖 p431.

Orthopaedic interventions
(See 📖 p433)
Although orthopaedic management of some types of musculoskeletal deformity may be deferred, hip and spinal deformities can benefit from early intervention. Severity of CP and age at pulling to stand are useful indicators of risk for hip subluxation/dislocation.

Physiotherapy interventions
(Also see 📖 p179)
- Physiotherapy programmes are aimed to prevent deformities and encourage the development of functional and independent skills/abilities by setting to improve:
  - Postural alignment.
  - ROM in all the joints.
  - Joint alignment and positioning.
  - Muscle control and strength.
  - Mobility.
  - Cardiovascular fitness.
- There are 3 main types of physiotherapy—Bobath approach, conductive education, musculoskeletal approach.
- There are great number of 'therapeutic motor intervention programmes' that have been tried for children with CP such as conductive education, electrical stimulation, strength training, biofeedback, hippotherapy, saddle riding, pelvic positioning, swimming programmes, functional physical therapy, sibling education programme,and Vojta therapy.

Occupational therapy
(Also see 📖 p188)
- The therapist focuses on hand skills, adaptive equipment, and sensory modulation.
- Help with assessment and provision of aids for bathing, toileting, seating, mobility, transfer, hand skills, self-care, sensory modulation activities, etc.
- CIMT: unaffected limb is intermittently restrained with the aim to promote the use of affected limb. Has a benefit when used in hemiplegia.

Orthotic interventions
(Also see 📖 p220)
- Optimal orthotic management involves liaison with the child's PT, OT, and, where necessary, orthopaedic surgeon.
- Orthoses are used as an adjunct to therapy, botulinum toxin, baclofen, orthopaedic and neurosurgical procedures.
- The evidence suggests that orthoses reduce equinus, increase speed and stride length, and consequently improve gait efficiency and stability.

Speech and language therapy interventions (📖 p205)
- SLT focus on communication (verbal, non-verbal, and assisted).
- Can advice on the role of assisted communication devices.
- Would help in assessment of feeding and swallowing difficulties (videofluoroscopy).
- Hence can offer advice on most appropriate feeding utensils, seating position, consistency of food/liquids, devise specific programmes to improve oral movements, to desensitize the oral area, etc.

Consultations
- Neurologist: seek opinion of neurologist if other neurological disorders suspected and for management of seizures (📖 p240).
- Geneticist: consult geneticist if dysmorphic features, multiple organ abnormalities, or a FHx of a similar neurological syndrome is present (📖 p380).
- GI surgeon: refer for consideration of a gastrostomy/jejunostomy tube (📖 p86) to overcome feeding difficulties and manage undernutrition.
- Dietician: to meet caloric needs and nutritional deficiencies (📖 p87).
- Respiratory physician: refer for sleep study (for suspected obstructive sleep apnoea), frequent chest infections (aspirations), restrictive lung disease, etc. (📖 p90).
- Eye: optometrist for correction of refractive errors, ophthalmologist for eye signs if other neurological disorders suspected (📖 p274).
- Audiologist: hearing thresholds (📖 p300).
- ENT surgeon: tonsillectomy and adenoidectomy for OSA, can address drooling (📖 p92).
- Dentist: can advise on dental health and hygiene (📖 p165).
- Endocrinologist: to address pubertal issues and osteopenia (📖 p99).
- Clinical psychologist: can provide counselling to child (address emotional and behavioural issues) and family (address stress, resentment, guilt, parental discord, etc.).

- Rehabilitation engineer: has a role in assessment and provision of environmental control systems, adaptation of equipment/environment, computer access service, custom contoured toilet seat/chair/arm rest, etc.

Prognosis

- Wherever possible, aspire to integrate patients in education, occupation, and society in full.
- The morbidity and mortality of CP are proportional to the severity of CP and associated disorders. In general, quadriplegia >diplegia >hemiplegia >monoplegia.
- Though some form of cognitive impairment occurs in nearly 2/3 of patients, standardized cognitive testing is likely to underestimate their cognitive abilities because of expressive language/speech difficulties.
- Approximately 1:4 have minimal CP with no functional limitation in ambulation, self-care, and other activities. Another 1:4 are severely disabled and hence are non-ambulatory and require extensive care. The rest are moderately impaired with varying degree of limitations.
- Ability to sit by age 2 years is a good prognostic sign of later mobility and children who do not sit by 4 years are unlikely to ambulate.

Further resources

bibic (brain injuries and other neurological conditions): ☎ 01278 684060 🖰 http://www.bibic.org.uk

Capability Scotland: ☎ 0131 337 9876 🖰 http://www.capability-scotland.org.uk

HemiHelp: ☎ 0845 123 2372 🖰 http://www.hemihelp.org.uk

Scope Response (Scope): ☎ 0808 800 3333 🖰 http://www.scope.org.uk

The Children's Trust, Tadworth: ☎ 01737 365000 🖰 http://www.thechildrenstrust.org.uk

For aids and equipment:

Disabled Living Foundation (DLF): ☎ 0845 130 9177 🖰 http://www.dlf.org.uk

Fledglings (helps identify, source, supply practical and affordable aids/equipment): ☎ 0845 458 1124 🖰 http://www.fledglings.org.uk

For funding:

Family Fund: ☎ 0845 130 4542 🖰 http://www.familyfund.org.uk

Turn2Us: ☎ 0808 802 2000 🖰 http://www.turn2us.org.uk

Oral motor dysfunction

- GI problems are encountered in at least 1/3 of children with CP (see
  📖 p67):
  - Feeding and swallowing disorders (with associated chronic
    pulmonary aspiration (see 📖 p91)).
  - Regurgitation and vomiting (see 📖 p83).
  - Abdominal pain.
  - Constipation (see 📖 p84).
- Effective oral feeding requires the coordination of sucking, swallowing,
  and breathing and is the most complex sensorimotor process the
  newborn infant undertakes.
- Development of oral-motor skills mirrors general neurological
  maturation; those children with the severest general motor deficit
  (bilateral CP) are also those with the most severe degree of oral-
  motor impairment.
- Dysphagia (50% of children with CP) is closely related to the severity
  of the neurological impairment.
- OMD in CP is associated with significant morbidity and mortality;
  major consequences include:
  - Nutritional and growth deficits (see 📖 p86).
  - Drooling (see 📖 p92) and aspiration pneumonia.
- Nutritional impairment from limited food intake may be exacerbated
  by factors such as :
  - Impaired communication.
  - Immobility.
  - Medication.
  - Constipation.
  - Excess losses (vomiting and GOR).

Management strategies for OMD

- The aim of management is to reduce the risk of aspiration
  (see 📖 p91), dehydration, and poor nutrition.
- Involvement of a SLT to formulate an eating and drinking plan is
  essential. This will: Ensure optimum positioning of the child and carer
  during feeding by:
  - maximizing stability and minimizing abnormal reflexes to give good
    head control.
  - Establish consistent and appropriate feeding techniques.
  - Utilize oral control techniques to aid lip closure and jaw stability.
  - Determine the optimum texture of food and drink to ensure a more
    efficient and safer swallow.
  - Determine the choice of suitable utensils to achieve efficient and
    effective safe feeding.
  - Advise on appropriate oral sensorimotor therapy and desensitization
    especially in the hypersensitive orally-aversive child.
  - Address behavioural issues such as food refusal and ensure good
    communication between carer and child.

Assessment of the disabled child with feeding difficulties

Multidisciplinary team input (see 📖 p23) is essential and includes:
- Community or neurodisability paediatrician, paediatric gastroenterologist, paediatric surgeon paediatric radiologist, SLT, dietician, clinical nurse specialist, OT, PT, psychologist and SW.
- Open channels of communication with the child's family doctor, school, HV, and community nurse are essential.

Medical history

Include information on:
- Aetiology of the child's condition.
- Severity of general and oral-motor impairment.
- Presence of comorbid conditions and drug therapies: vomiting, chronic cough, constipation.

Feeding history

- Food intake should be recorded, including information regarding quantities and consistencies of food ingested, and spillage.
- Duration of mealtimes and mode of feeding are important.
- 24-hour food recall or 3-day food diaries can provide useful information about energy and micronutrient intake.

Caution in interpretation is required; families may overestimate amounts consumed by overlooking spillage or vomiting.

Growth history

- The child health record, hospital, community, or school records can provide an accurate weight history.
- Given the difficulties in obtaining accurate height measurements in children who cannot stand it may not be possible to obtain previous accurate height recordings.

Physical examination

To identify factors interfering with feeding ability, complications of feeding difficulties, and evidence of malnutrition:
- Muscle tone, truncal stability, and head control.
- Contractures, spasms, and abnormal movements all impact on feeding ability.
- Chronic lung disease resulting from chronic aspiration.
- Peripheral circulation and skin condition provides information on nutritional status and identifies those at risk of micronutrient deficiencies.

Anthropometry and nutritional status

Obtaining accurate weight and (especially) height measures is difficult in children with severe neurological impairment:
- Body weight measurement may require the use of wheelchair, sitting, or hoist scales.

- Triceps skinfold thickness (TST) is a relatively easy measurement to perform; there is good evidence to suggest that TST below the 10th percentile is a strong indicator of low body fat stores in children with CP (see 📖 p67).
- Supine length is only useful if the child can lie in a straight position with appropriate limb alignment.
- Upper arm length, lower leg length (tibial length), and knee height are appropriate alternative height measurements.
- Measurements should be plotted on an appropriate gender-specific growth chart; CP specific growth charts are available (see 🔊 http://www.lifeexpectancy.org).

Oral motor skills

Evaluation of oral motor movements both at rest and during feeding and management of jaw movements with input from SLT are central to any feeding plan:

- Assessment of jaw stability and movement of the lips, cheeks, and tongue.
- Tonic biting, jaw thrusting, and retraction make spoon-feeding difficult.

Investigations

These will be determined by the history and examination and may include:

- Videoflurosopy:
  - Invaluable in the assessment of feeding and risk of aspiration (see 📖 p91).
  - Provides useful information on optimum feeding position, rate of feeding, and suitable textures.
- Micronutrient assessment: iron status, zinc, vitamins A and D.
- Lower oesophageal pH monitoring and oesophageal impedance:
  - Where there is concern about GOR (see below) and gastrostomy feeding is contemplated.

Note that despite normal clinical history and preoperative radiological and lower oesophageal pH studies, GOR can become apparent in neurologically impaired children after gastrostomy tube placement.

Gastro-oesophageal reflux

- GOR occurs in 19–75% of CP cases. Causes include:
  - CNS dysfunction.
  - Hiatus hernia.
  - Adoption of a prolonged supine position.
  - Increased intra-abdominal pressure secondary to spasticity, scoliosis, or seizures.
- Recurrent vomiting is an objective hallmark of GOR (occurs >80%). Other clinical symptoms include:
  - Haematemesis.
  - Anaemia.
  - Rumination and regurgitation.
  - Peptic oesophagitis.

Management of GOR
Feeding regimen
If tube fed then change from bolus to continuous pump feeding and use of whey-predominant enteral milk formulae which have been shown to be associated with faster gastric emptying and (more controversially) less reflux.

Drug therapy
- Proton-pump inhibitors, e.g. omeprazole.
- Proton-pump inhibitors are superior to histamine type 2 receptor antagonists (H2RA) as they reduce meal-induced acid secretion which H2RAs do not.
- Although widely prescribed, evidence for the efficacy of domperidone is lacking.

Surgical approaches
These approaches are usually required when there is an indication for gastrostomy feeding and/or presence of significant GOR:
- Fundoplication (Nissen or Thal; now routinely performed laparoscopically). Children with neurological impairment have >2 times the complication rate, 3 times the morbidity rate, and 4 times the antireflux re-operation rate than non-neurologically impaired children.
- Major complications can occur:
  • Hepatic vein laceration.
  • Bowel perforation.
  • Tension pneumothorax.
  • Paraoesophageal hernia.
  • Small bowel obstruction.
- Surgical jejunostomy: endoscopic gastrojejunostomy.
- Nasojejunal feeding: placed radiologically.

Delayed gastric emptying (DGE)
DGE in 28–50% cases of GOR—more at risk of developing gas bloat and persistent retching after fundoplication.

Management of DGE
- Gastric scintigraphy is considered to be the most accurate method of diagnosis.
- As gastric emptying depends to some extent on food type, a change to a whey-predominant feed may be helpful.
- Consider a surgical gastric emptying procedure (e.g. pyloroplasty) for significant DGE. NB carries a risk of precipitating dumping syndrome.

Constipation
- Constipation is a common comorbidity in CP (prevalence of 24–74%). Represents a significant therapeutic challenge and standard treatment regimens may prove to be insufficient.
- Contributory factors include:
  • Prolonged immobility.
  • Skeletal abnormalities.
  • Extensor spasm or generalized hypotonia.
  • Abnormal bowel motility associated with certain neurological lesions.

- Diet: low fibre and fluid intake (often due to associated feeding difficulties).
- Drugs: anticonvulsants, opioid, antispasmodic, antihistamines, or aluminium antacid medications in disabled children may also predispose to constipation.
- Chronic constipation has been associated with:
  - Impaired quality of life.
  - Urinary symptoms (see ▣ p162): poorly voiding bladder, recurrent urinary tract infection.
  - GI manifestations:
    — Recurrent vomiting.
    — Chronic nausea.
    — Chronic or recurrent abdominal pain.
    — Early satiety.

Management of constipation

Management of chronic constipation aims to evacuate retained faeces followed by maintenance therapy to ensure defecation is regular and painless.

Medical treatment

Mild constipation and no evidence of megarectum or soiling ensure regular passage of soft stool:
- Dietary manipulations to increase fluid and fibre intake.
- In gastrostomy fed use a formula with added fibre.
- Drug therapy may also be needed:
  - Stool softeners e.g. lactulose—use of preparations containing polyethylene glycol (e.g. Movicol™) or paraffin oil should be used with great caution in children with neurological abnormalities and GOR due to the significantly increased risk of aspiration.
  - Stimulant medications e.g. senna—to ensure defecation occurs at least 3 times a week. Docusate sodium has both stool softening and stimulant properties
- In children with rectal impaction and megarectum:
  - Disimpaction should be attempted—sodium citrate or sodium acid phosphate enemas before commencing stool softeners and stimulant medication.

Surgical treatment

- Surgery is usually reserved for patients who have failed medical management especially those with spinal cord lesions (see ▣ p261).
- Malone antegrade continence enema (ACE) procedure:
  - ACE procedure has an 80% reported success rate.
  - Best results are achieved in children >5 years old with a neuropathic bowel or anorectal malformation who are highly motivated to remain continent.

Further resources

Artificial feeding—PINNT: ✆ http://www.pinnt.com

British Association for Parenteral and Enteral Nutrition: ☎ 01527 457850 ✆ http://www.bapen.org.uk

Colostomy Association: ☎ 0800 328 4257 ✆ http://www.colostomyassociation.org.uk

IA® (The ileostomy and internal pouch support group): ☎ 0800 0184 724 ✆ http://www.the-ia.org.uk

Management of nutritional compromise in the child with disability

- Nutritional intervention should aim to achieve:
  - Appropriate nutrition and growth within the limits of the child's neurological condition.
  - Improved overall growth and not simply improved weight should be the goal.
  - Increased weight due to fat alone has negative impact on general health and increases carer burden.
- Formulate individualized care plans taking account of:
  - Nutritional status.
  - Feeding ability.
  - Degree of motor impairment.
  - Energy requirement.
- Intervention is required when there is evidence of poor nutrition and/ or growth failure. This may involve:
  - Dietary supplementation with glucose polymers and/or long chain triglycerides.
  - Hypercaloric or high-energy density feeds.
- Gastrostomy tube (GT) feeding is indicated:
  - If oral feeding is unsafe.
  - When nutrition cannot be maintained orally (e.g. dependence on nasogastric tube (NGT) feeding).
  - Daily feeding time is prolonged (>3 hours per day).
- Careful tailoring of nutritional requirements is important with GT feeding in children with severe motor impairment who are particularly vulnerable to overfeeding.
  - Consider use of low-energy dense, micronutrient complete, high-fibre feed.
- Regular re-assessment is necessary to gauge response to nutritional intervention.
  - Infants and younger children require more frequent assessment.
  - Yearly assessment may be sufficient in older children.

Further resources

Artificial feeding—PINNT: ℘ http://www.pinnt.com
British Association for Parenteral and Enteral Nutrition: ☎ 01527 457850 ℘ http://www.bapen.org.uk

Energy and nutritional needs for children with disability

The lack of normative growth data for children with CP (see 📖 p67) and the variable contribution of individual factors to growth make the assessment and management of growth problems in CP challenging. This also applies to estimates of energy intake requirements:

- Accurately determining the energy requirement of a child with complex neurological disability is challenging.
- The energy recommendations and equations used to estimate energy requirement for healthy children cannot be confidently applied to children with neurodisability.
- Differences in body composition and energy expenditure mean that standard reference data for ideal nutritional input and optimal growth do not apply to children with CP.

The body composition of the child with severe CP differs from that of the average child:

- A decrease in body cell mass accompanies an expansion of the extracellular fluid volume.
- The relative immobility of the child with severe CP reduces fat-free mass (largely muscle but also skeletal mass) as well as energy expenditure.
- The reduced energy expenditure of children with CP is reflected in a lower dietary energy requirement—around 80% of current recommendations for neurologically normal children.

These body composition and energy requirements differences have consequences for nutritional management:

- Previous studies of children with CP have pointed to a positive energy balance associated with reduced energy expenditure and both high body fat mass and low muscle mass even if the children are fed with 80% of the estimated average requirements for energy.
- Most feeds used for enteral nutrition via gastrostomy are high-energy proprietary feeds (1.0 or 1.5kcal/mL) which are not formulated to meet the nutritional needs of immobile children with severe quadriplegic CP and its associated motor and neurological deficits.
  - Thus overfeeding becomes a real possibility, especially in gastrostomy-fed children who receive such energy dense feeds.
  - Low-energy (0.75kcal/mL) gastrostomy feeds have been shown to improve nutritional status without adversely affecting body composition.

❶ It is important that paediatric enteral feeds are formulated to meet the macro- and micronutrient requirements of children who are reliant on them to supply a major proportion of their intake.

- Any attempt to 'dilute' the existing proprietary feeds in order to reduce the calorie intake to a level commensurate with the energy expenditure of a child with a disability is likely to have an adverse impact on micronutrient intake.
- This also applies to attempts to use liquefied family diet as a gastrostomy feed where both macro- and micronutrient intake may be compromised by the 'watering down' required to administer the feed through the GT.

Feeding difficulties: assessment and management from a SLT perspective

SLTs assess a child's ability to eat food and drink fluids orally and swallow safely. They then advise on modifying textures and feeding techniques to ensure optimum feeding and safety (also see 📖 p81).

The following aspects are assessed:

Child's oral motor ability

Oral phase
- Coordinated movements of lips and tongue to break up, collect bolus and ready it for swallow.
- Developmentally this progresses from:
  - Suckle: tongue moves in and out of mouth in forward–backward motion (from birth).
  - Tongue movements: in up-and-down squashing action on hard palate (~6–8 months).
  - Lateral tongue movements with chewing (~9–12 months).

Pharyngeal phase
Initiating and completing swallow without gag, choke, cough, or aspiration.

Ability to tolerate different textures
- Puree: when weaning at 4–6 months.
- Thick semi-solid: 6–8 months.
- Mashed or lumpy consistency: 8–10 months.
- Soft solids, e.g. cooked root vegetables: 8–12 months.
- Easy chew, e.g. casseroled meat: 12 months.
- Hard to chew, e.g. raw apple: 15 months.
- Mixed textures, e.g. mince with vegetables, soup with chunks: from 12 months.

> ### Points to note
>
> - Textures must be matched to the child's oral motor development. Feeding with inappropriate textures can lead to risk of choking or aspiration.
> - Children can be introduced to chewing using dissolvable or easily squashed foods placed between the lateral teeth whilst encouraging mouthing on teethers or on specific chewing toys such as Chewy Tubes.
> - Many typically developing children in the 7–12-month age range dislike lumpy foods (gagging on these) and do better with single textures.

Feeding position
- This is a particular issue for children with neurological conditions such as hypotonia or spasticity (see 📖 p67).
- Inappropriate feeding position (e.g. reclining or head in extension) can result in risk of choking and aspiration (see 📖 p91).

- *Feeding upright* and with the *head in midline* can inhibit abnormal reflexes seen in CP (e.g. tongue thrust, gagging, jaw extension, bite reflex) and enable the child to feed more normally.

Features that should cause concern

- Gagging: on lumps is relatively common in children between 9–15 months but diminishes as better ability to chew and sort mixed textures is developed. It is also seen in GOR (see 📖 p83) or neurological conditions such as CP (see 📖 p67) where heightened oral reflexes exist.
- Choke/cough.
- Pharyngeal residue: audible 'bubbly' breathing which is not cleared by swallowing or coughing.
- Aspiration (see 📖 p91) which can be audible or silent.

Investigation

Videofluoroscopy carried out by radiologist and SLT is the gold standard assessment for aspiration and should be considered if the following are evident:

- Watering of eyes when swallowing.
- Excessive gagging.
- Effortful or slow swallow, i.e. swallow slow to initiate.
- Pharyngeal residue (bubbly breathing).
- History of chest infections.
- Weak or absent cough.

Sensory aversion

- Condition where children refuse oral food and sometimes this extends to toys or teethers.
- It is often seen after prolonged periods of reflux (see 📖 p83), NGT or force feeding but can also follow difficult feeding experiences, e.g. early breathing difficulties or in children with poor oral motor/sensory control.

SLT treatment strategies

- *Positioning* in midline to suppress abnormal reflexes in CP and to prevent choking due to the opening of airway (if head extended) or gagging in neurological intact children.
- *Pacing* of bottle feeding or feeding with solids to allow child time to breathe and deal with each mouthful/clear residue.
- Use of *appropriate textures* for child's level of development (often eliminating lumps and keeping textures similar reduces gagging).
- *Practise chewing* with teethers (e.g. Chewy Tube) held if necessarily by carers between premolars/molars.
- Use of *dissolvable food* placed between premolars to stimulate chewing movements.
- *Thickening fluids* often aids swallowing as bolus moves more slowly to allow time to trigger safe swallow—aspiration of thin fluids is more common than thicker semi-solids.
- *Messy play* with food and 'gooey' textures such as 'play dough' and 'finger paint' can help with sensory aversion (see 📖 p194).
- Encouragement for child to *feed themselves* is often very effective in children who have sensory issues.

Respiratory care of the child with disability

Children with developmental disabilities have a high degree of respiratory morbidity and mortality because of the following factors:
- Feeding/swallowing difficulties (see 🔲 p81).
- Aspiration of oral secretions (see 🔲 p91).
- Ineffective cough/clearance of secretions (see 🔲 p91).
- GOR (see 🔲 p83).
- OSA.
- Muscle weakness leading to chronic hypoventilation (see 🔲 p257).
- Chest wall deformities causing restricted lung expansion.
- Predisposing factors, e.g. lowered immunity in DS (see 🔲 p387), CLD in ex-premature, immobility after TBI causing orthostatic pneumonia etc.
- Medications, e.g. AED causing sedation.
- Comorbidities, e.g. intractable seizures (see 🔲 p240).

Obstructive sleep apnoea

Conditions associated with increased risk of OSA
- Tonsillar and adenoidal hypertrophy.
- Achondroplasia.
- Craniosynostosis.
- Neuromuscular (see 🔲 p257), e.g. DMD, SMA.
- CP (see 🔲 p67).
- Syndromes, e.g. DS, Beckwith–Wiedemann, PWS, Treacher Collins.
- Obesity.
- MPS (see 🔲 p155).
- Hypothyroidism.
- Choanal stenosis.

Consequences of OSA
- Sleep fragmentation (decreased intellectual functioning, decrements in dexterity, daytime sleepiness, disorientation, confusion, irritability, anxiety etc.).
- Increased work of breathing (failure to thrive (FTT)).
- Pulmonary hypertension.
- Intermittent hypoxaemia (reduced ventricular function, neuronal apoptosis, hampers neurocognitive potential—no one is sure of the mechanism—this is the same as sleep fragmentation).

Management
- *History taking*: enquire about snoring, gasps, heroic snorts in sleep, unusual sleeping position, headaches, behaviour, etc.
- *Physical examination*: examine nasal passages, size of tonsils, palate, plot height, weight, BMI, BP, listen for loud P2.
- *Investigations*: nocturnal PSG is gold standard, night oximetry, ENT referral for nasopharyngoscopy/laryngoscopy, ECG and ECHO—rarely.
- *Treatment*: tonsillectomy and adenoidectomy (T&As). This resolves the great majority of OSA.

- *Follow-up*:
  - Weight reduction.
  - PSG 6–8 weeks after T&A—if snoring persists.
  - Intranasal steroids, montelukast, continuous/bilevel positive airway pressure have been used to address OSA under the care of specialists.

Aspiration

- Could be:
  - Antegrade (while feeding/swallowing) or
  - Retrograde (secondary to GOR (see 📖 p83)).
- Consequences of aspiration:
  - Bouts of coughing, gagging, vomiting.
  - Exacerbation of wheeze.
  - Pneumonia (see 📖 p94).
  - Repeated silent aspirations lead to chronic bronchitis, bronchiectasis, reduction in lung function.
- *Antegrade* (excessive oral secretions, poor swallow etc.):
  - Swallowing requires coordination of oral, pharyngeal, laryngeal, and oesophageal muscles (see 📖 p88).
  - Aspiration can result from impaired coordination of any of the previously listed muscles.
  - It could occur before, during, or after a swallow.
  - Aspiration can occur even when child is NBM (nil by mouth).
  - Videofluoroscopy is the investigation of choice to detect antegrade aspiration and establish safe swallow.
  - Management could include small frequent feeds, thickening liquids, positioning head/neck, oral sensory therapy, stopping oral feedings and temporary NGT placement (also see 📖 p89). Placement of percutaneous endoscopic gastrostomy (PEG) tube is safe and effective medium/long-term solution (see 📖 p84).
  - PEG helps in reducing feeding times, attaining satisfactory growth, reduce silent aspirations and lower respiratory tract infection (LRTIs). Children who require PEG should undergo tests for GOR. Those positive for reflux could have antireflux surgery (e.g. Nissen's fundoplication) and PEG placement at the same time.
- *Retrograde* (secondary to GORD, see 📖 p83).

Ineffective cough/airway clearance

Conditions commonly associated with inadequate clearance of secretions
- Neuromuscular diseases, e.g. DMD, SMA, etc. (see 📖 p257).
- Severe kyphoscoliosis causing restrictive lung function (see 📖 p416).
- CP (see 📖 p67) and associated very limited ambulation/immobility.
- Intractable seizures with depressed consciousness (see 📖 p240).

Consequences of ineffective cough
Repeated LRTIs, bronchiectasis (rarely), loss of lung volume, hospitalizations.

Investigations
- Lung function tests, e.g. baseline forced vital capacity.
- Serial measurements to monitor.

Management
- Avoid infections where possible and treat infections promptly.
- Vaccinate against seasonal flu. Other vaccinations as schedule to minimize respiratory morbidity from other causes, i.e. infections (see 📖 p620).
- Manual cough assist (caregiver pressing on upper abdomen as you cough).
- Treat thoracic deformities where possible.

Drooling
- ~1-1.5L of saliva can be produced/day. 70% of it is produced by submandibular gland alone.
- Considered normal in children <4 years. ~30% of patients with CP (see 📖 p67) have difficulties with drooling.
- Effects of drooling can be:
  - Anterior (loss of saliva from the mouth).
  - Posterior (i.e. aspiration into the airways).

Conditions
a) Normal amount of saliva production
- Cognitively impaired children (impaired attention, motivation, understanding (see 📖 p117)).
- CP (poor lip seal, tongue thrusting, impaired swallowing, open bite, poor neck/head control etc.)

b) Excess saliva production
- Medications, e.g. anticonvulsants, tranquilizers, etc.
- GOR (see 📖 p83).
- Gingivitis and caries could increase drooling (see 📖 p165).

Consequences of drooling
- *Anterior:* frequent change of bibs, soiling of teaching/communication aids, barrier to social interactions, dehydration, skin breakdown around mouth, burden on caregivers, etc.
- *Posterior:* coughing, gagging, vomiting, silent aspirations, repeated LRTIs.

Management
- History:
  - Frequency (occasional/frequent/constant drooling).
  - Severity (mild/moderate/severe (soiled clothing)/profuse (clothing, equipment, tray soiled).
  - Number of bibs/day.
  - Impact on quality of life (barrier to social interaction, soiled IT equipment, etc.).
  - Hx of consequences as listed.
- Examination:
  - Identify factors contributing to drooling (poor head control, tongue thrust, large tongue).

• Head/neck control, perioral hygiene, tongue thrusting behaviours, size of tonsils, open bite, caries, gag reflex, examine ENT and cranial nerves).

Treatment
   • Treat if any of these is compromised—hygiene, comfort, social interaction and respiratory system.
   • *Non-medical measures* (oral motor training, behavioural therapy) if child/carer motivated and adequate cognitive function in child. Time consuming. Not much data about effectiveness.
   • *Medical* e.g. benztropine, scopolamine, and glycopyrrolate. Effective to a great extent. But antimuscarinic side effects common. Botulinum toxin injections into submandibular gland—very effective, but requires repeat at periodic intervals.
   • *Surgical*, only after trying previously listed measures for 6–12 months. Includes re-routing of submandibular gland, excision of submandibular and/or parotid duct ligation to address drooling. Submandibular duct re-routing could worsen aspiration into lungs especially in presence of unsafe swallow.

Common infections in children with disability

For treatment of common infections, see 📖 p621 for details.

Only some common infections that are more likely to be encountered in children with disability are mentioned here as an exhaustive more complete list of infections is outside the scope of this book.

Pneumonia

- It is usually impossible to distinguish viral from bacterial aetiology on the basis of specific signs and symptoms and treatment with antibiotics is recommended where pneumonia suspected clinically.
- Amoxicillin covers the commonest bacterial causes—particularly *Streptococcus pneumoniae*. Where there is the possibility of aspiration pneumonia (anaerobes likely) or for pneumonia following influenza infection (*Staphylococcus aureus* more common) then co-amoxiclav provides a better spectrum of activity. Additional treatment for atypical organisms (e.g. *Mycoplasma pneumoniae*) should be considered in the event of severe disease or treatment failure.
- Recurrent infections are very rarely due to immunological problems and factors such as nutrition (see 📖 p87), recurrent aspiration (see 📖 p91), poor clearance of secretions, and GOR (see 📖 p83) need to be considered.

Acute otitis media

- Frequently viral in origin.
- Bacterial causes mainly *S. pneumoniae* and *Haemophilus influenzae* although *Moraxella catarrhalis* and Group A *Streptococcus* also involved.
- Antibiotics appear to confer relatively modest benefits in terms of either:
  - Symptom resolution in addition to antipyretics/analgesics or
  - Prevention of mastoiditis given the rarity of this complication. See NICE guideline CG69 (2008).[1]
- Initial treatment with amoxicillin. Consider co-amoxiclav (or ceftriaxone if not absorbing oral medication) if treatment failure at 48 hours as activity against resistant *H. influenzae* and also *M. catarrhalis*.

Tonsillitis

- Frequently viral in origin.
- Group A *Streptococcus* is the major bacterial cause.
- 'Centor' criteria may help distinguish viral from bacterial tonsillitis (fever, exudate, lymphadenopathy, absence of acute cough). Viruses

---

1. For both acute otitis media (AOM) and tonsillitis the 2008 NICE guideline (CG69) on respiratory tract infection recommended a policy of no/delayed prescribing except where the child is i) <2 years of age with bilateral AOM, ii) suffering AOM with otorrhoea, iii) systemically unwell, iv) showing signs of severe illness (e.g. quinsy, mastoiditis), or iv) at risk of severe complications due to underlying chronic condition. The recommendation of no/delayed prescribing is based on data showing little symptomatic benefit against significant adverse events and a high 'number needed to treat' for any severe complication (quinsy/mastoiditis/rheumatic fever) given the low incidence of such complications.

may be more likely where coryza, cough, or diarrhoea. Suspected bacterial infection can be confirmed with throat swab culture.
- Antibiotics confer modest benefit in terms of either:
  - Symptom resolution or
  - Prevention of quinsy or rheumatic fever since very low incidence of these conditions. For post-streptococcal inflammatory conditions such as rheumatic fever delayed prescribing is not associated with any less efficacy in preventing these complications. See NICE guideline CG69 (2008).[1]
- Treatment with oral penicillin for 10 days is recommended treatment. High-dose amoxicillin twice daily likely to have better compliance and similar efficacy.

Cellulitis

- *S. aureus* and Group A *Streptococcus* are the major pathogens.
- Treatment is with flucloxacillin (this includes cover for Group A *Streptococcus* and there is no additional benefit to adding penicillin).
- Consider methicillin-resistant *S. aureus* (MRSA) in the event of treatment failure. Group A *Streptococcus* is invariably flucloxacillin sensitive.
- Recurrent skin/soft tissue infections (including folliculitis, impetigo, boils) may be due to colonization with a virulent clone of *S. aureus* and decolonization may be considered.

See 📖 p621 for details of treatment of common infections.

Further resources:

BNF for Children (🔗 http://bnfc.org/bnfc/index.htm)

The Red Book (🔗 http://aapredbook.aappublications.org)

The Blue Book (🔗 Manual of Childhood Infections—OSH Series)

Dermatological care of children with disability

- Children with disabilities and complex care needs are at least as susceptible to ordinary skin diseases as the rest of the child population.
- Furthermore, their individual circumstances can make them prone to additional problems.
- For common skin problems and their management, see Table 4.5.
- Specific skin problems in children with disability include:

Pressure ulcers

- Incidence is higher in certain settings like NICU and PICU.
- Certain groups of children are at higher risk including those with spina bifida (see 📖 p261), neurological disabilities (see 📖 p267), multiple medical conditions, and those in palliative care (see 📖 p105).
- Commonly affected areas include those over bony prominences especially back of skull, ear lobes, and sacral area, knees, heels, scapula, spinal processes, sacrum, and ischial tuberosities.
- Orthopaedic problems can create localized areas of ulceration as in club foot (see 📖 p422), other skeletal deformities (see 📖 p416), and casts.
- The following factors can increase the risk of developing pressure ulcers:
  - Poor sensory perception.
  - Poor nutritional intake for variety of reasons, e.g. prolonged periods of clear intravenous fluid infusion (see 📖 p82 and p86).
  - Poor physical activity and restricted mobility spending longer periods in a wheelchair or a bed.
  - Poorly fitting appliances like special seating or callipers (see 📖 p183).
  - Skin dampness, e.g. sweating, leakage of urine (see 📖 p162), etc.

Principles of management of pressure ulcers

General

- Prevention by removal of pressure.
- Frequent change of posture.
- Adjustment and proper fitting of appliances.
- Soft linen and caregiver education.
- Maintaining normal skin integrity by frequent cleaning and drying.
- Frequent checking contact sites with equipments/appliances.
- Infection prevention and treatment.

Specific

- Support from tissue viability team.
- Irrigation and debridement if needed.

Dermatological problems associated with gastrostomy

Hypergranulation tissue

- Granulation tissue protruding beyond skin level, due to foreign body, friction from moving tube, and moisture.

- Can have associated green, yellow, or serosanguinous discharge making it look like it is infected.
- Proper fitting of button, tube, and external bumper to minimize friction reduces the risk.
- Treatment by topical steroids, silver nitrate, or, in severe cases, surgical excision.

Skin irritation around stoma
- May be a consequence of hypergranulation tissue, leakage of formula, and secretions from gastric mucosa.
- Can be treated by applying barrier paste such as dimethicone.

Candidiasis
- Clinical manifestations include few pustules, satellite lesions, and slight erythema but can be more severe causing excoriation.
- Mild cases respond to topical antifungal (e.g. nystatin) while severe forms require systemic as well as local treatment.

Cellulitis
- Uncommon.
- Needs systemic antibiotics.

Table 4.5 Common skin problems and their management.

Condition	Features	Management
Cradle cap/ seborrhoeic dermatitis.	<3 months of age, erythematous, yellow scales. Scalp and eyebrows Not itchy or painful.	Usually clears with mild emollient. Olive oil. Medicated/mild infant shampoo.
Nappy rash.	Common Irritation from faeces, urine, or fungal. May be a sign of neglect.	Frequent nappy change. Barrier cream (zinc oxide). Antifungal (nystatin). Avoid scented wipes—irritation.
Atopic eczema.	Familial predisposition. Intensely itchy, disturbing sleep. Red inflamed skin with scratch marks. Signs of infection. Weeping. Crusting. Enlarged lymph nodes.	Avoiding aggravating factors, e.g. hairy animals, keeping nails short. Emollient bath oil, soap substitute cream. Regular and liberal emollient use. Topical steroids (e.g., 1% hydrocortisone) for exacerbations. (Beware of skin thinning with prolonged use). Wet wraps, support from eczema nurse. Support at school, e.g. not sitting next to radiators.

Peristomal skin care
- An ostomy is a surgically-made opening from the inside of an organ to the outside.
- Stoma is a Greek term for mouth or opening; in children may be temporary or permanent.
- Usual indications for stoma formation in children include imperforate anus, Hirschsprung's disease, necrotizing enterocolitis, ulcerative colitis, Crohn's disease, and trauma.

Three main types
- Ileostomy—usually placed in right iliac fossa.
- Colostomy—usually in left iliac fossa.
- Urinary diversion—either side.

Two main types of continence stoma
- Antegrade continence enema (ACE):
  - Usually in right iliac fossa.
  - To irrigate colon with enema and saline.
  - Common in children with spina bifida.
- Mitrofanoff:
  - Channel between urinary bladder and abdominal wall or umbilicus.
  - For intermittent bladder drainage.

Stoma care
- Prior to stoma placement consideration should be given to the use of appliances, wheelchair, jackets, etc.
- During care, privacy and dignity to be maintained.
- Child/parents should be trained in stoma care prior to discharge (see 📖 p18).
- Stoma care/community nursing team (see 📖 p545) should be involved early.
- Contact with effluent can cause irritant dermatitis and skin breakdown. It can occur if skin barriers or wafers are left for too long or incorrect size pouch used.
- Barrier creams specific for stoma should be used.
- Stoma may prolapse from time to time. Seek medical advice if irreversible, tense, or dark.
- Urinary diversion procedures increase risk of urinary infection (watch for offensive or cloudy urine).
- Drink plenty of fluid especially in hot weather and with loose stools to avoid dehydration.
- Don't use cotton wool to clean stoma or general barrier cream.
(Also see 📖 p162)

Further resources
All About Bowel Surgery website: ℰ http://www.allaboutbowelsurgery.com
Colostomy Association: ℰ http://www.colostomyassociation.org.uk
National Eczema Society: ℰ http://eczema.org

Bone health in children with disabilities

Bone consists of 3 types of cells within an extracellular matrix:

- *Osteoblasts*: synthesize bone matrix, respond to systemic factors such as cytokines, bone morphogenic proteins, sex steroids, vitamin D, and to mechanical factors. They also control *osteoclasts*.
- *Osteoclasts*: controlled by osteoblasts. Resorb bone. Activated by prostaglandins and parathyroid hormone (PTH) (via osteoblasts). Suppressed by calcitonin.
- *Osteocytes*: communicate with each other through long processes in the lacunae. Are thought to be sensitive to mechanical stresses.
- The *extracellular matrix* contains type 1 collagen and is mineralized mainly with calcium hydroxyapatite. Alkaline phosphatase derived from osteoblasts controls mineralization with calcium and is a marker of bone turnover. Vitamin D enables absorption of calcium from the small intestine.

Causes of osteoporosis in children

- Primary bone conditions:
  - Osteogenesis imperfecta (see 📖 p429).
  - Idiopathic juvenile osteoporosis.
- Metabolic conditions:
  - Rickets
  - Vitamin D deficiency.
  - GI malabsorption (inflammatory bowel disease/coeliac disease).
  - Liver disease.
  - Renal disease.
  - Cystic fibrosis.
  - Malignancy (leukaemia, lymphoma).
- Endocrine disorders:
  - Hyperthyroidism.
  - Hyperparathyroidism.
  - Growth hormone deficiency.
  - Increased glucocorticoids.
  - Reduced sex steroids.
- Other:
  - Disuse, e.g. cerebral palsy (see 📖 p67), spina bifida (see 📖 p261).
  - Drugs, e.g. heparin, anticonvulsants, steroids.
  - Eating disorders (see 📖 p356).
  - Lack of sun exposure.

- Disuse, lack of weight bearing, limited mobility, restricted diet, lack of sun exposure, and medications are main factors causing/contributing to osteoporosis in children with neurodevelopmental disorders such as CP.
- Osteoporosis is a silent but preventable condition.

- Recognition of these risk factors and prevention is the best line of defence against this condition. Screening should be considered.

Investigations

Children with 1 or more risk factor(s) or recurrent fractures or known low bone density should have the following investigations:
- Full blood count (FBC), erythrocyte sedimentation rate (ESR).
- Urea and electrolytes (U&Es), creatinine.
- Liver function test (LFT).
- Calcium, phosphate, alkaline phosphatase.
- PTH.
- Coeliac screen.
- Vitamin D levels.
- TSH.
- Consider bone density measurement (dual-energy x-ray absorptiometry (DXA) scan).

Treatment

- If possible, any underlying cause of secondary osteoporosis should be addressed.
- Vitamin D and calcium supplements should be given if there is a deficiency, and weight-bearing exercise encouraged if possible.
- Sun exposure is very important and 15min a day of sun exposure without sun tan lotion during the summer months (May–Oct) should be recommended.
- Bisphosphonates may be considered particularly in osteogenesis imperfecta, but the efficacy for this in children has yet to be substantiated and should only be given under expert supervision.
- Bone deformities may improve with growth and medical treatment of the underlying condition, but may otherwise require corrective surgery.

Prognosis

- Is good if poor bone mineralization is detected early and action is taken. Address diet (calcium and vitamin D intake), sun exposure, exercise/activity and medications (GP/paediatric endocrinologist) to increase BMD.
- Osteoporosis can have physical (repeated fractures), psychological (pain and distress), socioeconomic (poor quality of life, increased mortality/morbidity) consequences.

Rickets

Vitamin D deficiency results in hypocalcaemia which stimulates production of PTH. This in turn stimulates osteoclasts and calcium is mobilized from the bones. In addition the kidneys excrete phosphate and the result is poor bone mineralization. The result is bowing and deformity of bones. X-ray findings are of increased epiphyseal width and widened cupped metaphyses. Other forms of rickets such as hypophosphataemic rickets or vitamin D-resistant rickets should be excluded. Orthopaedic surgery may be required to address deformities.

Further resource

The National Osteoporosis Society: ☎ 0845 450 0230 🖰 http://www.nos.org.uk

Gynaecological aspects in children with developmental disabilities

- Every child, regardless of their level of cognitive, physical, or medical needs should receive adequate care towards their gynaecological and sexuality needs.
- Children with developmental disabilities have similar sexual desires as their non-disabled peers.
- Puberty could be early (e.g. neurofibromatosis (see 📖 p250), hydrocephalus (see 📖 p264)), delayed (e.g. PWS), or less vigorous and less sustained (e.g. DS (see 📖 p387)). Hence feelings of sexual adequacy, and doubts of ability to reproduce and parent can arise.
- Adolescents with disability are likely to have more risk-taking behaviours as they may want to prove that they are normal.
- Children with disabilities are at increased risk of sexual harassment, abuse, and incest (see 📖 p453).
- Gynaecological care includes:
  - Menstruation and all the options related to it.
  - Education about contraception and pregnancy.
  - Periodic breast examinations by patient or carer (useful if you are looking for signs of galactorrhoea (hyperprolactinaemia, oligomenorrhoea/secondary or primary amenorrhoea) or assessment of pubertal status etc.
  - Refer for cervical smears (Pap smear) and human papilloma virus (HPV) vaccine as required (see 📖 p620).
  - Explanation appropriate to their developmental ability regarding sexuality, dating, sexual abuse (see 📖 p453), sexually transmitted diseases (STDs (see 📖 p462)), self-care, hygiene, etc.

Factors complicating gynaecological care

Child factors
- Reduced cognitive abilities (see 📖 p117) making it difficult to explain treatment and obtain consent.
- Increased communication difficulties (see 📖 p208).
- Other issues, e.g. feeding tubes, colostomy (see 📖 p99), catheters.

Parental factors
- Lack of knowledge regarding sexual health aspects.
- Refusal to engage in provision of such care.
- Guilt.
- Overprotection leading to lack of independence.
- Low priority, e.g. seizures (see 📖 p240), feeding issues (see 📖 p81 and p88), etc. take their attention and time.

Societal factors
- Myth that children with disabilities have no sexual needs.
- Myth that they do not require sexual education.

Physician/health professional's factors
- Lack of training in this area.
- Fear of upsetting parents hence this topic is best avoided.

- Lack of examination skills.
- Lack of time as other medical needs take priority

Physiological and anatomical factors
- Variations in timing of pubertal changes.
- Orthopaedic problems, e.g. spasticity (see 📖 p431), joint deformities, kyphoscoliosis (see 📖 p416).
- Neurological factors, e.g. paraplegia, seizures, antiepileptic medications.

Management
- Enquire about issues such as sexual activity, contraception, menstruation, masturbation, etc. with sensitivity as part of your routine health reviews.
- Provision of information in these aspects will improve their competence. Help avoids unwanted pregnancy, sexual abuse (see 📖 p453), sexual exploitation, STDs (see 📖 p462), etc.
- Refer to:
  - GP, e.g. contraception, HPV vaccine.
  - Gynaecologist, e.g. amenorrhea, menstrual problems, unwanted pregnancy.
  - STD clinic, e.g. screening for STDs, treatment.
  - School health nurse (see 📖 p542)/teacher, e.g. education about emergency contraception, hygiene, or a
  - Special counsellor (see 📖 p348), e.g. issues about sexuality, sexual dysfunction, past history of abuse/incest.
- Provision of access to such resources will maximize child's life chances.
- Holistic care should be extended to all—capable or incapable.

Assessment and management of pain

Assessing pain
- Ask the child (supplement questions by using body charts, pain scales, 'faces scale', etc.); younger and intellectually disabled children (see 📖 p117) may not be able to describe pain easily.
- Ask the family or carers.
- Assess it directly: observe heart and respiratory rate, pallor, sweating, quietness or crying, withdrawal, wincing, etc. Use FLACC (face, legs, activity, crying, and consolability) scale.
- Use a behaviour rating scale such as the Paediatric Pain Profile (PPP) as many children with life-limiting illness have intellectual impairments making communication more difficult.

Managing pain in children
- Use the WHO principles:
  - By the mouth (start with oral medication).
  - By the clock (every 3–6 hours rather than on demand).
  - By the ladder (the 3-step analgesic ladder).
- ▶The key principle is 'the right drug, in the right dose, at the right time'.
- Using opioids. See the ACT website for detail:
  - The correct dose is the dose that limits pain without causing significant side effects.
  - Give standard dose of morphine 4–6-hourly plus prn dose for breakthrough pain as 50–100 % of regular dose up to 2 doses per day.
  - Increase dose by up to 25–50% per day until pain is relieved.
  - Once pain is relieved switch to a sustained relief dose of the same daily total and add prn dose up to 1/6 of the daily dose

❶ Remember other causes of pain, e.g. neuropathic pain, increased intracranial pressure (see 📖 p264), anxiety (see 📖 p354), side effects of medication, incidental cause such as toothache or colic.

Further resources
ACT: ✌ http://www.act.org.uk/symptomcontrol
Action for Sick Children (pain management): ☎ 0800 0744 519 ✌ http://www.actionforsickchildren.org
British Pain Society ☎ 020 7269 7840 ✌ http://www.britishpainsociety.org
Paediatric Pain Profile ✌ http://www.ppprofile.org.uk
WHO pain ladder: ✌ http://www.who.int/cancer/palliative/painladder/en

The role of the hospice

- How best to help terminally ill young people and their families will depend upon personal circumstances, family beliefs and wishes, and the vagaries of local service provision.
- Hospices for young people began with the Helen House hospice (now Helen and Douglas House) in Oxford. Helen House opened in 1982 as the world's first children's hospice. Douglas House opened in 2004 as the world's first hospice specifically for young adults aged 16–35.
- Hospice provision across the UK is patchy and unpredictable, especially for young people. For many families wishing to use a specialist young person's hospice, there is the added difficulty of long journeys to an unfamiliar city or town.
- There are roughly 40 specialist children's hospices in the UK, linked via 'Together for Young Lives' the umbrella organization formed by the amalgamation of ACT (Association for Children with Life Threatening Conditions) and Children's Hospices UK in 2011.

Further resources:

ACT (Association for Children's Palliative Care) ☎ 0845 108 2201 ✆ http://www.act.org.uk
Children's Hospice UK: ☎ 0117 989 7820 ✆ http://www.childhospice.org.uk
'Together for Young Lives': ☎ 0845 108 2201 Email: info@togetherforshortlives.org.uk

Key principles in caring for the dying child

- Involve the child in the planning process.
- Use 'parallel planning'—it is often not possible to predict when a death will happen; children are very resilient.
- Good communication is critical. This takes time, but it is the key to success.
- Every family is different, has different priorities, and responds differently.
- Parents who have a relationship directly to each other rather than 'through the child' and who sustain this are best equipped to cope.
- Many different medications help, not just the obvious things like opiates and anxiolytics. The further resources listed have good sections on medications.
- Use the team—including the full range of therapists, chaplains, etc.
- Life goes on for other children—both for other children in the family, hospital or hospice and visitors. Father Christmas may be visiting while a child is in the terminal phase.
- Dying is a journey for the whole family, including siblings and grandparents, aunts and uncles.

An end of life plan
- The child and family should be helped to decide on a plan and should be helped by the medical team to achieve their wishes.
- ACT summarizes the purpose of the plan as: to think through the child's wishes, and the family's, to think through possible problems that may occur and plan for them, and for the doctor, 'to hope for the best and prepare for the worst'.

After the death has happened
- Respect the family's wishes.
- Allow them to grieve and to prepare for burial or cremation in their own way.
- Do not say 'you must' or 'you should' do particular things—for example, hold or see the body. Families have their own preferences and traditions.
- Some families may wish to use a 'cool room' available in many hospices, which allows them to spend time with the child. The room is maintained at around 4–8°C; a body can be held in a cool room for over 24 hours—practice varies between different hospices. A child's body can usually be kept in a cool room for up to 5 days with appropriate temperature control and air conditioning.

The 'stages of bereavement'
- Earlier models of a linear pattern of bereavement (denial, anger, bargaining, depression, and acceptance) associated particularly with Elizabeth Kubler Ross, have been followed by other models reflecting a more complex process.

• A useful example is Richard Wilson's model of bereavement as a process like travelling down a river—with various events and barriers such as whirlpools and rocks along the way. The traveller down this river may become stuck, get delayed, etc.

Further resources

ACT (Association for Children's Palliative Care) ☎ 0845 108 2201 🖰 http://www.act.org.uk
Children's Hospice UK: ☎ 0117 989 7820 🖰 http://www.childhospice.org.uk
'Together for Young Lives': ☎ 0845 108 2201 Email: info@togetherforshortlives.org.uk

Pervasive developmental disorders

- The term autism spectrum disorder (ASD) is generally used to describe a group of PDDs characterized by qualitative abnormalities in reciprocal social interactions and communication and by restricted and repetitive patterns of interests and behaviours (Table 4.6).
- These include
  - Autism (also see 🕮 p327).
  - Asperger syndrome (also see 🕮 p329).
  - PDD-not otherwise specified (PDD-NOS).
  - Rett syndrome (see 🕮 p403).
  - Childhood disintegrative disorder.
- Autism and Asperger syndrome are the most commonly recognized conditions by common public and represent prototype disorders from this group.
- Spectrum of these disorders includes children across the range of severity and intellectual ability. Notably children with higher intellectual functioning ('high functioning') may still have significant functional impairment.

Table 4.6 Common presenting features of children with ASD at different ages.

	Pre-school	Primary school	Secondary school
Communication difficulties.	Failure to respond to name. Failure to point or wave. Language delay or regression. Echolalia.	Limited or excessive talking at others. Frequent repetition of set phrases. Odd or inappropriate prosody.	Flat or odd intonation. Unusual ways of making themselves understood. Taking things literally.
Social interaction difficulties.	Lack of responsive smile. Poor eye contact. Preference for solitary play. Lack of turn taking. Lack of pretend play.	Temper tantrums. Lack of response to greetings and smiles.	Long standing difficulties in behaviour and social communication. Lack of awareness of personal space. Difficulty with social situations and rules.
Stereotypic and restricted behaviour.	Unusual attachment to object, toys, etc. Unusual sensitivity to textures, sounds, and other stimuli. Hand flapping, tip-toe walking.	Over- or under-reactive to sensory stimuli. Preference for routines and structures.	Unusual profile of skills and deficits. Preference for narrow and specific interests.

Prevalence

- Leo Kanner in 1943 described autism in children with shared pattern of behaviours including social remoteness, stereotypy and echolalia. Autism prevalence has been a focus of intense media and public interest over the last few years.
- Many reports including estimates based on epidemiological studies indicate an increase in prevalence of ASD. The overall prevalence of ASD in children is regarded to be ~1%.
- Factors responsible for increase in prevalence are unknown but possible explanations include:
  - Changes in diagnostic criteria.
  - Different ascertainment methods.
  - Conceptualization to a spectrum rather than a core categorical condition.
  - Diagnostic substitution.
- ASD is 3–4 times more common in boys, especially at the higher functioning end of the spectrum.

Diagnosis

- Diagnosis of autism can be made between the ages of 2 and 3 although it can be difficult in 'high-functioning' children on the spectrum.
- Lack of a specific biological marker or 'test' means that identification relies heavily on detailed clinical, developmental history, and observations.
- Earlier referrals whilst welcome, may pose challenges to diagnostic reliability and capability to indicate prognosis.
- Availability of various screening instruments to identify autistic behaviours has made it possible to diagnose some of these children as early as 18 months of age. However, despite high positive predictive value, modest sensitivity limits their use for general population screening.
- Potential benefits and disadvantages of early diagnosis are listed in Table 4.7.

Table 4.7 Potential advantages and disadvantages of early diagnosis.

Advantages	Disadvantages
IQ gains. Reduction in symptom severity. Identification and provision of SENs is easier when diagnosis is made. Amelioration of secondary negative consequences of social and communication deficits. Parental awareness of increasing risk in subsequent children. Timely access to information, services, and support.	Uncertainty of diagnosis at young age. Difficulty with assessing cognitive potential and predicting educational needs if assessed at a young age.

Screening and diagnostic tools for ASD

Screening tools for ASD
- The Checklist for Autism in Toddlers (CHAT) for children 18–24 months of age.
- The Modified Checklist for Autism in Toddlers (M-CHAT) for children 16–30 months of age.
- The Social Communication Questionnaire (SCQ) for children 4 years and older.

Diagnostic tools for ASD
- Autism Diagnostic Interview-Revised (ADI-R).
- Autism Diagnostic Observation Schedule-Generic (ADOS-G).
- Childhood Autism Rating Scale (CARS).
- Gilliam Autism Rating Scale (GARS).
- Diagnostic Interview for Social and Communication Disorders (DISCO).
- Developmental, Dimensional and Diagnostic Interview (3di).

Criteria

Internationally recognizable criteria are available for autistic disorders, developed by:
- American Psychiatry association (DSM-IV) and
- WHO (ICD-10) (Box 4.2).

Box 4.2 ICD-10 criteria for autism[a]

A. Abnormal or impaired development is evident before the age of 3 years in at least one of the following areas:
1. Receptive or expressive language as used in social communication.
2. The development of selective social attachments or of reciprocal social interaction.
3. Functional or symbolic play.
B. A total of at least six symptoms from (1), (2), and (3) must be present, with at least two from (1) and at least one from each of (2) and (3):
1. Qualitative abnormalities in reciprocal social interaction are manifest in at least two of the following areas:
a. Failure adequately to use eye-to-eye gaze, facial expression, body posture, and gesture to regulate social interaction.
b. Failure to develop (in a manner appropriate to mental age, and despite ample opportunities) peer relationships that involve a mutual sharing of interests, activities, and emotions.
c. Lack of socio-emotional reciprocity as shown by an impaired or deviant response to other people's emotions; or lack of modulation of behaviour according to social context; or a weak integration of social, emotional, and communicative behaviours.

   d. Lack of spontaneous seeking to share enjoyment, interests, or achievements with other people (e.g. lack of showing, bringing, or pointing out to other people objects of interest to the individual).
2. Qualitative abnormalities in communication are manifest in at least one of the following areas:
   a. Delay in or total lack of, development of spoken language that is not accompanied by an attempt to compensate through the use of gesture or mime as an alternative mode of communication (often preceded by a lack of communicative babbling).
   b. Relative failure to initiate or sustain conversational interchange (at whatever level of language skills is present), in which there is reciprocal responsiveness to the communications of the other person.
   c. Stereotyped and repetitive use of language or idiosyncratic use of words or phrases.
   d. Lack of varied spontaneous make-believe or (when young) social imitative play.
3. Restricted, repetitive, and stereotyped patterns of behaviour, interests, and activities are manifest in at least one of the following areas:
   a. An encompassing preoccupation with one or more stereotyped, restricted patterns of interest that are abnormal in content or focus; or one or more interests that are abnormal in their intensity and circumscribed nature though not in their content or focus.
   b. Apparently compulsive adherence to specific, non-functional routines or rituals.
   c. Stereotyped and repetitive motor mannerisms that involve either hand or finger flapping or twisting, or complex whole body movements.
   d. Preoccupations with part-objects or non-functional elements of play materials (such as their odour, the feel of their surface, or the noise or vibration that they generate).

[a]Data from World Health Organization (1992). *The ICD-10 International classification of mental and behavioural disorders: Diagnostic criteria for research.* Geneva: WHO.

Associated disabilities/medical conditions

- In addition to social and communication difficulties, children with ASD are at higher risk of various neurodevelopmental and behavioural disorders (Table 4.8).
- Their identification and appropriate management should be an important component of overall management strategy.

Table 4.8 Table showing comorbid conditions with ASD and their management.

Coexisting condition	Management
Mental health and behaviour problems. Anxiety. OCD. Depression Phobias. ADHD. Aggressive or self-injurious behaviour.	Support from mental health team for behavioural and psychopharmaceutical treatment.
Sleep difficulties.	Sleep hygiene measures. Consider melatonin.
Neuromotor problems. Coordination difficulties. Tics.	Occupational therapy assessment and support. Behaviour therapy. Neuroleptics.
Epilepsy.	Neurological assessment, EEG, anticonvulsant treatment.
Learning difficulty (75%).	Educational support.

Aetiology

- Not clearly known. Probably multifactorial.
- Strong possibility of genetic predisposition. Relative risk of a second child with autism 20–50 times than the population base rates.
- 'Theory of mind'—a possible psychological mechanism.
- Tends to occur more frequently than expected among individuals who have certain medical conditions, including:
  - Fragile X syndrome (see 📖 p403).
  - NF1 (see 📖 p250).
  - Tuberous sclerosis (see 📖 p251).
  - DS (see 📖 p387).
  - Angelman syndrome (see 📖 p396).
  - Williams syndrome.
  - Congenital rubella syndrome.
  - Untreated PKU.
  - Cytogenetic abnormalities such as maternal duplication of 15q1–q13 and deletion and duplication of 16p11.

Assessment

- A full and comprehensive assessment is vital to make an accurate diagnosis of ASD.
- It is important to have a clear and established referral pathway and easy and prompt access to specialized assessment services. Recently published guidelines by NICE in the UK has clearly laid down the pathway for recognition, referral, and diagnosis of C&YP on the autism spectrum.
- A comprehensive assessment by the multidisciplinary team could include assessments from the following professionals depending on the need:
  - Educational/clinical psychologist (see 📖 p531).
  - Specialist teacher or an early year professional (see 📖 p544).
  - Community paediatrician (see 📖 p2).
  - Child and adolescent psychiatrist (see 📖 p319).

- SLT (see 🕮 p200).
- OT (see 🕮 p188).
- PT (see 🕮 p176).
- ASD family support worker (see 🕮 p547).
- Social worker (see 🕮 p546).

Key components of diagnostic assessment of ASD
- Information already available in various settings should be collated to avoid repetition by child and family.
- Detailed history from carers including information about birth, developmental Hx, FHx, and current level of functioning (see 🕮 p6).
- ASD-specific history (see Box 4.3). Use of a semi-structured interview instruments like Autism Diagnostic Interview–Revised (ADI-R) can provide a framework to improve accuracy and reliability of diagnosis.
- Physical examination (see 🕮 p9) should include focus on dysmorphic features, neurocutaneous stigmata (including Wood's lamp examination), and neurological assessment (keeping in mind unusual sensitivity of some of these children to touch and personal space) in addition to routine paediatric assessment.
- Routine vision (see 🕮 p271) and hearing test (see 🕮 p299).
- Observations: a semi-structured standard observation tool like Autism Diagnostic Observation Schedule (ADOS) is designed to create planned social occasions ('presses') in which a range of social initiations and responses is likely to appear rather than relying on their spontaneous manifestation.
- Communication, speech, and language assessment should include communication strategies, social interaction and joint attention, learning potential, preferred learning style, as well as receptive and expressive competencies.
- Cognitive assessment: (see 🕮 p213) there are many standardized test available.
- Occupational therapy assessment especially if coordination difficulties and sensory issues (see 🕮 p194).
- Behaviour and mental health assessment especially to identify coexisting disorders (see Table 4.9).

Box 4.3 Autism-specific history

- Poor eye contact.
- Emotional inappropriateness.
- Inappropriate social responses to smile/hello.
- Repetitive, stereotypic routines/behaviours.
- Any loss of language or social skill.
- Hypersensitivity to noise and other stimuli.
- Lack of pointing to share interest (pointing for needs may be present in children with ASD).
- Difficulty sharing/playing with other children.
- Unusual hand/body movements, walking on tiptoes.
- Lack of nodding/shaking of head.
- Lack of pretend/imaginative play.
- Does he enjoy peek-a-boo/hide-and-seek games?

Investigations
- Identifiable medical disorders are only present in about 10–15% of autistic disorders.
- Yield from investigations may be higher in selected subgroup of children including those with SLD, dysmorphic features, or abnormal neurology and investigations should be planned based upon these (Table 4.9).

Table 4.9 Suggested investigations for ASD

Investigation	Indication/rationale
FBC including film.	Restricted diet to exclude iron deficient anaemia.
Karyotype including fragile X.	Significant language delay or LD.
Testing for Rett syndrome gene mutations (*MECP2*).	LD, regression, or clinical phenotype (see 📖 p403).
Thyroid functions and PKU screening.	If not tested at birth.
Metabolic investigations.	None routinely. Consider if clinical presentation suggestive (LD, fits, recurrent vomiting, etc.) (see 📖 p155).
EEG.	Only if clinical features suggestive of epilepsy (see 📖 p240).
Brain imaging (MRI).	Abnormal neurology, epilepsy.

Differential diagnosis
- LD (see 📖 p117).
- Language disorders. Children with receptive language problems may also have imaginative play and social interaction difficulties (see 📖 p202).
- Attachment disorders (see 📖 p346).
- Deafness (see 📖 p296).
- Acquired aphasia with epilepsy (Landau–Kleffner syndrome) (see 📖 p240).
- Selective mutism.

Interventions
ASDs are lifelong neurodevelopmental disorders and currently there are no aetiology based treatments available.

Approaches, therapies, and interventions

Behaviour interventions
- Applied behaviour analysis (Lovaas):
  - Teaching linguistic, cognitive, behavioural, and self-help skills by breaking them down into small tasks.
  - Preferably <5 years of age.
  - Parent mediated with support from helpers and professional consultants.
  - Involves 40hr/week of intensive therapy for 2 or more years.
  - Clear benefit in some areas like IQ in short term but probably less than originally thought.

- More effective in children with higher IQ and better baseline functioning.
- Behaviour interventions address a wide range of behaviours (e.g. self-injury and aggression) and improve adaptive skills (see 📖 p210).

Service-based interventions
- TEACCH:
  - Help to prepare people with autism to work more effectively at home/school/community.
- SPELL framework:
  - Structure, Positive, Empathy, Low arousal and Link.
- Day life therapy of Higashi:
  - Systematic education through group dynamics, modelling, and physical activity.

Skill-based interventions
- Makaton:
  - Communication system using combination of symbols, gestures, signs words, and speech.
  - Based upon the principle of better visual comprehension in autism.

Speech and language therapy including alternative/augmentative communication (see 📖 p208)
- Aim to maximize communication potential.

Social stories
- Improves social understanding.
- Help to see things from other's perspective.
- Involve short description of a particular situation, event or activity including information about what to expect and why.

(Carol Gray: 🕸 http://www.thegraycenter.org/social-stories/what-are-social-stories.)

Parent training
- Limited evidence to suggest beneficial effect for both children and parents (see 📖 p371).

Psychotherapy
(See 📖 Psychotherapy p373)

Pharmacotherapy

General considerations
- Existing pharmacotherapeutic agents not effective for core symptoms of ASD.
- Medicines may be useful to address comorbid symptoms and as an adjunct to educational, behavioural, and developmental interventions (Table 4.10).
- Overall assessment of child's environment (both at school and at home) and daily routine (e.g. sleep) is mandatory before considering

pharmacological intervention. Non-pharmacological approaches should be considered before starting medications.
- Potential benefits and risks from medications should be carefully considered before starting treatment.
- Clear goals and end points should be agreed with parents/young person to stop treatment.
- Pharmacological treatment should only be undertaken by clinicians with appropriate experience and expertise.
- Some of the medications used are not licensed for use in children.

Table 4.10 ASD medications

Medications	Indications
Risperidone	Short term use for aggression, tantrums, and self-injury (see 📖 p369).
Methylphenidate	Attention difficulties and hyperactivity (see 📖 p126).
Melatonin	Sleep problems persisting despite behavioural interventions (see 📖 p373).
Antiepileptic medications	Epilepsy (see 📖 p240).

Education
(See 📖 p533)
- Appropriate educational placement and provisions should be planned according to their intellectual ability, needs, and strengths to optimize child's functioning.
- Children may attend mainstream or special schools.
- Teaching strategies and techniques should be tailored to individual children taking into account their difficulties with verbal and non-verbal communication, social understanding and behaviour, inflexible thinking, and sensory perception and responses.
- Can process visual information better than that given orally.
- Should be taught in a structured and errorless way with predictable routines and timetables.
- More able children can succeed in subjects using technical and mathematical language like science, engineering and IT.

Outcome
- Long-term outcome usually difficult to predict in individual cases because of wide spectrum of cognitive, linguistic, social, and behavioural functioning.
- Across the spectrum, <1/4 live independently as adults.
- 1 in 7 adults with autism in UK are in full time employment.
- Poor outcome in those with lower IQ.
- Usual ongoing difficulties in the areas of communication, social relationships, and independence.

Asperger syndrome
(See 📖 Mental health p327 and p329)
- A form of ASD.
- Can be a hidden disability.

- Fewer problems with spoken language.
- Usually average or above average intelligence.
- Can be associated with specific learning difficulties like dyslexia (see 📖 p147) and dyspraxia (see 📖 p136).
- Preference for routines and structures and areas of special interest and detailed knowledge like numbers, dinosaurs, space science, etc.
- In long term may develop psychiatry symptoms like paranoia, depression (see 📖 p350), OCD (see 📖 p334), and alcohol abuse (see 📖 p367).

Pathological demand avoidance (PDA)

- Increasingly recognized to be a part of autism spectrum.
- High anxiety with feeling of losing control leads to avoiding demands made by others.
- Can be enigmatic and charming when feeling secure and in control.
- Better communication and social interaction than other children on spectrum.
- Much better with role play and mimicry.
- Sudden and rapid mood swings.
- Strategies useful for autism and Asperger syndrome may not help those with PDA.
- May appear sociable and empathetic on surface but fail to see bigger picture with pathological obsession to be in control.
- Over- or under-sensitivity to sensory stimuli (see 📖 p194).
- Real difficulty controlling temper with prolonged tantrums and violent outbursts.
- Extreme anxiety may lead to school refusal (see 📖 p522).
- Respond better to indirect and negotiative style to give them a sense of control.

Further resource

Pathological Demand Avoidance Syndrome Contact Group: ℘ http://www.pdacontact.org.uk
The National Autistic Society: ☎ 0845 070 4004 ℘ http://www.autism.org.uk and http://www.autismdirectory.org.uk

Learning/intellectual disabilities

Terminologies

- Various. Mentally retarded (in US until now), intellectual disability (ID) (US and internationally), global developmental delay (GDD) and learning disability (LD) (in UK).
- GDD is usually used to describe children <5 years of age with significant deficits in 2 or more developmental domains (see 📖 p36) as IQ testing is less reliable in this age group. All these terms are synonymous and have been used interchangeably.
- The term ID is being used increasingly as it aligns better with emerging emphasis being placed on functional behaviours and contextual factors (see 📖 p63).
- These entities share common features and represent defects or disorders in learning.
- ID is the most prevalent major neurodevelopmental disorder.
- The age at which a developmental problem is first suspected usually correlates well with the severity of ID.

Definitions

- ID is a static encephalopathy that encompasses a broad spectrum of functioning and disability ranging from mild ID to profound ID.
- ID has been defined as cognitive and adaptive skills assessed at >2 sd below mean.
- The Department of Health in the UK defines LD as reduced ability to:
  - Understand new or complex information.
  - Learn new skills (impaired intelligence).
  - Cope independently (impaired social functioning) starting before adulthood and with a lasting effect on development.
- DSM-IV uses the term 'MR' instead of 'ID', which it defines by 3 coexisting criteria:
  - Significant sub-average intellectual function (2 sd below the mean, i.e. IQ of 70 or less).
  - Significant limitations in adaptive behaviours (i.e. impairment in communication, activities, and skills of daily living).
  - Onset before the age of 18.
- ID has been categorized into gradations of severity (based on results from standardized IQ tests):
  - Mild: IQ between 50–69. Accounts for up to 80–85% of ID cases.
  - Moderate: IQ between 35–49.
  - Severe: IQ between 20–34.
  - Profound: IQ <20.
  - Unspecified: not testable but presumed low (i.e. <70).

Aetiology

- Any condition that interferes with brain development and maturation can cause ID. Hence ID has multiple aetiologies (Table 4.11).
- ID can be grouped together according to the time of insult.
- Prenatal causes (mostly genetic) account for most cases of ID.
- Prenatal causes also account for most number of severe cases of ID.

Table 4.11 Aetiology of intellectual disability

Prenatal	Perinatal	Postnatal
DS. Fragile X. Rett syndrome Mutations, e.g. ARX. TORCH infections. Teratogens e.g. alcohol. Environmental toxins, e.g. lead. CNS malformations. Metabolic, e.g. hypothyroidism. Neurocutaneous, e.g. TS, NF. PKU.	Extreme prematurity. HIE. Infections, e.g. GBS. Trauma. Intracranial bleed.	Trauma (accidental and NAI). Near drowning, i.e. hypoxia. Intracranial infections. CNS tumours. Severe malnutrition. Environmental toxins, e.g. lead, mercury, radiation, etc.

Risk factors
The following factors predispose to ID and are responsible for most cases of mild ID:
- Higher maternal age.
- Low maternal education (risk of ID up to 7 times greater if <12 years of education).
- Multiple births.
- Socioeconomic deprivation (see 🕮 p513).
- Poor educational provision (see 🕮 p520).
- Remote rural population.
- Under-stimulation.
- Child neglect and maltreatment (see 🕮 p449).
- Parents with LD/ID.
- Parents with substance misuse (see 🕮 p367).

Prevalence
2–3% of children have ID. This excludes children with SpLD.

Clinical presentation
- The more severe the disability, the earlier it is recognized.
- Impairment of self-help and self-care skills are more likely to be the presenting feature of ID than low IQ.
- ID can present at any time in childhood or adolescence in the following ways:
  - Delay in understanding, reasoning (see 🕮 p54).
  - Language delay (see 🕮 p52).
  - Behavioural problems (see 🕮 p340).
  - Poor self-care skills (see 🕮 p49).
  - Failure on Development screening in primary care (see 🕮 p57).
  - Deficits in social or community interaction.
  - Reduced academic ability (see 🕮 p520).
  - Problems at leisure or work place (see 🕮 p325).
- Developmental screening tests such as DDST-II, SOGS, Parents' Evaluation of Developmental Status (PEDS), etc. can be used in

primary care to identify and refer children to secondary care for further detailed assessments (see 📖 p36).

Common comorbid conditions

- The more severe the ID the more likelihood of these comorbid conditions.
- These are commonly under-diagnosed, mostly under-treated.
- Comorbidities have adverse impact on child's functioning, quality of life, rehabilitation, etc.
- The comorbidities are as follows:
  - CP and motor handicaps (see 📖 p67).
  - ASD (see 📖 p107).
  - Epilepsy (see 📖 p240).
  - ADHD (see 📖 p126).
  - Visual impairment (see 📖 p275).
  - Hearing impairment (see 📖 p296).
  - Mental Health, e.g. depression, aggression, anxiety, OCD, tics, (see 📖 p325) etc.
  - Behaviour—challenging behaviour (see 📖 p369), self-injurious, self-stimulating, etc.
- Up to half of the ID population will have significant impairments in communication. Half of those with moderate to severe ID have mental health problems (see 📖 p325). One-third of those with mild ID will have mental health problems.

Diagnosis

- Early diagnosis is optimal.
- Ideally neurodevelopmental disabilities are diagnosed over time rather than at a single clinical encounter.
- A multidisciplinary assessment is recommended (see 📖 p23).
- Identification of a cause helps in genetic counselling, focused interventions, more tailored treatments, surveillance for possible complications, and specifying a prognosis.
- Diagnosis involves:
  - *Detailed history* (see 📖 p6) from parents, teachers, etc. Obtain information on developmental milestones, comorbidities, self-care skills, behaviour, sleep, medications, FHx that covers 3 generations using open-ended questions, pregnancy and birth Hx, etc.
  - *Examine:* (see 📖 p9) height, weight, OFC, and plot. Head to toe examination looking for dysmorphic features, skin signs, congenital malformations, neurological assessment, signs of abuse/neglect, etc.
  - Accurate assessment of *neurodevelopment* on a standardized test (see 📖 p36) , e.g. GMDS, Bayley, British Ability Scales (BAS) will inform you of the 'degree' and 'profile' of ID. This is an important step in the evaluation and aids in estimating the natural history of ID.
  - *Speech and language assessment:* cognitive skills are an extension of language testing evaluated by the child's grasp of specific concepts. Report should comment on language, pragmatics, semantics, speech, literacy, as appropriate (see 📖 p202).
  - *Occupational therapy assessment:* hand function, visual perceptual skills, sensory profile for SPD (see 📖 p188 and p194).
  - Get *vision, hearing,* and *dental health* checked.

- Professionals from multidisciplinary team, e.g. physiotherapy, psychologist, continence advisor (see ☐ p162), wheelchair service (see ☐ p186) as required.
- Professionals from partner agencies (see ☐ Chapter 16), e.g. get reports from social services, education as required.

Investigations

The results of full Hx and detailed examination should guide you as to which investigations need to be performed. Evaluation of a child with ID is a time- and labour-intensive process. Hence a staged approach is recommended:

1. Karyotype should be performed in all cases. Genomic microarray analysis (chromosomal microarray) is increasing the diagnostic yield in unexplained ID and hence undertaken where available/possible.
2. Fragile X caused by a mutation of the CGG triplet repeat in the *FMR1* gene should be considered especially in those with FHx of ID/features of fragile X (see ☐ p403).
3. Additional genetic testing carried out based on clinical suspicion e.g. *MECP2* for Rett (see ☐ p405), etc.
4. Metabolic testing especially if Hx of episodic decompensation, developmental regression, dysmorphic features, organomegaly, or FTT. Review the results of the newborn screening (Guthrie card). Serum AAs, urinary organic acids, ammonia, lactate, and TFTs to be done first, before complex and higher-order metabolic testing is undertaken (☐ p124 and p157).
5. Lead, only if there are risk factors for lead toxicity.
6. Neuroimaging (MRI) especially if abnormal head size, shape, or motor signs. CT scan only if calcification or bony abnormalities are suspected.
7. EEG, only if, fits, faints or funny turns are present. Not done routinely.
8. Referral to geneticist if Hx of consanguinity, unexplained neonatal deaths, miscarriages, regression of milestones, dysmorphic features, etc.

Management

▶*Mission is to optimize health, promote functioning and community participation by supporting social and behavioural competencies across the lifespan.*

- ICF model describes both functioning and enablement by allowing the professional to describe body structures/functions, activities, participation, environmental, and personal facilitators and barriers (see ☐ p63).

Principles
- Each child with ID has unique strengths and difficulties in intellect and adaptation.
- The challenge is to find out exactly the child's current functioning in various domains to be able to address which supports are needed.
- Hence management should be multidisciplinary and holistic (see ☐ p23).
- Interventions should start early (see ☐ p59) and be sustained.
- Use strategies that are synchronous with child's interests.
- Most children with ID respond best to multisensory information or information presented both visually and auditory.

- Involves interagency communication.
- Must address the 'transition' to adult services (see 📖 p171).
- All health, education, and social care staff must accord with the Disability Discrimination Act 1995.

Practice
(Level of support/ rehabilitation required will depend on severity of ID and comorbidities.)

- Develop '*Health Action Plan*': advice on nutrition, exercise, sexual health, disease prevention, address existing health needs, anticipate future health problems, etc.
- '*Annual health checks*': immunisation, health promotion, vision, hearing, dental health, physical (including activities undertaken, mobility, posture), syndrome-specific checks, review medication, continence, sleep, behaviour, areas of risk, emotional and mental health, sexual health, healthy lifestyle (alcohol, smoking, drugs), etc. Treat conditions such as hypothyroidism, hydrocephalus, cataracts, hearing impairments, constipation, sleep disorders, seizures, etc.
- *Mental health/Child and Adolescent Mental Health Service (CAMHS* (see 📖 p325) *team:* to address behaviours (to improve socialization, communication and conduct), by offering psychological support, cognitive behaviour therapy (CBT), family therapy, counselling and support (see 📖 Chapter 9).
- *Physiotherapy*: for mobility, postural support, daily activities, stretches and ROM (see 📖 p179).
- *Speech and language therapy* (see 📖 p200): for communication passport, Makaton, picture exchange communication system (PECS), communication aid, swallowing and feeding assessment as required, social stories,
- *Occupational therapy*: provision of equipment, adaptations, sensory modulation activities (see 📖 p188).
- *Aids and appliances*: think of access, wheelchair, continence materials, vision aids, communication devices, voice output aids, engineering aids, adaptations, (see 📖 p191) etc.
- *Medications*: stimulants for ADHD, risperidone for aggression after consulting psychiatrist.
- *Social services* (see 📖 p546): refer for assessment of housing, benefits, respite care, employment and vocational opportunities, home hazard assessment, funding adaptations (see 📖 p514).
- *Education services:* write to them for statement of SEN, planning appropriate education setting, 1:1 teaching assistant, supervision during play/dining, inclusion, annual reviews, (see 📖 Chapter 15) etc.
- Referral to *special programs*, e.g. Hanen (effective communication skills), early bird (ASD), EYSENIT/portage (pre-school education (see 📖 p544)), parenting enablement courses (see 📖 p371) etc.
- *Employment support agencies*, e.g. connexions, arrange work experience, apprenticeships etc.
- *Social support*: involve voluntary agencies (see 📖 p547); access to community facilities, short breaks for carers, transport, etc.
- *Prepare for 'transition'* to adult services, key worker to coordinate services and monitor successful transition to independent living (see 📖 p171).

- *Parental partnership:* Involve them throughout. Provide support, information of self-help/support groups (see below).

Prognosis

▶It is important to question why a child has a neurodevelopmental disability at least once for each child. Every attempt must be made to answer this question using the management process, described above.

- The outcome of ID depends upon:
  - Aetiology (e.g. hypothyroidism, PKU, or DS).
  - The degree of ID (mild ID more likely to find employment and live independently and severe ID likely to need high level support).
  - Presence of comorbid conditions (e.g. challenging behaviour or aggression).
  - Social factors (e.g. caregiver support, parental education, socioeconomic circumstances).
  - Environmental factors (availability of appropriate education and rehabilitation services).
- The ID group as a whole will have greater health needs than the general population.
- Four times more likely to have a preventable cause of death.
- Majority of individuals with ID can live in community settings.

Further resources

Brainwave: ☎ 01376 505290 🖰 http://www.brainwave.org.uk
Cerebra: ☎ 0800 328 1159 🖰 http://www.cerebra.org.uk
ENABLE Scotland: ☎ 0141 226 4541 🖰 http://www.enable.org.uk
Mencap: ☎ 0808 808 1111 🖰 http://www.mencap.org.uk

Investigation of learning difficulties/ developmental delay

Why investigate?

- Investigation can help in diagnosis and diagnosis can help in counselling of recurrence risk.
- Diagnosis helps in giving a prognosis.
- Management of associated medical conditions and identification of secondary disabilities.
- Specific therapeutic interventions.
- Preventive programmes, e.g. metabolic decompensation could be avoided.
- Limits further unnecessary testing.
- Resources follow a label.
- Empowers families, e.g. deciding about family planning, jobs, career, etc.

When to investigate?

- Global delay: delay in 2 or more developmental domains.
- Significant: 2 or more sd below the mean on developmental assessments (see 📖 p36).
- Severe (IQ <50) or profound delay (IQ <20).
- 'DD plus' (see 📖 Second-line investigations p124).
- Do not investigate in isolated cases of speech and language or fine motor delay, mild DD with no associated features or children with SpLD.

Continued follow-up is important in global delays as regression may be slow or new features may emerge with time.

How to investigate?

An approach to aetiological evaluation

- Thorough Hx (see 📖 p6).
- Physical examination: detailed head-to-toe check including neurology. Plot head circumference, height, weight. Look for dysmorphic features, neurocutaneous disorders, etc. (see 📖 p9)
▶An aetiology is evident in ~1/3 cases from Hx and examination.
- Developmental assessment: developmental diagnosis is cornerstone for treatment. The testing results could reveal delay, dissociation, or deviance. Developmental assessment could help in formulating a list of differential diagnosis.
- Clinical observations: attention, behaviour (phenotype), activity, etc.
- Hearing: refer for hearing thresholds in all cases (see 📖 p300).
- Vision: refer for assessment of vision and eye in all cases (see 📖 p271).

First-line investigations

Investigations are not a substitute for Hx or examination. 1ˢᵗ-line tests should be considered in all cases of developmental delay where a likely cause is unclear after a thorough Hx and examination.

- Genetic: karyotype and fragile X screen.
- Blood: FBC, U&E, LFT, TFT, bone profile, CK, lactate, ammonia, urate, blood gases, glucose.
- Urine: glycosaminoglycans, organic acids, amino acids.

Second-line investigations

These tests should be considered in '*developmental delay plus*' scenarios, i.e. where GDD is associated with other features as mentioned under genetic, imaging, metabolic and neurophysiology subheadings.

Genetic

- Routine karyotype and fragile X screen would pick up abnormalities in ~1–3% cases.
- Consider a referral to geneticists if DD is associated with the following features (see 🕮 p384):
  - Congenital abnormalities.
  - Dysmorphism.
  - Abnormal growth (head circumference, height, weight).
  - Prenatal onset of growth retardation.
  - Sensory impairment (vision or hearing).
  - Unusual behaviour (self-harm, obsessions with food, etc.).
  - FHx of significant developmental delay.
- Newer techniques such as:
  - Subtelomeric deletion/rearrangements by microarray CGH could increase the yield further to ~17%.
  - Microarray CGH could become a 1st-line investigation in near future as the cost goes down and availability of this facility widens.

Imaging

- The yield from neuroimaging studies is considerably increased when DD is associated with one of the following features:
  - Abnormal head shape or size.
  - Focal neurological signs.
  - Cutaneous markers.
  - Seizures.
  - EEG abnormalities etc.
- MRI: consider if CNS malformations, cerebral atrophy, delayed myelination, white matter disease, post-ischaemic lesions, neurocutaneous disorders are suspected.
- CT scan: consider if intracranial calcification or bones/skeletal abnormality is suspected.
- Skeletal survey: consider in disproportionate stature or significant short stature.
- Imaging studies can pick up abnormalities in ~40–60% of children with DD plus above feature(s).
- Advances in neuroimaging e.g. proton magnetic resonance spectroscopy (MRS) (helpful in measuring the biochemistry of the brain) and diffusion tensor imaging (DTI) (helpful in knowing the position of the white matter tracts) would further enhance our ability to identify causes of GDD in the coming years.

Metabolic

Consider if DD is associated with one of the following:

- Consanguinity
- Family hx of developmental delay.
- FTT
- Regression or developmental arrest
- Coarse features
- Organomegaly

Investigations for IMD (see 📖 p156): these should be carried out after discussion consultation with a metabolic unit/lab.

Neurophysiology

Consider EEG if DD is associated with 1 of the following:

- Hx or examination suggests presence of epilepsy.
- Certain cases of speech and language delay (Landau–Kleffner syndrome).
- Regression or developmental arrest.
- Imaging/genetic/IMD investigations suggesting a neurodegenerative disorder.

Conclusion

- Accurate identification leads to appropriate interventions.
- 'Why does this child have DD?' should be asked at least once for every child.
- Just as every case of DD is unique, so is the list of investigations undertaken in each one. Tests should be guided by comprehensive Hx, clinical scenario, stepwise approach, and networking with specialist colleagues.
- An aetiology could be found in a majority of cases of GDD by systematic approach and the listed suggestions.
- Re-evaluation should be considered after a period of time (e.g. 5 or 10 years) if this approach/tests fail to identify a cause for GDD. A better appreciation of dysmorphic features with time coupled with advances in imaging/genetics might provide answers.

Attention deficit hyperactivity disorder

- A neurobehavioural developmental disorder.
- ADHD is a heterogenous condition of children who are inattentive, impulsive, and active at levels higher than expected for their mental and chronological age.
- ADHD sufferers actually have difficulty 'regulating' their attention, e.g. pay too much attention on too many things.

Incidence

- 3–5% of children globally.
- Boys:girls = 2–4:1. Boys show more aggressive/externalizing behaviours and girls show more inattentive and internalizing ones.
- Lifespan condition: 30–50% of these will continue to have difficulties in adulthood.
- ~ 4.7% of American adults live with ADHD.

Aetiology

- *Multifactorial*: ADHD is most likely caused by a complex interaction of genetic and environmental factors.
- *Genetic:*
  - Twin studies indicate that this disorder is highly heritable. Genetics are a factor in about 75% of cases.
  - Many arise from a combination of various genes which affect dopamine transporters, D2, D4, DAT1, DRD4, etc.
  - Numerous susceptibility genes, each of small effect size, contribute to the symptoms.
  - Many have a parent or close relative with a similar condition.
- *Environmental:*
  - 10–20% of the variance in ADHD symptoms can be attributed to environmental factors.
  - In rare instances, pregnancy or birth complications, prematurity, trauma to the CNS, meningitis/encephalitis are thought to result in ADHD.
  - Maternal depression and social disadvantage maintain/exacerbate rather than cause ADHD.
- *Diet:*
  - Symptoms of some children get worse with certain artificial food colourings and additives e.g. sodium benzoate etc. But this is not the main cause of ADHD.
  - Parents/carers frequently report that certain foods/drinks could make the child more hyperactive.
- *Social factors:*
  - Relationships with caregivers have a profound effect on attention and self-regulatory abilities. E.g. studies of foster children reveal high number of them have behaviours which could be described as ADHD.
  - Poor parenting is not the cause but can make the symptoms worse.

- *Neurochemical:*
  - A variety of recent pharmacological, imaging and neuropsychological studies have suggested that the attention problems are due to dysfunctions of ventral catecholaminergic (dopaminergic and noradrenergic) pathways projecting to prefrontal and frontal cortex.
- *Neuroanatomical:*
  - Structural and functional neuroimaging studies of the brain in patients diagnosed with ADHD have implicated the prefrontal cerebral cortex and its innervations of subcortical regions such as caudate-putamen, nucleus accumbens, and amygdaloid complex in the pathophysiology of ADHD.
  - MRI studies have revealed that the more severe the symptoms of ADHD were, the smaller their frontal lobes, caudate nucleus, and cerebellum were likely to be.

There are various *theories* to describe the causation of ADHD. Some of them are:
- *Low arousal theory:* states that people with ADHD need excessive activity as self-stimulation because of their state of abnormally low-arousal.
- *Evolutionary theory:* Hunter vs Farmer. Hunters are adept at searching, seeking, and risk taking and less adept at staying put and managing complex tasks over time.

Comorbidities
Nearly half of children with ADHD could also have 1 or more of the following conditions:
- Learning difficulties (specific and global) (see 📖 p117 and p145).
- Autism (Asperger syndrome, ASD) (see 📖 p107).
- Communication disorders (receptive, expressive, and mixed) (see 📖 p202).
- Behavioural disorders (oppositional defiant disorder, OCD, etc.) (see 📖 p340 and p369).
- Conduct disorder (📖 p334).
- Tourette syndrome (📖 p332).
- Anxiety/mood (📖 p354).
- Sleep disorders, e.g. delayed sleep phase syndrome (📖 p168).
- Substance-related disorders (📖 p367).
- Developmental coordination disorder (📖 p136).
- Sensory processing disorder, e.g. sensory defensiveness, sensory seeking, etc. (📖 p194).

Associated features
The following features are frequently associated with ADHD and are frequently confused with symptoms of ADHD:
- Sleep disturbance (📖 p168).
- Non-compliant behaviour (📖 p334).
- Aggression (📖 p334).
- Temper tantrums.
- Clumsiness (📖 p136).

- Literacy problems (📖 p147).
- Emotional outbursts.
- Thoughts 'whirling'.

History

- ADHD manifests differently at different ages.
- Obtain information from more than one setting, such as school.
- A detailed history of daily functioning with specific examples, onset of problems, situations, and current/ongoing concerns should be elicited.
- History taking should also include:
  - Strengths and weaknesses.
  - School: work performance/educational concerns (see 📖 p520).
  - Social skills and friendships.
  - Home and family interactions.
  - FHx (ADHD, LD, drugs, alcohol, abuse, death, divorce etc.).
  - Pregnancy/birth/early developmental history.
  - Medications and substance abuse (see 📖 p367).
  - PMHx: any hepatic, heart, renal, CNS disease, glaucoma, etc.
- Screen for the comorbidities.
- As executive functioning (EF) is the major task of frontal lobes check whether the EF tasks such as planning, organization, sequencing of behaviours, response inhibition, and self-regulation are affected.

Physical examination

- Search for coexisting conditions or differential diagnosis that make the diagnosis more difficult or complicate treatment planning.
- Examination should include:
  - CVS: pulse, BP.
  - Growth: height, weight.
  - Head circumference: microcephaly, macrocephaly (see 📖 p231).
- Behaviour: comment on impulse control, fidgeting, attention.
- Skin: neurocutaneous disorders (see 📖 p250) and dysmorphic features (see 📖 p384).
- Neurology: focal neurological signs, epilepsy (see 📖 p240), etc.
- Developmental/psychometric assessment (to identify LD, SpLD (see 📖 p145)).

Investigations

- Investigations are guided by the Hx and physical examination.
- Developmental assessment (any evidence of discrepancy between IQ and ability).
- Rating scales, e.g. Conner's TRS/PRS, Barkley HSQ/SSQ, and Child Behaviour Checklist (CBC), etc.
- Other psychometric and educational testing as warranted.
- If LD (see 📖 p117) is present then investigate accordingly (see 📖 p123).
- Imaging investigations, i.e./MRI head, only if abnormal physical examination.
- Suspicions of seizures then consider an EEG.
- ECG: only if Hx of palpitations, FHx of QT interval abnormality, heart disease, etc.
- FBC: if you suspect bone marrow dysfunction on methylphenidate.
- LFTs: only if there is Hx of liver dysfunction.

- Screen for substance abuse when suspected in a teenager/early adulthood.

Diagnosis

❶ Diagnosis should not be based just on scoring the rating scales.
- There is no diagnostic, objective, or confirmatory test. Diagnosed on the basis of a recognizable behaviour pattern.
- As part of the diagnostic process it is crucial to assess:
  - Child/young person's needs.
  - Clinical assessment.
  - Coexisting conditions.
  - Social/family circumstances.
  - Information on educational/academic/occupational impairment.
- Use either:
  - DSM-IV (used in US, worldwide. Uses more broader and inclusive definition) or
  - ICD-10 (used by WHO, Europe. Uses a narrower diagnostic category) criteria checklists.
  - The difference between the two is that all children must be hyperactive to fulfil the ICD-10 definition. For diagnosis by the DSM-IV, criteria for inattention or hyperactivity/impulsivity must be met.
- For diagnosis:
  - The child/young person should meet the DSM-IV or ICD-10 criteria and
  - Have at least moderate degree of social, psychological, educational, or occupational impairment
- Determining severity of ADHD is a matter for clinical judgement based on the information obtained.
- Diagnostic criteria (Boxes 4.4 and 4.5) is most valid for boys aged between 6–12 years. Girls and adolescents could present with less typical features.

Box 4.4 ICD-10 criteria: attention deficit/hyperactivity disorder—F90 Hyperkinetic disorders

G1 Inattention

At least six of the following *symptoms of attention* have persisted for at least six months, to a degree that is maladaptive and inconsistent with the developmental level of the child:
(1) often fails to give close attention to details, or makes careless errors in school work, work or other activities;
(2) often fails to sustain attention in tasks or play activities;
(3) often appears not to listen to what is being said to him or her;
(4) often fails to follow through on instructions or to finish school work, chores, or duties in the workplace (not because of oppositional behaviour or failure to understand instructions);
(5) is often impaired in organizing tasks and activities;
(6) often avoids or strongly dislikes tasks, such as homework, that require sustained mental effort;

(7) often loses things necessary for certain tasks and activities, such as school assignments, pencils, books, toys or tools;
(8) is often easily distracted by external stimuli;
(9) Is often forgetful in the course of daily activities.

G2 Hyperactivity

At least three of the following *symptoms of hyperactivity* have persisted for at least six months, to a degree that is maladaptive and inconsistent with the developmental level of the child:
(1) often fidgets with hands or feet or squirms on seat;
(2) leaves seat in classroom or in other situations in which remaining seated is expected;
(3) often runs about or climbs excessively in situations in which it is inappropriate (in adolescents or adults, only feelings of restlessness may be present);
(4) is often unduly noisy in playing or has difficulty in engaging quietly in leisure activities;
(5) exhibits a persistent pattern of excessive motor activity that is not substantially modified by social context or demands.

G3 Impulsivity

At least one of the following *symptoms of impulsivity* has persisted for at least six months, to a degree that is maladaptive and inconsistent with the developmental level of the child:
(1) often blurts out answers before questions have been completed;
(2) often fails to wait in lines or await turns in games or group situations;
(3) often interrupts or intrudes on others (e.g. butts into others' conversations or games);
(4) often talks excessively without appropriate response to social constraints.

G4

Onset of the disorder is *no later than the age of seven* years.

G5 Pervasiveness

The criteria should be met for *more than a single situation*, e.g. the combination of inattention and hyperactivity should be present both at home and at school, or at both school and another setting where children are observed, such as a clinic. (Evidence for cross-situationality will ordinarily require information from more than one source; parental reports about classroom behaviour, for instance, are unlikely to be sufficient.)

G6

The symptoms in G1 and G3 cause *clinically significant distress or impairment* in social, academic, or occupational functioning.

G7

The disorder does not meet the criteria for pervasive developmental disorders (F84.–), manic episode (F30.–), depressive episode (F32.–), or anxiety disorders (F41.–).

Reproduced with permission of the World Health Organization, *International Statistical Classification of Diseases and Related Health Problems (ICD-10)*, 10th edition, (1992). Available online at http://apps. who.int/classifications/icd10/browse/2010/en#/F90.1

Box 4.5 DSM-IV criteria for ADHD

Readers can access DSM-IV (and soon to be launched DSM-V) criteria for ADHD by visiting the American Psychiatric Association website or by visiting the CDC web page listed here: ℞ http://www.cdc.gov/ ncbddd/adhd/diagnosis.html

Differential diagnosis

The following can present as ADHD:
- ODD (📖 p334).
- CD (📖 p334).
- Autism/ASD (📖 p107).
- Hearing impairment (📖 p297).
- Vision impairment (📖 p275).
- Sleep impairment (📖 p168).
- Child abuse (📖 p440).
- Epilepsy (📖 p240).
- Anaemia.
- Thyroid problems.
- Lead poisoning.
- Substance misuse (📖 p367).
- Anxiety/mood disorder (📖 p354).
- Learning difficulties e.g. global LD/specific LD-causing 'secondary inattention' (📖 p117).
- *Secondary inattentiveness:* is situational to setting that overburdens the cognitive ability of children, e.g. with LD.
  - Even SpLD (see 📖 p145), e.g. dyslexia, dyscalculia, dysgraphia, can give rise to inattentiveness.
  - Some children with high IQ will perform poorly or may become disengaged from schoolwork, demoralized, or depressed because the assigned class work is too simple, uninteresting, or unchallenging.
  - Hence it is important to carry out *'cognitive screening' or 'developmental testing'* (see 📖 p36).
- Children with ASD (see 📖 p107) may be mistaken as having ADHD for several reasons: temper tantrums, repetitive behaviours, stereotyped mannerisms (misinterpreted as restlessness or hyperactivity), avoidance of eye contact (misinterpreted as inattention), inattention to activities outside of their circumscribed preoccupations, etc. However, it is important to bear in mind that both ASD and ADHD can coexist.
- ADHD children can be impulsive, erratic, domineering, and intrusive whereas children with ASD appear as remote, aloof, and eccentric.

Other conditions that trigger behaviour resembling ADHD

- Death or divorce in the family.
- Parent's job loss.
- Problems with school work (📖 p520).
- Poor parenting for parenting (see 📖 p371) attachment difficulties (📖 p346).
- Bullying (📖 p342).
- Physical illness.
- Medical conditions such as:
  - Fragile X (📖 p403).
  - TS (📖 p401).
  - NF (📖 p400).
  - Smith Magenis.
  - Thyroid disorders etc. These conditions can also accompany ADHD.

Management: general principles

- Allow the child/young person to give his/her account. Involve child and family in decision-making. Get their agreement/cooperation (see 📖 p16).
- Encourage parental participation in self-help/support groups.
- Provide information on self-instruction materials and positive parenting techniques.
- Balanced diet, regular exercise, along with elimination foods that worsen behaviour help.
- Good communication between home, school, and health professionals is crucial for success.
- Typical uncomplicated history and normal physical examination = then start treatment (behavioural ± medication according to the degree of impairment).
- Smooth transition to adult services is necessary for continued monitoring and success in adulthood (📖 p171).

Management without medication

- Is considered in mild, mild to moderate, or moderate impairment with ADHD as 1st-line treatment.
- NICE recommends offering following interventions as 1st-line treatment:
  - Parent-training/education programme.
  - Behavioural interventions in classroom provided by teachers.
  - Social skills training offered to children/young person.
- There is good evidence for the effectiveness of behavioural treatments in ADHD. The following cognitive therapies/interventions should be considered/offered before the use of medications in a child with moderate difficulties with ADHD (see 📖 p373):
  - Psycho-educational input.
  - Cognitive behaviour therapy (CBT).
  - Family therapy.
  - Interpersonal psychotherapy (IPT).
- The behavioural interventions should consist of (see 📖 p210):
  - Reinforcing the wanted behaviour.
  - Decreasing the behaviour you don't want (negative reinforcement).
  - Setting house rules, routine, structure, time table, visual cues, etc.

- Avoiding trouble: play, planning ahead, problem solving.
- Participation in a support group, obtaining peer feedback is helpful.
- School interventions (see 📖 p524): pastoral support, encouragement, regular feedback, modifications, e.g. sitting in the front of the class, away from windows/doors, short breaks between activities, appropriate seating, working in small groups, etc. are very useful.

Management: medications

- Are considered as 1st-line treatment in moderate-to-severe or severe impairment with ADHD.
- Drugs should preferably be part of a comprehensive package of care with social, psychological/behavioural, educational advice, and interventions.
- Children with additional mental health needs/complex needs should preferably be reviewed and followed-up in close collaboration with colleagues in CAMHS (see 📖 p325).
- Before starting medications:
  - Review Hx (mental health, social/family circumstances, comorbidities).
  - Physical examination (height, weight, BP and HR. FBC, LFT, ECG if indicated).
- Start medications at low dosage and gradually increase the dose as required.
- Monitor side effects, effects and risk of abuse especially with stimulant medications.
- If *poor response* to treatment, consider:
  - Reviewing the diagnosis.
  - Considering and dealing with comorbidities.
  - Providing psychological/behavioural interventions.
  - Checking treatment adherence (see 📖 p375).
  - Checking parental/child motivation.
  - Increasing the dose of the existing medication to the maximum tolerated level.
  - Trying other medication i.e. atomoxetine if methylphenidate has been tried.
  - Referral to specialist/tertiary CAMHS (see 📖 p319).

Stimulants:

Methylphenidate
- Not licensed for children <6 years
- It is a controlled medication. Risks for stimulant misuse and diversion present.
- Recommended as 1st-line treatment for:
  - ADHD without significant comorbidity.
  - ADHD with conduct disorders.
- Sustained/modified-release preparations are preferred as:
  - Single dosing is convenient.
  - Compliance/adherence to treatment is better
  - No need for administration at school hence reducing stigma.
  - No need to store and administer controlled drug in school etc.

- Short-acting/immediate-release could be considered during:
  - Initial trial and titration—helps determine correct dose.
  - Where increased flexibility in dosing regimens is required.
  - Occasionally as a top-up dose in the evening to enable homework etc.

Dexamphetamine
- Do not use as a 1st-line treatment. More potent stimulant than methylphenidate.
- Acts by blocking the reuptake of noradrenaline and dopamine.
- Used only after methylphenidate and atomoxetine have been tried and failed.
- Use limited to experienced professionals, e.g. specialist/tertiary CAMHS.

Non-stimulants
Atomoxetine
- Selective noradrenaline reuptake inhibitor.
- Not licensed for children <6 years.
- Should be considered when ADHD:
  - Is associated with tics, Tourette syndrome, anxiety disorders.
  - Risk of stimulant misuse or diversion is present.
  - Methylphenidate is ineffective at maximum tolerated dose.
  - Side effects of methylphenidate preclude its use.
- Monitor for side effects: agitation, irritability, suicidal thinking, self-harming behaviour, rare idiosyncratic liver disease.

Other medications
- These medications are prescribed rarely and for good reason! Use should be limited to very experienced professionals such as tertiary CAMHS.
- Clonidine:
  - Central alpha agonist.
  - Treat hyperactivity, tics, delayed sleep phase.
- Antidepressants, e.g. imipramine:
  - Inhibits reuptake of noradrenaline and serotonin.
  - Rarely used in treatment of ADHD in children.

Why treat ?
Untreated sufferers have high incidence of:
- Low self-esteem.
- Poor relationships with parents, peers, and partners.
- Progressive school failure (see 📖 p520).
- Poor educational and employment outcomes (see 📖 p344).
- Increased chance of injuries, accidents, driving offences.
- Convictions, assaults, drug/alcohol abuse are common.
- Intergenerational low human capital.

Prognosis

- Hyperactive symptoms may decrease with age. Inattentive symptoms are likely to remain in to adulthood. Low self-esteem is common even in adulthood.
- Children with ADHD are difficult to bring up and are liable to develop educational, behavioural, and conduct or emotional problems and suffer from low self-esteem.
- Outcome is likely to be better if:
  - Child has no comorbidity (or the comorbidities are investigated and treated).
  - Child/care givers/teachers are given information, support and advice (see below).
  - Adherence to treatment continues.

Support groups/patient information

- Provide parents/carers and children with information on:
  - Causation.
  - Therapeutic approaches to managing.
  - Medical information re: medicines, controlled medications, storage, holidays, airport laws.
  - Local and national support groups.
  - Support websites, etc.
  - List of books/booklets for parents, teachers, and siblings.

Further resources

Adders.org: ♒ http://www.adders.org
ADDISS: ☎ 020 8952 2800 ♒ http://www.addiss.co.uk
CHADD (Children and Adults with Attention Deficit/Hyperactivity Disorder) (leading US organization): ♒ http://www.chadd.org
Hyperactive Children's Support Group: ♒ http://www.hacsg.org.uk
Living with ADHD: ♒ http://www.livingwithadhd.co.uk

Developmental coordination disorder

- Historical terms associated with DCD:
  - Dysfunction of attention, motor function and perception (DAMP).
  - Clumsy child syndrome.
  - EHC problem.
  - Apraxia.
  - Ideomotor dyspraxia.
  - Developmental dyspraxia.
  - Minimal neurological dysfunction.
  - Mild CP.
- In essence, DCD means an impairment or difficulty in planning, organizing, and executing movements in the absence of a neurological or intellectual impairment. This has an impact on schooling and social functioning secondary to the difficulties in carrying out ADL.
- According to APA (DSM-IV) the following criteria need to be met to qualify for a diagnosis of DCD:
  - Motor coordination substantially below chronological age.
  - Motor coordination substantially below measured intelligence. If IDs are present, motor deficit is in excess of cognitive deficit.
  - Significantly interferes with academic achievement or adaptive function.
  - Disturbance not due to a general medical condition, e.g. myopathy or neuropathy.
  - Does not meet the criteria for a PDD (see 🕮 p107).

The 2006 Leeds Consensus statement (🕸 http://www.dcd-uk.org/diagnosis_c-d.html) states that 'It is inappropriate to exclude the possibility of a dual diagnosis of DCD and a pervasive developmental disorder, and both should be given if appropriate'.

- There is little difference between the DSM-IV definition and the WHO definition. The WHO labels this condition as 'Specific Developmental Disorder of Motor Function' (SDDMF). Both the diagnoses include a discrepancy factor between IQ and motor delay.
- DCD can be *classified* into:
  - Ideational DCD (affects planning and coordination).
  - Ideomotor DCD (affects fluency and speed of motor activities).

Prevalence

- Approx 5–6% of children may qualify for a diagnosis of DCD.
- The prevalence ranges from 5–15% in all the studies.
- 2–3% are likely to be more severe and the rest are on a continuum.
- Boys 3–4 times more likely to be affected than girls.

Risk factors

- FHx.
- Preterm birth.
- Extremely low birth weight.
- Exposure to teratogens in pregnancy, e.g. alcohol.
- Negative sociodemographic factors and environmental disadvantages may further compound the problem and/or worsen chances of enablement.

Causation

Various theories have been proposed.
- Internal modelling deficit (IMD): inability to accurately generate internal models of motor planning and execution.
- Possible sources of neuropathology: cerebellum, parietal lobe, corpus callosum, and basal ganglia. Cerebellar dysfunction is likely to be an important but not the sole cause.

Factors underpinning motor function

- Attention.
- Executive function, e.g. impulse control.
- Memory and cognition.
- Praxis (refers to planning and sequence necessary to perform the action).
- Vision (visual tracking, visual perception).
- Proprioception (reception of stimuli from muscles and tissues that results in a sense of body position).
- Sensorimotor feedback (aural, kinaesthetic, vestibular) impede or enhance the motor postures and movements.

Impairment or dysfunction in any of these areas will cause motor/coordination difficulties.

Common comorbidities

- ADD/ADHD (📖 p126).
- Dyslexia/reading disability (📖 p147).
- ASD (📖 p107).

Presenting features

Any of the ADL could be affected. Commonly present with:
- Slow, laborious, and immature handwriting.
- Difficulty in playing ball games, i.e. poor catching/throwing.
- Ambidextrous.
- Difficulty with dressing, undressing. Left–right confusion, wear clothes inside out/back to front.
- Messy eating. Preferring to eat with hands rather than fork or spoon.
- Shy from sports or physical activity. Poor at running, jumping, and team sports.
- Significant emotional and behavioural problems. Refuses to go to school, physical complaints to avoid work, tearful, anxious, depressed, isolated, withdrawn.

Assessment

- Hx and examination can rule out presence of physical or neurological condition causing incoordination.
- Neurodevelopmental testing (see 📖 p39) can confirm presence or absence of significant coordination difficulties by ability to provide percentiles, motor quotient, and sd.

History
- Results of previous scans, metabolic tests, genetic analysis if any.
- Parent and teacher behaviour questionnaire (SDQ).

- Pregnancy (teratogens, complications, TORCH infections/screen.
- Birth Hx (gestation, complications, birth weight, resuscitation required, special care, etc.).
- Acquisition of developmental milestones usually delayed (e.g. age of walking).
- Has the child lost any skills?
- Personal-social/adaptive skills, e.g. dressing, eating, tying laces, self-care etc.

Worsening of coordination difficulties and regression or loss of existing skills (see ☐ p253) would be inconsistent with the diagnosis of DCD.

Physical examination
- Any dysmorphic features? Examine head to toe (see ☐ p384).
- Growth (height, weight, head circumference) and plot them on centile charts.
- Neurological examination (assess cranial nerves, posture, tone, muscle bulk, muscle strength, deep tendon reflexes, primitive reflexes, involuntary movements, cerebellar functions, stressed gait, etc.). Stressed gaits = walking on the toes, heels, sideways, and backward.
- Developmental soft signs (refer to fine motor and social skills milestones (☐ p46 and p49)) and plot child's attainment).
- Vision. Correction of any refractive error (see ☐ p286).
- Hearing. Confirm hearing thresholds. Treatment of OME (see ☐ p306).
❶Presence of weakness, profound hypotonia, hypertonia, or ataxia would be incongruent with the diagnosis of DCD.

Neurodevelopmental assessment (see ☐ p36)
- Do gross and fine motor function assessment on GMDS-ER, Bayley, Bruininks-Oseretsky Test of Motor Proficiency, Test of Motor Impairment, etc.
- Administer motor tests, calculate quotients, and compare with standard scores. A score below the 5th centile would confirm evidence of significant coordination difficulties in gross and fine motor areas.
- M-ABC is widely used to screen for movement difficulties in school and can be completed by teachers.

Management
- Have a 'multifaceted' and 'holistic' approach to enablement.
- Treatments/therapies which incorporate the below are likely to be more successful.
  - Engage/motivate the child, i.e. child-centred.
  - Address functional activity, e.g. handwriting/drawing.
  - Are repetitive, i.e. practice and long term.
  - Goal directed, e.g. learning to ride bicycle.
  - Reward, i.e. SMART targets that give a sense of accomplishment.

Occupational therapy (see ☐ p188)
Following approaches have been in use to address coordination difficulties, namely:
- CO-OP (cognitive orientation to occupational performance)—can result in significant improvements in motor skill acquisition:

- The key feature is 'dynamic performance analysis' which looks into the difficulties child encounters while performing an activity. Use a problem-solving approach.
  - 'Goal–Plan–Do–Check'—child is taught a framework for solving motor-based performance problems.
  - 'Domain specific strategies'—uses a number of motor-based, child chosen activities such as cycling, using cutlery, handwriting, ball games, etc.
- SIT (sensory integration therapy): the theory is that certain motor deficits can be treated by controlling sensorimotor behaviour and thus promoting sensory integration. Can be useful in children with PDD/ASD.
- Specific skills approach: one of the most effective approaches. Emphasizes repetitive training of specific motor skills/task specific strategies.
- Motor imagery training: has shown promising results in small studies.
- OTs can also give advice on seating, access, modifications to the cutlery/dressing/writing materials, work surface etc. which is usually found very helpful by children and carers.

Physiotherapy (see 🕮 p176)
Can help with advice and modifications on posture, gross motor skills, and exercises.

Community/neurodevelopmental paediatrician
Identify and address comorbidities which compound the difficulty and impact on the treatment given, e.g. methylphenidate use for children with ADHD and DCD is shown to improve coordination and ADHD symptomatology.

School (see 🕮 p524)
- Educational/occupational interventions, e.g. teachers and teaching assistants can provide daily exercises as shown by the OT which would be effective in the majority of children.
- Provide scribe for important work or exams.
- Giving extra time for completing examinations.
- Actively encouraging and involving the child in team sports.
- Career counselling etc.

Psychologists
Counselling to address low self-esteem, shyness, and provide coping strategies.

Educational psychologists/neuropsychologists
Can identify associated co morbidities such as dyslexia, mild LD, etc. and give advice on appropriate interventions/modifications to the curriculum.

Adaptations to the environment (Also see 🕮 p191 and p193)
- Access to keyboard/laptop for work.
- Velcro instead of shoe laces.
- Fasteners instead of buttons.
- Rubber grip holders for pencils, chunky crayons, modified forks/spoons.
- Adjustments to chair/desk height, inclination, etc.

Support groups
Provide information about support, run courses, activity camps, advice on activities to practise, advocacy, raising awareness.

Prognosis

- DCD usually persist into adulthood, i.e. lifelong. Hence likely to lead to poor social and occupational outcomes.
- Children with DCD are more likely to show social isolation, emotional and behavioural problems, and low self-esteem compared to their peers.
- Children with DCD are also more likely to have aversion to physical exercises, have higher body fat, be obese, and suffer from poor cardiorespiratory fitness.
- With early identification (see 🕮 p59) followed by early multidisciplinary (see 🕮 p23) intervention the prognosis for social integration, self-esteem, emotional adjustment, and educational achievement is likely to be good.

Further resource

Dyspraxia Foundation: ☎ 01462 454986 ✎ http://www.dyspraxiafoundation.org.uk

Apraxia of speech

Terminologies
Apraxia of speech (AOS) has also been known in the past as:
- Articulatory dyspraxia.
- Verbal dyspraxia.
- Oromotor dyspraxia.
- Speech apraxia.
- Broca's aphasia etc.

Definition
- 'An impairment of motor speech control which leads to errors in sequencing, timing, coordination, initiation, and vocal tract shaping.'
- 'Articulatory errors' and 'prosodic abnormalities' are the hallmarks of AOS.
- Prosodic abnormalities include abnormal rhythm, stress and intonation of speech.

Pathophysiology
- In order to produce oral speech sounds, the nose must be closed and the velum (soft palate) must lift to close off the nasopharynx. With this closure the speaker is able to build up air pressure required to produce oral sounds (velopharyngeal (VP) competence).
- If this closure is not possible because of conditions such as cleft-lip, cleft-palate, short soft palate, enlarged tonsils, irregular tonsils, adenoidectomy, apraxia of speech, neuromotor disorders then VP incompetence or VP dysfunction ensues.
- Neuropsychology (see 🕮 p213): children with AOS show deficits on a range of phonologic tasks, including phoneme awareness and phonologic memory which are also common in reading disability and language impairment.

Presenting features
- Effortful 'trial and error' groping with attempts at self-correction.
- Persistent dysprosody, i.e. abnormal resonance, voice.
- Articulatory inconsistency on repeated productions of the same utterances.
- Obvious difficulty initiating utterances.
- Pausing between syllables and words is common.
- Difficulty imitating mouth movements.
- Use of vowel sounds, grunting, or single syllables.
- Omission of words in sentences.

Characteristic examples of AOS
The following examples are common in children with phonological delay and AOS children tend to have more severe difficulties:
- Omissions: 'I go to school on the bus' could become 'a do doo da'.
- Substitutions: 'I saw a little lamb'—'I saw a wittle wamb' b and/or d for all other consonants e.g. ba for Dad, sad, car etc.

- Distortions: difficulty in articulating differences between s, sh, ch; a for other vowels, e.g. ba for bed, bus, or bee.
- Extra sounds: 'animal'—'animamal or amimamal'.

Comorbidities

- Emotional and behavioural problems ~50%.
- ADHD ~19% (📖 p126).
- Anxiety disorders ~10% (📖 p354).
- Externalizing disorders, e.g. ODD, CD ~7% (📖 p334).
- Reading disability—dyslexia (📖 p147).
- Coordination problems—dyspraxia (📖 p136).

As a rule of thumb, a child's social and emotional development correlates well with his/her language development.

Assessment of speech and language

Language typically develops in predictable fashion and assessment of language should be a central part of every child visit (see 📖 p52).

History
Enquire about:
- Verbal comprehension and listening skills.
- Attention skills (e.g. stories, TV).
- Understanding of speech—1/2/3 step commands.
- Verbal expression: expressive speech, use of body language, facial expression eye contact, lip reading.
- Ask how much of what he/she says, do they understand (intelligibility of speech)?
- Any hearing concerns?
- ENT problems?
- Breathing/feeding problems at birth.
- Social skills.
- Communicative intent.
- Behaviour: any frustration/anger/tantrums, awareness? Teased? Friends?
- Speech:
  - 1,2,3,4,5-word sentences(in/out of context).
  - First recognizable word, when?
  - Amount of therapy/variety/previous tests.
  - Paucity of babbling, speech sounds, i.e. quiet child.
- Child care: nursery, playgroup, amount of home stimulation.
- Education: SEN/Statement/schooling/education psychology/concerns
- Mouth/oro-motor:
  - History of feeding difficulties in infancy.
  - Choking on food, dribbling, chewing, biting, swallowing.
  - Licking, sucking through straw, blowing bubbles.
  - Popping tongue out.
- Developmental Hx:
  - Coordination, running upstairs, kicking, pedalling.
  - Writing, buttoning, dressing/undressing, right/left-handed.
  - Other professionals involved?

- FHx: LD, speech and language delay, dyspraxia.

Examination
- Atypical facial expressions or lack of variety.
- Efforts to produce sounds are immature, laboured, and ineffective.
- Gap between receptive and expressive language abilities.
- Placement of lips, teeth, tongue during speech.
- Velum (soft palate).
- Facial movements (eye closure, blowing, smiling, coughing, whistling, licking, clenching, jaw etc.).
- Examine oral cavity and ENT: rule out submucous cleft, anatomical abnormalities.
- CNS: examine cranial nerves.
- Fine motor and performance skills.
- Observe and comment on (see 📖 p202):
  - Attention.
  - Behaviour.
  - Communicative intent.
  - Voice quality.
  - Syntax.
  - Semantics.
  - Prosody.
  - Pragmatics.
  - Non-verbal communicative skills.

▶Children rarely have a single LD. Multiple LDs (see 📖 p145) can be expected because reading, spelling, listening, speaking, and writing all involve manipulations of the same linguistic system. Children who have difficulty with reading are likely to have difficulty with spelling and speaking.

Speech sounds
- MSE (motor speech evaluation) includes a collection of words, phrases, and sentences that are sensitive in identifying and eliciting the deficits seen in AOS, i.e. articulation and prosodic abnormalities.
- Difficulty blending consonants and vowels.
- Inconsistent articulation of same words.
- Restricted set of consonants used.
- Difficulty in producing repeated sounds, e.g. Pitta/pitta/pitta etc.

Treatment
- Oro-motor exercises (breath control, air stream, lip shaping, tongue movements, facial movements, voice).
- Vocal play, babbling, single vowels/consonants.
- Practising single sounds, e.g. using Jolly phonics.
- Sequencing exercises (vowels and consonants), e.g. Nuffield dyspraxia programme.
- AAC: signing, use of symbol or picture communication, VOCAs, non-verbal (see 📖 p208 and p225).

Prognosis
- The course of language development determines prognosis.
- Non-verbal intelligence is the most important variable.
- Language impairment confined to expressive phonology is associated with low risk of later language/reading problems.
- Persisting language deficits at 5.5 years—poorer outcome (language/literacy/education).

Specific learning disabilities

- SpLD are a diverse group of conditions characterized by:
  - Difficulty of the child to attain, retain, and/or retrieve information proficiently.
  - Resulting in the child failing to achieve reading, writing, or mathematics skills at an age-appropriate level.
  - Despite average or above average cognitive abilities.
- Children rarely have a single LD.
▶Multiple LDs can be expected because reading, spelling, listening, speaking, and writing all involve manipulations of the same linguistic system e.g. children who have difficulty with reading are likely to have difficulty with spelling and speaking.

Aetiology

Is complex. Interaction of the following:
- Genetics. Highly heritable:
  - Found in clusters in families.
  - Likely autosomal dominant inheritance.
  - For example, various genes have been identified for developmental dyslexia such as 1p34–36/*DYX8*, 2p11–16/*DYX3*, 3p12–q13/*DYX5*, 6p21.3–22/*DYX2* etc.
- Environment, e.g.:
  - Low literacy levels in parents.
  - Poverty.
  - Absence of reading materials.
  - Living with <2 parents.
  - Prematurity, low/very low birth weight.
  - School absenteeism (see 📖 p344 and p522).

Predisposing factors/comorbidities

- Family history of SpLD/LD.
- Neurological conditions, e.g. CNS trauma/infection/irradiation, epilepsy.
- Neurodevelopmental disorders, e.g. ADHD (see 📖 p126), ASD (see 📖 p107), language disorders.
- Genetic/syndromic, e.g. fragile X (see 📖 p403), Klinefelter (see 📖 p393), etc.
- Chronic medical conditions (with frequent hospitalizations).

Types of SpLD

- Difficulty in reading and spelling (developmental dyslexia, 📖 p147).
- Difficulty in mathematics (developmental dyscalculia, 📖 p151).
- Difficulty in some or all aspects of writing, i.e. organizing and expressing thoughts, visuospatial (e.g. copying) difficulties (developmental dysgraphia, 📖 p150).

Outcome
- SpLD are common, pervasive and long term. They are an important cause of academic failure (see 📖 p520).
- Individuals with SpLD are more likely to:
  - Drop out of higher education.
  - Have lower job satisfaction.
  - Have difficulties in forming stable relationships etc.

Developmental dyslexia

Definition

- Is a specific learning disability characterized by difficulties with written language, both spelling and reading despite intelligence, motivation, and education opportunities.
- It is not an ID, occurs at all levels of intelligence including highly gifted.
- World Neurology Congress in 1968 stated: 'a disorder in children, who despite conventional classroom experience, fail to attain the language skills in reading, writing, spelling commensurate with their intellectual abilities'.
- ICD-10 describes this under 'Specific Developmental Disorders of Scholastic Skills' and defines this as "Disorders in which the normal patterns of skill acquisition are disturbed from the early stages of development. This is not simply a consequence of a lack of opportunity to learn, it is not solely a result of mental retardation, and it is not due to any form of acquired brain trauma or disease".

Pathophysiology

- Prevalence worldwide. Boys are 3–4 times likely to be referred, though epidemiological studies show equal number of poor readers in both sexes.
- The cause/combination of causes is likely to involve the following areas of the brain:
  - Broca's area–inferior frontal gyrus (word articulation).
  - Parieto-temporal region (word analysis).
  - Occipito-temporal (word form).

Presenting features in a preschool child

- Delay in speaking.
- Difficulty learning nursery rhymes.
- Trouble learning to recognize letters/alphabets.
- Frequent mispronunciations.
- Difficulty playing rhyming game with words.
- Strong FHx of reading, spelling, and literacy difficulties.

Presenting features in a school child

- Pointers in speech and language:
  - Difficulty in pronouncing long and complicated words.
  - Non-fluent speech, i.e. stuttering, stammering, hesitancy, etc.
  - Use of imprecise language.
- Pointers in reading:
  - Slow progress in reading skills/phonics.
  - Difficulty in reading unknown, new, or unfamiliar words.
  - Significantly poor spelling.
  - Difficulty in consistently sounding out words.
  - Reading is slow, effortful, and laboured.
  - 'He/she is not doing well in school'.
  - 'Slow reader', i.e. fail to recognize words automatically.
  - FHx of reading, spelling, and literacy difficulties.

Common comorbidities
- ADD/ADHD (□ p126).
- DCD (□ p136).
- Short-term memory problems (see □ p213).
- Poor organizational skills.
- Behavioural difficulties: low self-esteem, CD, ODD (□ p334).
- Anxiety, depression, withdrawal (□ p350 and p354).
- Multiple LDs are to be expected as reading, spelling, speaking and writing all involve manipulation of the same linguistic system (□ p145).

Work-up/diagnosis
- Developmental dyslexia is diagnosed by history, observation of educational progress and psychometric assessment of reading ability.
- Distinguished from other disorders that cause reading difficulties by its distinct deficit in phonologic processing. Listening to a child reading aloud an age appropriate book helps in identifying.
- Refer to either:
  - Educational psychologists (see □ p531).
  - Neuropsychologists (see □ p215).
  - Child psychologists.
  - Teachers with specialist expertise in reading disability.
- These professionals would use tests such as:
  - Dyslexia Screening test (Preschool and Junior versions).
  - Test of Phonologic Processing in Reading.
- The 'dyslexia tests' measure child's phonologic abilities by assessing:
  - Decoding (accuracy of reading).
  - Fluency of reading (phonologic awareness).
  - Comprehension.
  - Pseudoword or nonsense word reading.
  - Word rhymes (ability to identify).
  - Rapid naming of pictures or symbols.
  - Elision (say stream without 'r').
  - Blending of sounds/words e.g. can/dy/?
  - Segmenting, e.g. bat 'bbb' 'aaa' 'ttt' etc.
  - Digit memory, e.g. say 4–2–9–1, ask them to repeat.

Management
- Early identification/screening of 'at-risk' children.
- Prevention programmes e.g. 'Sure Start' help. Explicitly teaching children about segmenting and blending words is effective.
- Rule out impairments in general cognition (see □ p42 and p213), vision, and hearing.
- Referral to SEN services at Local Education Authority (□ p524).
- Provision of extra time in assessments.
- Scribe or 'note taker' for important assignments.
- Taping classroom lectures.
- Effective intervention programmes that target phonemic awareness, phonics, comprehension strategies, format of tests, e.g. short essays.

- Involve an *educational psychologist* for remedial instruction (see 📖 p533 and p537), compensatory strategies, multisensory instruction, software programs (spell check, grammar check, word processing, etc.), organizational strategies (timelines, binders, coloured sheets, etc.).
- Identify and treat comorbidities.

Further resources

Dyslexia Action ☎ 01784 222300 🖑 http://www.dyslexiaaction.org.uk
The British Dyslexia Association ☎ 0845 251 9002 🖑 http://www.bdadyslexia.org.uk

Developmental dysgraphia

- It is difficulty with writing regardless of the ability to read.
- It is not due to ID.
- The DSM IV (the sourcebook for mental health diagnoses) identifies a 'Disorder of Written Expression' as 'writing skills (that)…are substantially below those expected given the person's…age, measured intelligence, and age-appropriate education'.
- Many types have been described: dyslexic dysgraphia, motor dysgraphia, spatial dysgraphia, etc.
- WHO describes this condition as a 'Writing disorder' (ICD-10 code F81.1).

Presenting features

- Handwriting difficulties: swapping upper case/lower case letters, illegible writing.
- Huge number of errors in grammar, syntax, and occasionally spelling.
- Visuospatial difficulties resulting in difficulty in using lines and space.
- Slow, effortful, and ineffective writing.
- Difficulties in organizing and expressing thoughts in writing.
- Difficulty in copying from board/text.
- Find written work tiring and stressful. Many complain of pain in the hands.
- No difficulties in reading, spelling, or giving answers verbally unless there is accompanying dyslexia.
- Need not necessarily have difficulties in other fine motor and gross motor coordination skills unless there is comorbid DCD (see 🕮 p136).

Assessment

- Get 'hearing' (see 🕮 p296) and 'vision' (see 🕮 p271) assessed.
- Examine neurology (see 🕮 p228): tone, power, reflexes, movements, cerebellar function. Look for neurocutaneous stigmata, dysmorphic features.
- Developmental assessment (see 🕮 p36) to rule out 'global delay/ ID'(see 🕮 p117).
- Refer to OTs (see 🕮 p188) and/or educational psychologists (see 🕮 p531) to assess and confirm.
- Assessment for comorbid conditions such as dyslexia (see 🕮 p147), DCD.

Remediation

- Occupational therapists/teachers can offer a handwriting programme, e.g. Handwriting Without Tears®.
- Use of pre-lined paper. handwriting practice.
- Extra 1:1 support. Small groups. Provide encouragement. Motivate.
- Use of a keyboard/laptop for written work in class.
- Teachers giving copy of lectures/class work.
- Use of note-takers/scribe for important work such as exams or providing answers on Dictaphone.
- Extra time to complete the task especially in exams/assessments.
- Computer can assist with spell check, grammar check, voice recognition software, word recognition, etc.

Prognosis

- Is better if there are no other SpLD such as dyscalculia (see 🕮 p151) or dyslexia.
- The incidence of emotional and behavioural disorders appears to be less compared to other SpLD (see 🕮 p145).

Developmental dyscalculia

- The DSM-IV has the following diagnostic criteria for 'Mathematics Disorder': "Mathematical ability, as measured by individually administered standardised tests, is substantially below that expected given the person's chronological age, measured intelligence, and age-appropriate education, which significantly interferes with academic achievement or activities of daily living that require mathematical ability' (American Psychiatric Association, 1994, Section 315.1).
- Department for Education and Skills in UK describes this as: a condition that affects the ability to:
  - Acquire arithmetical skills.
  - Understand simple number concepts.
  - Grasp numbers intuitively.
  - Learn number facts and procedures etc.
- WHO ICD-10 F81.2 describes this condition as a 'Specific disorder of arithmetical skills'.
- Comorbidities are the rule rather than exception, i.e. dyscalculia is more likely to accompany other SpLD such as dyslexia, dyspraxia, dysgraphia.

Pathogenesis

- Parietal lobe (considered important in numeracy, judgement of size and shape, written language, etc.) is most commonly implicated.
- The heterogeneous nature of this disorder and the accompanying varied comorbidities makes it unlikely to be a single-lobe disorder. Frontal (executive function attention and working memory) and temporal (auditory perception, language comprehension, verbal categorization, long term memory) regions have also been implicated.

Presenting features

- Depend on presence/absence of:
  - Comorbidities, e.g. dyslexia (see 🕮 p147), DCD (see 🕮 p136).
  - Emotional and behavioural disorders.
  - Amount of intervention/tuition/coaching/stimulation the child has been exposed to.
- Children can present with difficulties in:
  - Mastery of basic computational skills of addition, subtraction, multiplication, and division.
  - Calculating, budgeting, sometimes even at a basic level.
  - Navigating, reading analogue clocks, conceptualizing time/duration.
  - Right/left orientation, visuospatial orientation, multistep problems.
  - Remembering/retrieving of mathematical concepts, rules, formulae, and sequences.
  - Correctly deciphering the language of maths.

Assessment

- Collate reports from teachers on child's academic and social functioning.
- Check 'hearing' and 'vision'.
- Developmental tests to rule out 'global delay/ID' (see 🕮 p117).

- Assess neurology (see 📖 p228) e.g. signs of neurocutaneous disorders
- Examine to look for chronic medical conditions, dysmorphic features, etc.
- Consider referral to educational psychologists (see 📖 p531) or occasionally neuropsychologists (see 📖 p215) who can carry out standardized arithmetic, reading and writing tests.
  - They also collate information from teachers, parents and other health professionals on FHx of LD/SpLD, socioeconomic status and educational interventions already tried, etc. before making a diagnosis.

Remediation and rehabilitation

- For success it is crucial to address the following:
  - Comorbid conditions.
  - Behavioural/emotional difficulties and self-esteem issues.
- Involve the family. Explain the implications of the diagnosis and interventions available to child, family, and school.
- Accommodation and modification to the child's curriculum and environment. Some examples are:
  - Small group/1:1 teaching by teachers experienced in remedial education.
  - Repetition and plenty of practice.
  - Access to computer and calculator.
  - Set small targets. Frequent feedback and use of rewards to maintain motivation.
  - Extra time for exams.
  - Career counselling.

Prognosis

- We live in a society that is becoming increasingly literate and numerate. Hence difficulties in numeracy, arithmetic skills, and literacy can have a negative impact on social, educational, and occupational outcomes.
- Prognosis is better with:
  - Early identification.
  - Better tuition/remedial teaching.
  - Involvement of family.
  - Accommodation of difficulties.
  - Adjustment/acceptance of the diagnosis.
  - Playing to one's strengths/positives.
  - Choosing an appropriate course for further education.
  - Career counselling.

Further resources

Dyscalculia (help through dyslexia associations).
Dyslexia Action ☎ 01784 222300 🖱 http://www.dyslexiaaction.org.uk
The British Dyslexia Association ☎ 0845 251 9002 🖱 http://www.bdadyslexia.org.uk

Inherited metabolic disorders

- IMDs are conditions characterized by:
  - A lack of a specific enzyme, a cofactor, or a transport protein.
  - Leading to either toxic accumulation or deficiency of an end product.
  - Causing disruption of energy production, energy utilization, or progressive damage to organs due to disruption of normal physiological and biochemical pathways.
- ~500 IMDs have been identified. Moreover, many of these conditions vary in their onset, severity, and in the way they are inherited. Hence a detailed summary of IMD is beyond the scope of this book!
- Also many of these IMD present in neonatal period or infancy. Some could present anytime till adulthood.
- Most IMD present to neonatologists, neurologists, or acute paediatricians. A smaller proportion present to community paediatrics masquerading as developmental delay or regression.
- Professionals should be able to suspect/recognize IMD and make onward referrals to tertiary centres for further investigations and management.
- Specific treatment is available for an increasing number of IMDs.

Incidence

- Individually rare. Collectively ~1:1000–1:1500.
- PKU~1:13000, mitochondrial disorders ~1:5000, lysosomal storage disorders ~1:5000, medium chain acyl dehydrogenase deficiency (MCADD) ~1:8000.

Inheritance

- IMDs are generally single-gene disorders.
- Most common mode is AR. Hence higher incidence/prevalence in populations with high consanguinity.
- Modes: AR (e.g. galactosaemia), X-linked recessive (e.g. Hunter syndrome, ornithine transcarbamylase deficiency, Menkes syndrome), AD (e.g. familial hypercholesterolemia), mitochondrial (e.g. MELAS, MERFF).

Types of IMD

Disorders of:
- Carbohydrate metabolism e.g. glycogen storage diseases (GSDs).
- Fatty acid oxidation, e.g. MCAD.
- Amino acid, e.g. PKU.
- Purine metabolism, e.g. Lesch–Nyhan syndrome.
- Urea cycle, e.g. ornithine transcarbamylase deficiency.
- Mitochondria, e.g. pyruvate dehydrogenase deficiency.
- Peroxisomal, e.g. Zellweger syndrome.
- Lysosomal storage disorders, e.g. MPS, Tay–Sachs, Niemann–Pick disease.
- Metal, e.g. Wilson, Menkes disease (copper), PKAN (iron).
- Others, e.g. hypothyroidism.

Clinical presentation

- Severe variants present in the neonatal period or early infancy. Less severe cases could present anytime.
- Clinical presentation depends on the severity of enzyme deficiency, the nature and rate of the accumulating toxic metabolite, and the severity of disruption of energy metabolism.
- Presentation also depends on timing of the insult/trigger in many cases. Illness, fasting, unaccustomed exercise, certain medications, childbirth, surgery could trigger a decompensation and uncover IMDs.
- IMD can present in following ways:
  - *Neurological* (acute encephalopathy, weakness, abnormalities of tone, ataxia, peripheral neuropathy, paraparesis, delirium, hallucinations, agitation, coma, seizures, neuropsychiatric manifestations, e.g. self-injury in Lesch–Nyhan disease, ADHD in Sanfilippo syndrome).
  - *Gastrointestinal* (FTT, poor feeding, vomiting, e.g. organic acidurias, hepatomegaly, e.g. GSD, hepatosplenomegaly, e.g. lysosomal storage disorders).
  - *Haematological* (neutropenia, e.g. GSD, pancytopenia, e.g. Gaucher disease, megaloblastic anaemia, e.g. disorders of B12 metabolism).
  - *Renal* (nephrolithiasis, e.g. cystinuria, RTA, e.g. mitochondrial disorders).
  - *Musculoskeletal* e.g. exercise intolerance, muscle pain and cramps in metabolic myopathies.
  - *In infancy* as sudden infant death syndrome, apparent life-threatening event, e.g. MCAD deficiency or as critically ill neonate.
  - *Biochemical* (hypoglycaemia, ketosis, hyperammonaemia, metabolic acidosis, lactic acidosis, etc.).

Abnormal biochemistry could accompany any of these system disorders or these biochemical abnormalities could be found unexpectedly in a child with a mild illness.

Neurodevelopmental disorders and inherited metabolic disorders

- IMDs account for ~1–5% cases of DD.
- Developmental delay in IMD is:
  - Usually global, not specific or isolated skill delay (see 📖 p117).
  - Usually progressive.
  - Usually associated with 'DD plus' i.e. central/peripheral nervous system disease, cardiomyopathy, dysmorphology (see 📖 p123), etc.
- Have a low threshold to investigate those children where DD presents with other features in Hx or examination.
- There are >200 IMDs which could result in DD.
- IMD could present as DD, regression, mild to profound LD, autism (see 📖 p107).
- Conditions causing DD, e.g. lysosomal storage disorders, urea cycle disorders, peroxisomal disorders, mitochondrial disorders, etc.

History

- Pregnancy: decreased fetal movements, e.g. Zellweger syndrome, non-immune hydrops, prolonged labour, previous miscarriages, HELLP syndrome, neonatal encephalopathy could all be a signs of IMD.
- PMHx: recurrent vomiting, dehydration, hypoglycaemia, seizures, abnormal movements, hospitalizations, stepwise deterioration.
- FHx: consanguinity, thrombotic events, DD, deaths in infancy, affected siblings.
- Enquire about growth (FTT), diarrhoea, lethargy in the morning, DD, unusual odours (organic acidurias), protein aversion (urea cycle disorders).

Examination

- Height (tall in homocystinuria, short in MPS disorders), OFC (small in untreated PKU, large in Canavan disease), weight.
- Hair (sparse and kinked in Menkes disease).
- Skin (hirsute in MPS, eczema/alopecia in biotinidase deficiency).
- Dysmorphic features (marfanoid habitus in homocystinuria, coarse features in MPS, etc.).
- Eyes (cataracts, e.g. galactosaemia, cherry red macula in Tay–Sachs disease, Kayser–Fleischer ring in Wilson disease, corneal clouding in MPS).
- Ears (conductive hearing loss in MPS).
- Mouth (gingival hypertrophy in MPS).
- Abdomen (hepatosplenomegaly in LSD).
- Neurology (assess tone, power, reflexes, abnormal movements, cognitive development). E.g. dystonia in Lesch–Nyhan syndrome and organic acidaemias, hypotonia in mitochondrial and peroxisomal disorders, etc.
- Behaviour (e.g. challenging in Sanfilippo syndrome, autistic in Smith–Lemli–Opitz syndrome, self-mutilation in Lesch–Nyhan syndrome).
- Skeletal dysplasias (lysosomal and peroxisomal disorders).

Investigations

▶Good detailed Hx (milestones) is the single most important investigation (will differentiate static vs progressive).

Why investigate?
- Identify treatable condition (urea cycle defects, aminoacidurias, biotinidase deficiency, dopa-responsive dystonias, pyridoxine deficiency, Wilson disease, Refsum disease etc.).
- Genetic implications.
- A support group.
- Leverage with resources.
- An explanation to parents etc.

Baseline

Undertake if DD is present with other features in Hx:
- FBC.
- Blood gas (to check for metabolic acidosis and respiratory alkalosis).
- Ammonia (do not use tourniquet. Transfer bloods to lab on ice).
- U&E (to calculate anion gap).
- LFTs.
- TFTs.
- Uric acid (high in Lesch–Nyhan syndrome).
- Lactate (no tourniquet, transfer bloods on ice).
- CK.
- Blood glucose.
- Urine (amino acids, organic acids, glycosaminoglycans).

See Table 4.12.

Interpretation of the results from the baseline tests should take the following guidance into account.

Table 4.12 Interpretation of baseline tests[a]

Test Abnormality	Comments and Possible Causes of Abnormal Results
↑ Creatinine Kinase	Muscle Injury. Muscular Dystrophy. Fatty Acid Oxidation Disorders.
Lactate ↑	Excessive screaming, tourniquet pressure. Gluconegenetic disorders. Disorders of Pyruvate metabolism. Mitochondrial Disorders
	Is urine lactate increased? } If yes suggests elevation of plasma alanine increased? } lactate.
↑ Ammonia	Sample contamination. Sample delay in transport/processing. Specimen haemolysed. Urea Cyle disorders. Liver Dysfunction.
Urate	An abnormally high or low result is significant. Glycogen Storage disorder ↑. Purine disorders ↑. Molybdenum Cofactor deficiency ↓.

[a] Reproduced with permission from 'Best Practice Guidelines for the Biochemical Investigation of Global Developmental Delay for Inherited Metabolic Disorders (IMD)', Green A (2006) The National Metabolic Biochemistry Network, http://metbio.net

Further investigations
- Guided by history, examination findings, and baseline tests.
- Best done in a specialist setting where there are facilities for ordering these tests and interpreting them appropriately.
- If specific clinical features then discuss with metabolic team before ordering tests.
- There are 'profiles', i.e. bunch of tests for each scenario, i.e. hepatosplenomegaly, hydrops, cherry-red macula, etc. (Table 4.13):
  - Brain MRI scan. MRI abnormalities in inborn errors of metabolism are usually symmetrical.
  - Plasma AAs (quantitative).
  - VLCFA, plasmalogens and phytanic acid.
  - White cell enzymes for lysosomal disorders.
  - Plasma and urine creatine.
  - Lumbar puncture (glucose, protein, protein, glycine, serine, alanine, OA, neurotransmitters, lactate, pyruvate).
  - Echocardiography (cardiomyopathy in fatty acid oxidation disorders).
  - Eye (refer to ophthalmologists).
  - X-rays for skeletal abnormalities.

Table 4.13 Developmental delay plus (B, blood; C, cerebral spinal fluid; P, plasma; U, urine).[a]

Disorder	Test
Hypotonia	
Peroxisomal disorders	VLCFA (P)
Biotinidase deficiency	Biotinidase assay (P)
Purine/pyrimidines disorders	Urate (B) and (U)
	Purine/pyrimidines (U)
Neurotransmitter deficiencies	Biopterins (B) and (C)
	Neurotransmitters (C)
Fatty acid oxidation defects	Acylcarnitines (P)
Organic acid disorders	Organic acids (U)
Neurological regression	
Biotinidase deficiency	Biotinidase (P)
Mucopolysaccharidoses	Urine glycosaminoglycans (U)
	White cell enzymes (B)
Neuronal ceroid lipofuscinosis	Vacuolated lymphocytes, NCL enzymes, mutations (B)
Other lysosomal disorders	White cell enzymes (B)
	Oligosaccharides (U)
Mitochondrial disorders	Lactate (B) and (C)

Table 4.13 (Continued)

Disorder	Test
	Respiratory chain enzymes (muscle and skin)
	Mitochondrial mutations/deletions (B and muscle)
Neurotransmitter deficiencies	Neurotransmitters (C)
	Biopterins (B) and (C)
Organic acid disorders	Organic acids (U)
	Acylcarnitines (P)
Eye signs	
Peroxisomal disorders	VLCFA (P)
Disorders of cholesterol synthesis	7-dehydrocholesterol, cholesterol (B)
Mitochondrial disorders	Lactate (B), CSF lactate
Congenital disorders of glycosylation	Transferrin isoforms (B)
Sulphite oxidase deficiency	Urate (P), sulphites (U)
Homocystinuria	Homocysteine (P)
	Amino acids (homocystine) (U)
Lysosomal storage disorders	Glycosaminoglycans (U)
	White cell enzymes (B)
Cerebrotendinous xanthomatosis	Bile acids (U)
Severe seizure disorder	
Sulphite oxidase deficiency/ molybdenum cofactor deficiency	Urate (P)
	Sulphites (U)
Biotinidase deficiency	Biotinidase
Neuronal ceroid lipofuscinosis	Vacuolated lymphocytes, NCL enzymes, mutations (B)
Non-ketotic hyperglycinaemia	Amino acids (P and U)
Creatine deficiency	24-hour creatine:creatinine, specific metabolites
	MRS brain

(Continued)

Table 4.13 (Continued)

Hepato(spleno)megaly	
Lysosomal storage disorders	Glycosaminoglycans (U)
	White cell enzymes (B)
	Oligosaccharides (U)
Urea cycle disorders	Ammonia
	Amino acids (P) and (U)
	Orotic acid (U)
Bile acid disorders	Bile acids (U)
Glycogen storage disorders	Lactate (B), glucose profile, cholesterol, triglycerides
Developmental delay plus dysmorphism	
Smith–Lemli–Opitz syndrome	7-dehydrocholesterol, cholesterol (P)
	Cholesterol precursors (P)
Other cholesterol precursor disorders	
Peroxisomal disorders	VLCFA (P)
	Plasmalogens
	(XR epiphyses)
Congenital disorders of glycosylation	Transferrin isoforms (P)
Mucopolysaccharide disorders and other storage disorders	Glycosaminoglycans (U)
	White cell enzymes (B)

[a]Reproduced from Cleary MA et al. Developmental Delay: when to suspect and how to investigate for an inborn error of metabolism. *Arch Dis Child* 2005; **90**:1128–32 with permission from BMJ Publishing Group Ltd.

Diagnosis

- Reliant on having a high index of suspicion in the earlier given clinical scenarios, ordering appropriate tests and
- Considering referral to units with specialist expertise in IMD.
- Diagnosis will help in offering specific treatment.
- Also helpful in counselling and enables clinicians to give a prognosis.

Management

- An increasing number of IMDs are being included in the newborn screening programmes.
- Early recognition is likely to prevent progressive neurological damage in many cases.
- Requires specialist expertise in IMD and intensive care facilities especially during acute decompensation. Mortality and morbidity is higher if poorly treated during acute illness.
- In the acute situation, the child might need:
  - Ventilator support.
  - Fluid resuscitation.
  - Treating of hypoglycaemia (IV 10% dextrose).
  - Hyperammonaemia (medications).
  - Acidosis (bicarbonate).
  - Reversal of catabolism (insulin infusion).
  - Renal replacement therapy (dialysis).
  - Empiric antibiotics till cultures are negative.
  - For emergency management guidelines see ℘ http://www.bimdg.org.uk.
- Specific long-term treatments might include:
  - Dietary education and compliance is crucial. Special diets, e.g. phenylalanine free in PKU.
  - Provision of cofactors, e.g. pyridoxine in pyridoxine-dependent seizures.
  - Enzyme replacement therapy, e.g. MPS correcting deficiency, e.g. thyroxine in hypothyroidism.
  - Stimulating alternative metabolic pathway, e.g. benzoate for urea cycle defects, penicillamine for Wilson disease.
  - Organ transplantation, e.g. liver transplant in GSD, bone marrow transplant in metachromatic leucodystrophy.
- Close follow-up to monitor growth, cognitive development (see 📖 p36), and physical health.
- Enablement:
  - Housing, e.g. adaptations for ramps, railings, hoist, downstairs toilet/ shower/bed (see 📖 p191), etc.
  - Aids, e.g. wheelchairs, glasses, hearing aids, etc.
  - Appliances, e.g. orthoses (see 📖 p220), splints, special mattress, etc.
  - Education, e.g. statement of SEN, home schooling (see 📖 p524 and p534).
  - Leisure, e.g. access to swimming, entertainment activities, etc.
- Social support, e.g. help with respite, transport, benefits, allowances, etc (see 📖 p514).

- Refer affected families to geneticists for counselling regarding recurrence risks (see 📖 p380).

Further resources

Inherited Metabolic Diseases: ☎ 0800 652 3181 🖰 http://www.climb.org.uk
Mucopolysaccharidoses Society: 🖰 http://www.mpssociety.co.uk
National Society for Phenylketonuria (UK) Ltd.: ☎ 020 8364 3010 🖰 http://www.nspku.org
🖰 www.bimdg.org.uk (for emergency management)

Incontinence in children with developmental disabilities

Problem

- Control of bladder and bowel function is influenced by genetic, neurodevelopmental, social (parental expectations), environmental (starting preschool), and physiological (ability to sit) factors. Most children are continent by 3 years of age.
- ~85% of children with tetraparesis and ~2/3 of children with an IQ <50 suffer from daytime/night-time wetting.
- ~1:10 children with developmental disabilities have normal fluid intake.
- Late toilet training in children with LD (see 📖 p117) is associated with an increase in urinary incontinence and child's reluctance to engage with toilet training later.

Causes

- Central: CP (see 📖 p67), severe ID, TBI (see 📖 p267), cerebral malformations.
- Local: spina bifida (see 📖 p261), spinal cord defects, myelomeningocele, Hirschsprung disease, anal atresia/stenosis.
- Behavioural: ASD (see 📖 p107) (resistance to change).
- Consider sexual abuse (see 📖 p453) as a possibility.

Contributory/predisposing factors

Constipation

- Causes: poor diet, reduced fluids intake, decreased mobility, non-erect positioning, low tone, inability to communicate pain/discomfort, medications, etc. all contribute towards establishment of significant and long-standing constipation (see 📖 p84).
- Consequences: pain, bleeding, anal fissures, poor feeding, behavioural problems, social stigma (overflow incontinence), psychological distress to family, megacolon, urinary incontinence, bowel obstruction.

Poor fluid intake

- Causes: swallowing difficulties (see 📖 p81 and p88), inability to communicate thirst, reduced access to drinks, inability to fetch a drink, considered a low priority (vs medications, feeds, etc.), lack of appreciation of importance of fluid intake in parents/carers, etc.
- Consequences: insufficient hydration over a period of time causes small capacity bladder (bladder deficit) leading to urinary incontinence. There is good correlation between maximum voided volume and bladder continence. Also poor hydration can contribute to sustaining constipation which is well correlated with urinary and faecal incontinence.

Associated developmental disabilities

For example, ADHD (see 📖 p126), DCD (see 📖 p136), communication difficulties (see 📖 p208), Epilepsy (see 📖 p240) can interfere with acquisition of skills required for continence.

Consequences of incontinence
- Impact on the child: low self-esteem, social isolation, long-term psychological consequences (see 📖 p363).
- Impact on family: stigmatization, parental stress, siblings discord, significant burden of care (see 📖 p27).
- Impact on society: huge financial implications from provision of additional carers and aids. Social exclusion.

Toilet training
- Indicators of readiness-child's ability to stay dry for 1–2 hours.
- Benefits of early toilet training—more chance of becoming continent. Better social functioning and parental well-being. Less burden physically and financially.
- Steps of toilet training:
  - Sitting on the toilet (or potty) regularly, especially after meals.
  - Addressing well-balanced diet and good drinking habits.
  - Toilet habits-pulling pants up/down, sitting on the toilet, handwashing.
  - Moving on to washable underwear and trainer pants.
  - Rewards, praise, encouragement for using the toilet.
- Techniques:
  - Shaping (increasing proximity to toilet).
  - Fading (reducing presence of nappy).
  - Operant conditioning (modification of voluntary behaviour by positive or negative reinforcement).
  - Other measures: soft music and distractions, blowing bubbles, etc. while seated on toilet.

Management
- General measures: adequate fluids and balanced diet are crucial. Normalization of fluid intake has good correlation with bladder continence.
- Multidisciplinary liaison:
  - OT: advice on access to toilet, seating, clothing, self-care skills, (see 📖 p191) etc.
  - Continence nurse advisor: can help with fluid intake charts, behavioural modification, toilet training methods, supply of absorbent products, advice on bedding, enuresis alarms, etc.
  - Psychologist: address low self-esteem in child, psychological support to the family (see 📖 p373).
  - SLT: use of social stories and PECS system to communicate needs around toileting (see 📖 p208).
  - School: consistency and good communication between home and school.
- Medical measures: treat constipation with laxatives (e.g. lactulose), stimulants (e.g. senna) and osmotic agents (e.g. polyethylene glycol/ Movicol®).
- Surgical measures: appendicocaecostomy (MACE procedure) for chronic treatment resistant constipation (see 📖 p98).
- Adaptations: clothing alterations.

- Aids: nappies or pull-ups. The choice depends on the level of independence in toileting, discreetness in changing, fit, appearance, etc. Pull-ups can assist with toileting and pad changes. Nappies are easy to change especially if child has callipers, adapted footwear, etc. Since diapers are more absorbent they are preferred for night-time use.

Prognosis

- Likelihood of continence is directly proportional to the degree of LD and degree of physical mobility.
- Children with moderate LD and moderate disability in mobility can be expected to be continent by 3–4 years.
- Children with severe to profound disability in learning and mobility are less likely to become continent after 8 years.

Further resources

ERIC (Education and Resources for Improving Childhood Continence) ☎ 0845 370 8008
🖰 http://www.eric.org.uk
PromoCon: 🖰 http://www.promocon.co.uk
The Bladder and Bowel Foundation: ☎ 0845 345 0165 🖰 http://www.bladderandbowelfoundation.
   org

Dental health in children with developmental disabilities

Problem
- Children with disability are 4–5 times more likely to have dental problems vs non-disabled peers.
- They are less likely to receive preventive and restorative dental care.
- Dentists report communication problems and carers report non-cooperation of the child as significant barriers to oral care.
- Poor access to dental services who can manage children with complex needs.

Predisposing factors to poor dental care
- Child factors: fear of examination, inability to comprehend the need for treatment, dry mouth (e.g. mouth breathing), medications (syrups), difficulty in swallowing/feeding, inability to communicate sensation in the mouth, involuntary tongue thrusting, sensory integration difficulties with brushing.
- Parent/carer: competing priorities with other health needs, lack of awareness of importance of early dental care, difficulty in accessing suitable services.
- Service: lack of training in special needs, lack of adequate number of dentists in special needs dentistry, negative attitudes, inadequate provisions for socially excluded groups.

Common dental conditions in children with special needs
- Halitosis: caused by mouth breathing, chronic sinusitis, bronchitis, GI disturbances, periodontitis (gum disease), certain foods, etc.
- Malocclusion: crowding, misalignment, gap between upper and lower set of teeth makes provision of care difficult.
- Dental caries: secondary to inadequate brushing, poor hygiene, medications containing sugar, GORD (see 📖 p83).
- Tooth anomalies: eruption could be delayed e.g. DS (see 📖 p387) delayed by 2 years. Also could be variations in shape, size, and number of teeth.
- Xerostomia (dry mouth): mouth breathing, medications, salivary gland problems could cause this.
- Bruxism (habitual grinding and clenching of teeth): secondary to boredom, anxiety, pain, malocclusion, etc. Consider bite guarding splint or referral to orthodontics.
- Oral trauma: more common. Secondary to falls, seizures, lack of protective reflexes, etc.
- Periodontitis: caused by plaque formation. More teeth are lost due to periodontitis than tooth decay.
- Infections: herpetic gingivostomatitis (HSV), oral thrush (candida), etc.
- Bleeding gums: could be first sign of gum disease. Scurvy, bleeding disorders, phenytoin use.
- Pica: eating of non-edible substances can damage teeth and gums.

Consequences of poor dental health

- Inability to receive adequate nutrition.
- Halitosis, missing teeth, and periodontal disease add a further barrier to social interaction/acceptance.
- Build up of bacteria in the mouth can impact on general health.
- Frequent dental pain can have impact on sleep, behaviour, general well-being, and hence on quality of life.

Prevention

- Good oral care (twice daily brushing after meals, dental floss) and hygiene (mouthwash or rinsing with plain water) can prevent dental disease.
- Start brushing after the first tooth eruption. Use fluoride toothpaste.
- Involve OT and/or SLT to help with positioning, equipment, and oral desensitizing techniques (see 📖 p88 and p194).
- Resistance to brushing could be overcome by: good support, comfortable head position, well-lit location, using brush with soft/ultra soft bristles, brushing while seated in front of a mirror, brushing as a family, letting the child play with brush, oral massaging, lots of praise, being patient, etc.
- Fear of dental practices can be managed by gradual introduction to the premises, short appointments.
- Regular dental visits help prevent dental emergencies and gum disease.
- Balanced diet, sugar-free medications, and physical activity where possible.
- Education of patients and parents/carers should be undertaken early.
- Preventive dentistry will minimize the need for dental extractions, operative interventions, etc.

Management

- CBT in selected cases could address dental phobias (see 📖 p373). Listen to parents/carers.
- Undertaken by community dental services or specialist dental hospitals where dentists trained in special needs are available.
- Measures to restrain should be explained and agreed with parents/carers before the procedure.
- Good analgesia and use of conscious sedation should be offered when required. Small proportion of children might require general anaesthetic.
- Sealants for dental cavities, tooth extraction and restoration for dental caries.
- Consider artificial saliva for dry mouth.
- HSV stomatitis: analgesic mouthwashes/spray (e.g. Difflam®) and oral acyclovir for 5 days.
- Candidiasis: Treat with nystatin pastille, suspension, or gel.

Further resources

Association for Rehabilitation of Communication and Oral Skills: ⌨ http://www.arcos.org.uk
British Dental Health Foundation: ⌨ http://www.dentalhealth.org/
British Society for Disability and oral Health: ⌨ http://www.bsdh.org.uk
National Institute of Dental and Craniofacial Research, National Institute of Health: ⌨ http://www.nidcr.nih.gov
Scope Response (Scope): ☎ 0808 800 3333 ⌨ http://www.scope.org.uk

Sleep disorders and management

- Sleep disorders are very common in typically developing children, up to 20–30%.
- Sleep disorders are very prevalent in children with neurodevelopmental and psychiatric conditions.
- Process of sleep regulation and sleep consolidation is influenced by a combination of biological, behavioural, environmental, and neurodevelopmental factors.

Types of sleep disorders

- Primary sleep disorders:
  - Dyssomnias (a disturbance in the quality, quantity, or timing of sleep), e.g. bedtime resistance, delayed sleep onset, frequent awakenings, primary hypersomnias, idiopathic insomnia, narcolepsy, etc.
  - Parasomnias (deviated behavioural or physiological events that occur during sleep), e.g. sleep walking, night terrors, nightmares.
- Sleep disorders secondary to medical conditions, e.g.:
  - CNS (cerebral palsies (see 🛄 p67), epilepsies (see 🛄 p240)).
  - Respiratory (asthma, OSA (see 🛄 p90)).
  - CVS (pulmonary oedema due to heart failure, see 🛄 p90).
  - GI (colitis).
  - Skin (atopic dermatitis).
  - Skeletal (juvenile rheumatoid arthritis).
  - Eye (blindness (see 🛄 p275)) etc.
- Sleep disorders secondary to psychiatric/mental health conditions: e.g. anxiety (see 🛄 p354), depression (see 🛄 p350), phobias, post-traumatic stress disorder (PTSD (see 🛄 p365), ADHD (see 🛄 p126), ASD (see 🛄 p107), etc.
- Substance induced (see 🛄 p367) sleep disorders: e.g. alcohol, cocaine, opioids, amphetamines, caffeine, sedatives, etc.

▶ Behavioural sleep disorders constitute a major proportion of all causes of sleep difficulties/disorders.

Causes of behavioural sleep disorders

Can be classified into:

- Child factors, e.g. difficult temperament, developmental delay.
- Parental factors, e.g. poor parenting (see 🛄 p371), poor sleep hygiene, maternal depression.
- Environmental factors, e.g. noisy neighbourhood, overcrowded household, shared bedroom.

Consequences of sleep disorders/deprivation

- *Child:*
  - Short term: irritability, tiredness, daytime somnolence, hyperactivity, behavioural problems, prone to accidental injuries.
  - Long term: negative impact on neurocognitive functioning, learning, educational attainments, emotional and behavioural disorders, overweight/obesity, drug abuse.

- *Family:* significant impact on family functioning, parental well-being, marital discord, increased incidence of child neglect and abuse, poor quality of life.
- *Society:* reduced chances of employment, family breakdowns, antisocial behaviours, increased dependence on state benefits/support.

Assessment

History taking
- What exactly is the problem? i.e. bedtime refusal, difficulty in falling asleep or staying asleep, daytime behaviour/sleep, etc.
- Enquire about severity (hours of sleep), frequency (number of awakenings/per night/per week), and duration of the sleep difficulties (months/years etc.).
- Explore predisposing factors (e.g. developmental delay), precipitating factors (e.g. recent house move, illness in family, etc.), and perpetuating factors (poor sleep hygiene, erratic routine).
- Elicit the impact/consequences of the sleep disorder.
- Child (concerns from nursery/pre-school, behaviour, daily routine, medical problems).
- Parent (education, motivation, behavioural techniques, co-sleeping, mental health).
- Family (number of persons in household, relationships, number of bedrooms, family routine).
- Environment (room temperature, access to TV/computer games/toys in bedroom, noise, light, activities of siblings, neighbours, etc.).
- Comorbidities (ADHD, ASD, LD, epilepsy, depression, etc.).

Physical examination
- Growth (height, weight, OFC).
- Look for dysmorphic features (see 🕮 p384), craniofacial anomalies, neurocutaneous (see 🕮 p250) signs, signs of metabolic disorders (see 🕮 p153).
- Complete system review including chest and neurology (see 🕮 p228).
- Developmental assessment (see 🕮 p36). Note behaviour, affect, alertness/attention.
- ENT (size of tongue, tonsils, maxilla, etc.).

Investigations

- Review 'sleep log/diary'.
- Request audio-visual recording, e.g. capture snoring, night terrors on home video/mobile phone.
- PSG: consider in OSA, narcolepsy, breathing, and neurological disorders.
- Multiple sleep latency test: helps assess speed with which one falls asleep. Useful in assessing narcolepsy, daytime sleepiness, etc.

Management of sleep difficulties

Behavioural
Evidence based and effective.
- Establish good sleep hygiene:
  - Consistent bed time/ awake time in the morning.
  - Consistent sleep routine (giving warm bath, soft music, warm glass of milk, read a book in bed/bedtime story, 'lights off', quiet time/low

noise activities for 1–2 hours preceding, no TV/computer games 1–2 hours prior to sleep).
• Daytime physical activity/exercise is likely to have a positive effect.
• Diet: avoid caffeine. Avoid heavy meal just before bed.
• Sleep programmes:
  • Graduated extinction (involves ignoring bed-time crying for increasing length of time).
  • Unmodified extinction (involves putting child to bed at a predetermined time and letting child develop self-soothing skills and falling asleep).
  • Scheduled awakening (involves parents waking up the child before the child's expected awakenings and gradually withdrawing this over time).

Pharmacological
• Consider only after or with behavioural interventions.
• To be considered only for children with neurodevelopmental disabilities or medical problems and not for typically developing children.
• Use for short-term periods to help establish sleep routine. Medications are unlicensed for use in children < 18 years.
• Medications:
  • Melatonin—used to treat circadian rhythm disturbances. Evidence suggests a decrease in sleep latency and increase in overall sleep time in children with neurodevelopmental disabilities.
  • Ramelteon—selective melatonin receptor agonist. Used to treat insomnia in adults

Referrals
Referral to the following professionals may be required:
• Neurologist (narcolepsy, frontal lobe epilepsy, see 📖 p240).
• Respiratory physician (asthma, CLD, sleep apnoeas).
• ENT (OSA, see 📖 p90, floppy larynx, macroglossia).
• Dietician.
• Psychiatrist (ASD, depression, substance abuse).
• Psychologist (CBT, behavioural programmes, see 📖 p120 and p373).

Transition: moving from paediatric to adult services

The case for 'transition clinics'

- During the years of childhood and adolescence the patient and family have a supportive relationship with an identifiable lead clinician, the paediatrician. At around 18 this relationship is lost. Families often ask 'Who is in charge of his/her care now?' The simple answer is, very often, no one in particular.
- Increasing numbers of young children are surviving into adult years with technology-dependent conditions. In 2006 it was thought that in the UK there were around 6000 children in this category who had not yet entered adult services.
- The transition clinic is an attempt to meet the needs of the patient, his/her family, and the primary care physician. Conditions such as CP (see 📖 p67), spina bifida (see 📖 p261), hydrocephalus (see 📖 p264), sensory impairments (see 📖 p275 and p296), metabolic disorders (see 📖 p155), and static or slowly progressive neurodegenerative (see 📖 p253) conditions might lead to a referral to a transition clinic.

Good transitions: what young people say they want

- Active management of transition. Plan early and prepare for leaving children's services.
- Take account of how attitudes, thinking, and behaviour vary between individual young people.
- Involve young people in service design and delivery: provide opportunities to ask questions, express opinions, and make decisions.
- Provide accessible information about services, share information between services, ensure multiagency working, coordination, and accountability.
- Stress the importance of a trusted adult who can challenge and support them, act as advocate, and help develop self-advocacy skills.
- Establish a shared philosophy between adult and paediatric care.
- Adopt an individualized honest approach.
- Address loss of continuity of care at transition; ensure new relationships are established.
- Train professionals in adolescent health in both paediatric and adult sectors.

Source: *Transition: getting it right for young people* Department of Health/ Department for Education and Skills, 2006.

Running a transition clinic

The pattern described here follows a routine developed for a paediatric transition clinic covering Oxfordshire.

- The 'clinic paediatrician' familiarizes with the history before the clinic, and preferably would also have spoken with the paediatrician

referring the patient to the clinic. The history to date is reviewed and summarized with patient and their family participating as much as possible.
- Observation suggests that this process of reviewing and summarizing is itself therapeutically beneficial, allowing time to reflect on and reassess critical events such as operations, or periods of crisis like hospital emergency admissions.
- Adult disability specialists attending might include a whole range of therapists, according to the individual patient's needs. But to avoid overwhelming the family, the adult services are represented by a 'Consultant in Rehabilitation Medicine'.
- The clinic runs in roughly two halves, firstly summarizing past events and reviewing current problems, followed by a consideration of what adult services are available that might be helpful.
- A typical clinic may result in several referrals for further review typically to:
  - The wheelchair or seating clinic (see 🕮 p186).
  - The spasticity clinic (see 🕮 p431).
  - The adult learning disability services (see 🕮 p319 and p325).
  - A specialist college and so on.
- It is essential to offer follow-up to avoid the feeling of abandonment, which is inherent in this process of transition. An offer of a follow-up appointment by the rehabilitation physician in a few months time and a phone number to call if there is a crisis is helpful.

Schedule for a transition clinic

- Introductions.
- Explanation of the purpose of the clinic.
- Review of medical history especially key events.
- Review and list all agencies currently involved.
- Review of current, active problems. A 'biopsychosocial model' is paramount: medical, educational, social, and psychological matters are all considered.
- Referrals to appropriate agencies (e.g. tertiary specialist college, Connexions, counselling, wheelchair services).
- Arrangements for follow-up.
- How to get back in touch with adult disability team in time of emergency.
- Summary letter copied to agencies involved (with permission).

What needs to be addressed in transition clinic?

The philosophy of the clinic is a *'biopsychosocial approach'* (see 🕮 p63) to alleviation and enablement of the adolescent. There are many transitions spaced over just a few years towards the end of adolescence:
- 16 years: the right to smoke, sexually majority, leaving school.
- 17 years: the right to apply for a driving licence.
- 18 years: the right to vote, to drink alcohol, and to marry without parental consent. Many young people go to college or university at age 18.

❶ The age of 18 often carries with it a realization for the patient and the family of the gap between the experience of the disabled young person and their able-bodied peers, who may be heading off on independent holidays and are likely to be leaving home for university or training for a career. Awareness of the different prospects facing the patient with a complex disabling condition is often particularly profound at transition points such as the age of 18!

The clinic should consider all of the following *social concerns*, according to the ability of the patient:
- Educational needs.
- Relationship issues.
- Accommodation plans for the future.
- Driving.
- Vocation, plans to work, etc.
- Hobbies and interests.

Medical issues might include the following:
- Referrals to a wide range of adult clinics including neurology, specialist epilepsy services, spasticity clinic (see 📖 p431).
- Wheelchair and special seating review (see 📖 p183).
- Women's health services (see 📖 p101).
- Assessment of fitness to drive.
- Assessment of mental capacity relating to financial and other matters.
- Liaison with LD services.

Consults with allied professionals

Limitations are but boundaries created inside our minds.

Chinese proverb

Physiotherapy: assessment

Refer children with the following conditions to physiotherapy

- Long-term neurological, e.g. CP (see 🕮 p67).
- Syndromes, e.g. Down syndrome, (see 🕮 p387) Rett syndrome (see 🕮 p405).
- Neuromuscular, e.g. muscular dystrophy (see 🕮 p257).
- Developmental delay in gross motor skills (see 🕮 p44).
- Developmental coordination disorder (DCD) (see 🕮 p136).
- Hypermobility (see 🕮 p180).

Other conditions that may be treated in the community or alternatively in secondary/tertiary centres or musculoskeletal outpatient physiotherapy departments:

- Juvenile arthritis.
- Developmental orthopaedic conditions; Erb's palsy, talipes/clubfoot (see 🕮 p422), plagiocephaly (see 🕮 p231), torticollis, tip-toe walking.
- Long-term respiratory conditions, e.g. cystic fibrosis.

Assessment

Subjective

Abilities, concerns, and problems in the areas of:

- Impairments, e.g. pain.
- Activity limitations, e.g. mobility, self-care.
- Participation, e.g. how does child spend day, interests, sport, etc.
- Environment, e.g. equipment used.

Objective

Observation is made of the child's posture and movements in supine, prone, side lying, floor sitting, box sitting, and standing of:

- Position of head, upper limbs, lower limbs, shoulder girdle, pelvis, spine.
- Alignment of body parts to each other.
- Weight distribution.
- Symmetry/asymmetry.
- Tone, associated reactions, reflexes, involuntary movements, tremor.

Assess how child achieves the movements listed in Table 5.1 including predominant movement patterns and the ability to dissociate one movement from the rest of the body.

Range of movement/muscle power/deformity

May be measured of all muscles and at all joints but with attention to those listed in Table 5.2 for specific conditions.

Tone

- Assessed partly through observation of posture and movement in different positions.
- Through examination and palpation of muscle.
- By passive movement at different velocity.

Table 5.1 Movement assessment

Position	Movement
Supine	Head turning, lifting off supporting surface.
	Upper limbs to midline and crossing midline.
	Lower limb kicking, hands to feet.
	Rolling over either side to prone.
	Pivoting.
Prone	Freeing arms.
	Lifting and turning head.
	Forearm prop.
	Pivoting.
	Pushing up into 4 point kneeling.
	Crawling.
	Rolling over either side to supine.
Side lying	Maintenance of position.
	Hands to midline.
Lying to sitting	How the child achieves sitting actively.
	If unable to rise to sit independently, observation of pull to sit for; head control; fixation of pelvis; flexibility of hips; active assistance.
Floor sitting	Tailor sitting, side sitting, long sitting, and w-sitting.
	Head upright, turning and control.
	Maintenance with and without propping.
	Movement within and outside of base of support.
	Pivoting.
	Bottom shuffling.
Box sitting	Movement on and off box to floor.
	Maintenance of position with and without hand support.
	Movement within and outside base of support.
	Movement into standing.
Standing	Maintenance with and without support.
	Crouch.
	Single leg stance.
	Gait.
	Kick.
	Run.
	Hop.
	Jump.
	Stairs.

Table 5.2 Movement/muscle range in specific conditions

Condition	Measurement/muscle
CP with lower limb involvement	Two joint muscles; rectus femoris, hamstrings, gastrocnemius.
	Rotational profile; femoral neck anteversion, hip rotation, tibial torsion, foot posture.
	Leg length(measured from anterior superior iliac spine to medial malleolus).
CP with upper limb involvement	Pectorals, supinators, long finger flexors, thumb abduction.
CP	Individual isolated movement.
Lower limb developmental orthopaedic conditions	Rotational profile as above.
	Intramalleolar distance with knees touching.
	Intracondylar distance with malleolli touching.
Muscle weakness	Oxford scale (0–5).
	Timed rising from floor.
	Timed 10m walk.

Standardized tools for assessment (Table 5.3)

Table 5.3 Standardised assessment tools

Condition	Assessment
Talipes/club foot	Pirani score.
Neuromuscular disease	North Star.
CP	Gross motor function measure (GMFM).
	Functional mobility scale (FMS).
	Chailey ability levels.
	Migration percentage from hip X-ray.
	Shriners Hospital Upper Extremity Evaluation (SHUEE).
	Assisting Hand Assessment (AHA).
Developmental delay	Alberta Infant Mobility Scale (AIMS).
DCD	Movement ABC.
Hypermobility	Beighton Scale.

Physiotherapy: approaches to treatment

Cerebral palsy and long-term neurological conditions
(see 📖 p67)
- Aim: to encourage and increase the child's ability to move and function in as normal a way as possible whilst preventing contracture and deformity.
- Treatment may include:
  - 24-hour postural management in lying, sitting and standing. In the child with low ability this will be achieved through the use of suitable equipment such as sleep systems, wheelchairs, static supportive seating, and standing frames. Emphasis is on improvement of body alignment.
  - Stretches; active, passive, through use of position/equipment or orthotics. Targeting susceptible muscles.
  - Influencing tone through position, manual techniques, handling, facilitation, active movement.
  - Constraint-induced movement therapy—active use of the hemiplegic upper limb whilst the non-affected arm is restrained, e.g. by wearing a mitten/glove.
  - Strengthening.
  - Providing mobility aids; k-walker, rollator, tripod/quadripod sticks or walkers that offer trunk support such as Rifton Pacer.

Neuromuscular conditions (see 📖 p257)
- Aims: slow down rate of development of contractures/deformity. Preserve respiratory function. Promotion of activity and participation.
- Treatment includes:
  - Stretches; active, passive, through position/equipment or orthotics.
  - Exercise and activity without fatigue.
  - Appropriate introduction of aids/equipment.
  - Respiratory physiotherapy.

Developmental coordination disorder (see 📖 p136)
- Aim: improve core stability, hip stability, shoulder stability, bilateral integration, eye–hand coordination, eye-foot coordination, motor planning.
- Treatment may include:
  - Strategies for both home and school to compensate for problems.
  - Direct therapy/exercises targeting problems either individually or in a group.
  - Recommendations for suitable mainstream sport/clubs to generalize skills gained through therapy.
  - Recommendations of suitable games and equipment.

Developmental delay (see 📖 p57 and p117)
- Aim: promote gross motor development through play and daily activities.
- Treatment may include:
  - Progression through prone development, rolling, crawling, sitting, standing, and walking.

Hypermobility
- Aim: develop co-contraction around joints to promote gross motor skills, and prevent problems such as pain and joint subluxation/dislocation.
- Treatment: muscle strengthening programme.

Hippotherapy
- Also called therapeutic riding.
- This may be beneficial in a variety of neurological conditions such as CP.
- The 3-dimensional movement of the horses pelvis as it walks can affect a child's tone, alignment, balance, strength, and function.

Hydrotherapy
- Water properties can be used to provide an environment conducive for treating a variety of conditions.
- Water temperature, buoyancy, turbulence, and drag provide an alternative medium for treatment.
- Halliwick is a method of teaching swimming and water safety for both disabled and non-disabled children. The child is taught to achieve independence in water starting with breathing control and relaxation.

Gross Motor Function Classification System

The gross motor function classification system (GMFCS) is a valuable tool for classifying children with CP (see 📖 p67). If the question is 'Will my child walk?' this would help provide the answer. A child usually remains in one level and does not change levels and therefore, by looking ahead to the descriptor as they age, their prognosis can be determined. Professionals will be less accurate classifying a child when they are within the low end of the age band, e.g. at 1 year they still have a year to achieve more skills as the age band is 1–2 years.

- A 5-level classification for children with CP.
- Determine which level best describes the child's current gross motor abilities at their current age.
- Age bands:
  - <2 years
  - 2–4
  - 4–6
  - 6–12
  - 12–18.
- Distinctions between levels are made by; functional limitations; use of hand-held mobility aids; use of wheelchairs.
- Scale is ordinal.
- After 2 years of age GMFCS levels are stable and a child is not likely to change level.
- PTs and doctors do not require specific training to perform the assessment.
- The title for each level describes the main method of mobility after 6 years:
  - Level I: walks without limitations.
  - Level II: walks with limitations.
  - Level III: walks using a hand-held mobility device.
  - Level IV: self-mobility with limitations; may use powered mobility.
  - Level V: transported in a manual wheelchair.
- Developed by Robert Palisano, Peter Rosenbaum, Stephen Walter, Dianne Russell, Ellen Wood, and Barbara Galuppi in 1997.
- It was expanded and revised in 2007.
- In 2002, motor growth curves for children with CP were produced by plotting GMFM-66 (Gross motor function measure) against GMFCS.

Gross motor function measure

While the GMFCS is quick to use, the gross motor function measure (GMFM) takes up to an hour for an experienced assessor. This is a validated tool to assess function over time in children with CP but is has also been used in DS (see 🕮 p387). It was designed to be administered by PTs and the original tested 88 items while a shorter version tests 66 (GMFM-66). An overall score or percentage can be calculated for each child

Subsections
- Lying and rolling.
- Sitting.
- Crawling and kneeling.
- Standing.
- Walking, running and jumping.

Scoring key
- 0 = does not initiate.
- 1 = initiates.
- 2 = partially completes.
- 3 = completes.

Posture management and special seating

- Many young people with complex disabling conditions, primarily neurological in origin (see 📖 p67), require wheelchairs (📖 p186) and special seating provision to:
  - Maintain comfort.
  - Maximize function.
  - Minimize further deterioration.
  - Energy expenditure.
- People with physical disabilities usually tire more quickly than able bodied people and are less able to resist the forces of gravity. This needs to be considered when prescribing wheelchairs and seating.
- 'Off the shelf' seating systems offer a limited amount of accommodation of asymmetric body shape.
- Custom contoured seating (this is system where a mould is taken of the body and a bespoke seat manufactured to match this; a variety of materials are available, each having specific beneficial features) is beneficial.

Posture and mobility services

In some areas, a posture, independence, and mobility service (PIMS) (see 📖 p225) encompasses the wheelchair service (📖 p186). The extended services include:

- Assessment and provision of assistive technology for children (see 📖 p225).
- Assessing therapeutic positioning in lying, sitting, and standing.
- Considering supportive positions to restore symmetry and reduce destructive postures in the child with complex problems.

Posture and seating assessment: the key principles

- A thorough assessment requires input from:
  - Clinicians (typically OTs and/or PTs with specialist training in a seating course).
  - Clinical engineers with specialist expertise (see 📖 p225).
- This guarantees that the costly process of designing bespoke seating is justified by good clinical outcomes such as:
  - Maximizing functioning.
  - Minimizing clinical risks such as pressure sores.
  - Minimizing pain and spasticity.
- For example, a patient with CP (essentially a non-progressive condition) will experience deterioration due to spasticity, deteriorating skin, and increased pain if careful attention is not paid to seating.

Seating provision

- Pushchairs of buggies may be more suitable for the younger child.
- Consideration is given to the postural need of the child.
- Specialist seating systems may be provided for children requiring extra postural control and support.

Principles for achieving stability in seating
- Wide base of support.
- Recruit gravity to secure a position.
- Account for established structural asymmetries, e.g. scoliosis, kyphosis, pelvic asymmetries, hip joint range limitations, by matching body contours to support surfaces (seat cushion, backrest, etc.).
- Minimize distorting factors, e.g. gravitational pull on shoulders from weight of arms.

Principles of ideal seating position
- Feet hip width apart, ankle at 90° (right angle) and foot supported. Footrest height maintains femora horizontal.
- Knee flexed to 90°.
- Cushion horizontal under ischial tuberosity and then ramped from gluteal crease to support the femora horizontally.
- Sacral pad forward of back rest up to the lumbosacral junction to accommodate the greater width of the trunk at chest height.
- Trunk symmetrical; may require curved backrest with side supports.
- Head upright and in midline.

Fundamentals of posture/physical assessment
- Assessment of the pelvis is fundamental to good seating.
- The pelvis has 3 planes of motion:
  - Obliquity (lifting on one side).
  - Rotation (forwards on one side).
  - Tilt (the pelvis moves to either exaggerate or diminish the lumbar lordosis).
- Basic measurements at the assessment:
  - Seat width, depth, and height.
  - Armrest height.
  - Backrest height and angle.
  - Footrest height.
  - User's weight.
- For all patients, but especially those with diminished sensation, measurement of pressure at the interface between the body and the cushion is vital to minimize the risks of pressure ulceration. Pressure mapping systems are commercially available and are used in specialist seating centres.
- Typical deviations from the ideal posture:
  - Windswept hips.
  - Scoliosis (see 📖 p416).
  - Kyphosis.

Posture management
- It should be noted that management of posture in the wheelchair in isolation to other forms of support used in any 24-hour period is likely to be ineffective, regardless of the age of the individual (including babies!).

- Children can spend 10–12 hours of every day in their beds. If adequate support is not provided, posture in the wheelchair will be affected. As an example, for someone with flexion contractures in the hips and knees and lying on their back, the legs will tend to fall to one side or the other. This places a twist on the pelvis and the spine causing discomfort.
- The adoption of such sustained postures is likely to lead to the development of structural musculoskeletal changes and will, as a result, impact on wheelchair seating provision.

Training in posture management
Clinicians who wish to become specialists in this area can follow a variety of courses ranging from, for example, the 4-day course at OCE in Oxford to a major component of the Oxford Brookes University Master's degree in Rehabilitation.

Wheelchair services

- Wheelchair services are provided by local health authorities. Services, organization, and eligibility vary between locations. In some areas they are part of PIMS which may have a more all-encompassing role.
- Children generally need to be >30 months to be referred as before this age standard buggies can usually accommodate need.
- Referrals are accepted from healthcare professionals but some localities accept self-referral.

Role of wheelchair service

- Assessment of need.
- Recommendation of suitable chair.
- Explanation of funding options.
- Provision of chairs ± accessories.
- Training in use of equipment.
- Maintenance and repair of equipment.

Assessment

Assessment for a chair will include:
- Child's condition and level of ability.
- Where and when the chair will be used.
- The child's ability to use the chair themselves or whether others will be propelling them.
- Where children have more severe disability standard chairs may not be appropriate and more postural custom made support will be necessary.

Types of wheelchairs and accessories

- Manual:
  - Self-propelled.
  - Attendant propelled.
- Powered, either indoor (often called EPIC: electrically powered indoor chair), indoor/outdoor (EPIOC), or outdoor (EPOC):
  - Driven by occupant.
  - Driven by attendant.
- Tilt in space, either in manual or powered wheelchairs (utilizing gravity to maintain position).
- Other forms of posturally supportive seating:
  - Armchair.
  - Work station, e.g. for computer use, hobbies.
  - Classroom.
  - Dining.
- Accessories include: mobile arm supports, arm rests, trays, cushions, head supports, leg rests.
- Rain covers are *not* provided by the wheelchair service.

Funding options

Standard option
- Chair provided, maintained, and repaired free of charge.

Wheelchair voucher scheme
- Each local service chooses whether or not to use this scheme.
- Allows purchase of a non-NHS chair using the voucher to the value of the recommended chair and the family paying the difference.
- If this is done in 'partnership' the chair is purchased through an approved supplier. The wheelchair service will maintain and repair the chair (some of this cost will be reflected in a lower amount of the voucher).
- If the voucher is used 'independently', the family own the wheelchair and are responsible for its repair and maintenance.
- The voucher scheme increases the choice of chairs available to a child.

Training
- Training is provided for families in use of any equipment supplied, including safety issues.
- Some charities also provide skills training, e.g. Whizz-Kidz.

Maintenance and repair
- A wheelchair service has an associated approved repairer/maintenance service including deliveries, collections, modifications, and servicing.
- Service organization in UK: there are ~150 generic small-scale wheelchair services in England, with fewer larger centres in Scotland and Wales. In addition, there are a small number of highly specialist centres with expertise in managing the most complex seating problems, for example the Specialist Disability Service, Oxford Centre for Enablement (OCE), Oxford University Hospitals NHS Trust and the West Midlands Rehabilitation Centre, Birmingham Community Healthcare NHS Trust.

Further resources
Disabled Living Foundation (DLF) (impartial advice and information on all aspects of equipment): F 0845 130 9177 ℘ http://www.dlf.org.uk
Fledglings (helps identify, source, supply practical and affordable aids/equipment): 0845 458 1124 ℘ http://www.fledglings.org.uk
NHS directory of wheelchair services: ℘ http://www.wheelchairmanagers.nhs.uk/services.html

Occupational therapy: principles and assessment

Occupational therapy is a profession concerned with promoting health and well-being through occupation. It is the art and science of enabling people to actively participate in the day-to-day activities that are important to them despite illness, impairment or disability.

The aim of occupational therapy

To enhance participation in activities of everyday life within the areas of:
• Work/productive activities, e.g. school work (adult-directed activities).
• Play/leisure activities (child-directed activities).
• Self-care activities, e.g. ADLs.

Activities of daily living include:

• Toilet hygiene.
• Bathing/showering.
• Personal hygiene and grooming.
• Eating and feeding.
• Dressing.
• Functional mobility.
• Sleep and rest.

Instrumental activities of daily living (IADLS) are more complex ADLs needed for adult independence such as:
• Community mobility.
• Shopping, meal preparation, and clean up.
• Home management (e.g. laundry, cleaning, household maintenance).
• Health maintenance and safety/emergency responses.
• Financial management.

OT assessment

Ideally occurs within the child's natural environment (e.g. home and/or school) and consists of standardized (e.g. norm-referenced tests) and non-standardized assessment tools (e.g. observation, screening tests/questionnaires, parent/teachers interview, review of reports of other professionals), to gain relevant information about the child's:
• Abilities.
• Performance patterns and activity limitations.
• Contexts, e.g. home, school, childcare, and community settings taking into account physical, social, and cultural factors.
• Interaction between the child's abilities and the demands of the environment.
• Concerns/priorities of the child, parents/caregivers, and teachers.

Setting collaborative OT goals

Goals/objectives of OT intervention are often linked to:
• Specific performance limitations (e.g. short-term goals).
• Participation restrictions (e.g. long-term goals).

OT goals are developed in collaboration with the child, parents, and multi-disciplinary team and outline:
- The activities the child will perform.
- The environmental conditions.
- Any environmental modifications.
- Amount and type of activity assistance (adapting activities or providing additional adult support or equipment/assistive devices). See Table 5.4.

Table 5.4 Examples of fine motor difficulties and practical suggestions for children <5 years ▶Ensure child feels successful to maintain motivation

Fine motor skills	OT recommendations
Drawing/handwriting	Provide thicker, triangular barrelled pencils, chunky chalk, thick crayons/paint brushes, finger painting, trial of pencil grips.
	Encourage drawing/writing on vertical surface (e.g. wall, easel/chalkboard, magnetic/felt boards) or writing slope to improve wrist position for writing.
	Demonstrate drawing simple shapes (increasing in complexity), e.g. vertical line, then horizontal line, circle, cross, square, and wait for child to imitate.
	Appropriate handwriting programme, e.g. 'Write From the Start' or 'Handwriting Without Tears', etc.
Dressing	Encourage child to sit while dressing.
	'Backward chaining' approach to dressing—adult does the first step, e.g. adult pulls sock halfway off the foot, then child finishes the task by pulling sock off foot. Gradually reduce assistance until child completes whole task.
	Choose shoes with Velcro fasteners. Encourage unzipping before zipping up. Start with loose, large buttons first when ready (e.g. undoing pyjama/coat buttons).
Feeding	Ensure child is sitting in a stable position with feet supported, e.g. 'Tripp Trapp' chair.
	Adult to steady base of 2-handled cup as child brings to mouth, gradually reduce assistance then move to 1-handled cup then a beaker.
	<3 years encourage use of either spoon or fork only using 'hand-over-hand' then move hand to child's elbow to reduce level of help.
	Cut food to mouthful size and encourage child to stabilize bowl/plate with other hand.
	Use child-sized built up cutlery, e.g. 'Junior Caring Cutlery' to aid grasp. Introduce cutting with knife to cut 'Velcro fruit', 'play dough', or banana, etc.

(Continued)

Table 5.4 (Continued)

Fine motor skills	OT recommendations
Other play activities to develop manual dexterity	For more challenging fine motor activities, encourage child to sit at child-sized table rather than sitting unsupported on floor.
	Use 'play dough'/clay to strengthen hands by rolling, squeezing, squashing, etc. before using shape cutters.
	Large building blocks, e.g. 'Duplo' or magnetic or Velcro blocks before providing smaller construction toys, e.g. 'Lego'.
	Inset jigsaws with large handles.
	Thread beads onto dowel before threading onto shoelace/string.
	Pick up objects with tongs, teabag squeezers, etc. before snipping with scissors.

Occupational therapy: aids and adaptations

Occupational therapy assessment for equipment and/or home/school adaptations considers the following:

- Environment, space within the property, ease of moving from one room to another, door widths and thresholds, etc.
- Lifestyle and cultural context of the child/young person and family—perceptions of ease of transfers (acceptability of being lifted by parents).
- The opinions of the child/young person and family, being aware of perception of aesthetics, design, comfort, and perceived usefulness of adaptations/equipment.
- The other equipment already in use and need for complementary options.
- The cognitive abilities of the child/young person, physical stage of development, and need for appropriate positioning in line with 24-hour postural management.
- Will the proposed adaptations/equipment meet the child's needs and is it 'necessary, appropriate, reasonable and practical' as set out in the Housing Grants, Construction and Regeneration Act 1996.
- Is the family eligible to apply for a means-tested *disabled facilities grants* (DFG) from the district or city council for major adaptations to privately owned, rented and housing association properties?
- Will the child/young person be more integrated into the family life and have increased access to activities after provision of adaptations/equipment?
- Is recommended equipment adjustable for growth?

The OT works together with a range of professionals within:

- Health (e.g. paediatrician, physiotherapist (see 🕮 p176), SLT (see 🕮 p200), etc.).
- Education (e.g. teaching assistant, teacher, SEN coordinator (see 🕮 p531), EP, Properties and Facilities for adaptations to school buildings/grounds).
- District/county council (e.g. application for DFG).
- Voluntary Sector (e.g. charities who may provide additional funding).

OT intervention may include recommendations (Table 5.5) for:

- Standard or specialist equipment/assistive devices.
- Minor or major housing adaptations to the child's home/school environment.
- Information and advice to children and families about other sources of support.

Further resources

Disabled Living Foundation (DLF) (impartial advice and information on all aspects of equipment): F 0845 130 9177 🕾 http://www.dlf.org.uk

Fledglings (helps identify, source, supply practical and affordable aids/equipment): F 0845 458 1124 🕾 http://www.fledglings.org.uk

Table 5.5 Examples of adaptations and equipment/assistive devices which may be recommended

Potential barriers	Adaptations	Assistive devices
Entrances and exits (including access to car and garden)	Grab rails. Stair rails. Ramps. Built-up terrain to threshold height. In-home lift. ↑ door width. Door re-hinged to open in/out.	Lever door handle. Environmental control unit.
To improve safety for children who have reduced awareness of danger	Stable doors. Door handles raised to adult height. Safe fencing.	Sound monitors.
Bathroom	Low mounted sink. Level access shower with shower seat. Ceiling hoist. Grab rails.	Toilet seat reducer. Toilet step/footrest. Potty chair with postural support. Single lever faucets. Bath board/seat/lift. Mobile over toilet/shower chair. Mobile hoist. Hoisting bathing and/or toileting slings.
Bedroom	Downstairs bedroom. Ceiling hoist. Grab rails.	Bed rails. Firm mattress and/or specialized bed. Mobile hoist. Hoisting slings.
Kitchen	Lowered countertops/cabinets. Sliding drawers and organizers in cabinets.	Dining seating with postural support. Cutlery with built-up handles.
Living room	Ceiling hoist.	Seating with postural support. Mobile hoist. Hoisting slings.

Occupational therapy: enabling hand function, seating, etc.

Effective use of the hands to engage in a variety of occupations depends on a complex interaction of:

- Fine motor skills (see 📖 p46).
- Postural mechanisms (see 📖 p183).
- Cognition (see 📖 p54).
- Visual perception (see 📖 p213).

Link between postural ability and fine motor skills

- Tasks that require concentration and accurate fine motor skills necessitate stabilizing the body, work surface, and tools. Improved postural ability with increased shoulder and pelvic girdle control, leads to increased control of fine motor skills. No one correct sitting posture exists because no position is constant, nor should it be.
- Many variables influence the choice of body position and posture including:
  - The nature of the activity.
  - Convenience.
  - Requirements of speed, precision, and strength.
- Postural and motor ability are affected by a combination of factors including:
  - The maturational level of the nervous system.
  - Sensory integration.
  - Changes in lengths of muscles.
  - Selective muscle control for posture and movement.
  - Formation of bones and joints.
  - Biomechanical forces.
  - Nutrition.
  - Health.
  - Environmental factors.
  - The activity the child is engaged in.
- Postural management equipment, e.g. specialized seating, is designed to (see 📖 p183):
  - Promote normal motor control.
  - Support without restricting movement.
  - Improve practical ability.
  - Reduce the progression of deformity.
  - Improve the efficiency of complex cognitive tasks by reducing the need to focus attention on maintaining posture.

Sensory Integration

- Sensory integration theory hypothesizes that every human action involves integrated neurological processes from sensory, motor, and other cognitive and emotional systems.
- Sensory integration knowledge can be applied in different ways to different populations for different purposes. This has resulted in difficulties in drawing conclusions about the effectiveness of sensory integration intervention; however, there is evidence in the neuroscience literature to support the use of active, engaged, sensory-motor activities to enhance neuroplasticity (and emerging evidence that they support learning, memory, and problem solving).

Sensory Processing Disorder (SPD)

- Previously described as sensory integrative dysfunction—is not currently included in the DSM-IV.
- SPD is a neurological disorder characterized by poor detection, modulation, discrimination, or responses to sensory stimuli.
- This results in the brain having problems with sorting out, filtering, analysing, organizing, and connecting (integrating) sensory messages.
- When some aspect of sensory integration does not function efficiently, the child may experience stress in the course of everyday occupations because neurological processes that should be automatic or accurate are not.
- Common diagnostic groups who may exhibit signs of sensory processing disorder:
  - ASD (see 📖 p107).
  - ADHD (see 📖 p126).
  - CP (see 📖 p67).
  - Genetic conditions, e.g. fragile X syndrome (see 📖 p403), DS (see 📖 p387).
  - DD.
  - Visual impairment (see 📖 p275).
  - Hearing impairment (see 📖 p296).
  - Learning disabilities (see 📖 p117).
  - Traumatic brain injury.
  - Prematurity.
  - Environmentally deprived e.g. in cases of abuse/neglect.

Sensory processing disorder is usually manifested as either over-responsiveness (hypersensitivity) or under-responsiveness (hyposensitivity) specific to any, or a combination of the 7 senses:

Over-responsiveness (hypersensitivity)—'A little feels like a lot'

- The child who is over-responsive is overwhelmed by ordinary sensory input and reacts defensively to it, often with strong negative emotion and activation of the sympathetic nervous system.
- Over-responsiveness is characterized by 'sensation avoiding' with a tendency to avoid sensations, be fearful, distressed, cautious, negative, aggressive, or withdrawn (a 'fight or flight' response).
- This condition may occur as a general response to all types of sensory input, or it may be specific to one or a few sensory systems affected, e.g.
  - Tactile defensiveness.

- Gravitational insecurity.
- Over reactions to light, sounds, odours, and tastes.

Under-responsiveness (hyposensitivity)—'A lot feels like a little'
- The child who is under-responsive frequently fails to attend to or register relevant environmental stimuli.
- The child may seem oblivious to touch, pain, movement, taste, smells, sights, or sounds.
- This is characterized by either 'low registration' with a tendency to withdraw and be difficult to engage, or 'sensory seeking' behaviours—craving/seeking out intense sensory input, e.g. being constantly 'on the go', jumping from dangerous heights during play, preferences for very strong flavours in foods, etc.
- Children with under-responsiveness to tactile and proprioceptive input may also have difficulties postural control or praxis (ideation, motor planning and sequencing of movements), e.g. dyspraxia (see 📖 p136).

Aims of occupational therapy intervention in SPD
- To help children, parents, and teachers understand SPD and its impact on the child and their everyday life.
- To provide strategies enabling child to achieve optimal level of alertness, facilitating more effective engagement in everyday life activities at home, school and in community.
- To improve child's self-esteem by empowering child and family, decreasing frustration/stress levels (by addressing sensory difficulties) and improving participation in activities (occupations).

Occupational therapy recommendations for children with SPD

▶Occupational therapy recommendations for children with SPD should be very specific, according to the child's individual sensory profile (for examples see Table 5.6). Parent/carers should supervise all recommended activities, allow the child to do the activities in his/her own way, build on activities chosen by the child, and stop the activity if the child becomes distressed.

Sensory modulation

Sensory modulation refers to CNS regulation of its own activity. Sensory modulation problems may be identified when children fluctuate between the two extremes of over and/or under-responsiveness, even within the same sensory system, affecting the child's level of alertness.

Occupational therapy resources for parents

- *'The Out of Sync Child': Recognizing & Coping with Sensory Processing Disorder* by Carol Stock Kranowitz (revised edition 2006).
- *Sensational Kids: Hope and Help for Children with Sensory Processing Disorder* by Lucy Jane Miller (2006)
- *The Out-of-Sync Child Has Fun: Activities for Kids with Sensory Processing Disorder* by Carol Stock Kranowitz (2006)
- *The Ultimate Guide to Sensory Processing Disorder: Easy, Everyday Solutions to Sensory Challenges* by Roya Ostovar (2010)

Table 5.6 Occupational therapy recommendations for children with SPD

	Over-responsiveness	Under-responsiveness
Proprioception	(Not observed)	Lots of 'heavy work' activities, i.e. activities where muscles/joints are pushed/pulled, e.g. weight-bearing on hands and knees, jumping on a trampoline, pushing/pulling heavy wagon, digging, hammer toys/drums, tug of war, obstacle course, etc. Provide chewy necklace/bracelet or chewy tube. Offer sleeping bag or heavier blanket/duvet for sleeping.
Tactile	Avoid light/sudden touch—use firm touch instead. Offer firm 'bear hugs'. Offer firm head massage and/or wear tight fitting hat prior to hair washing/cutting. Offer child choices for texture/type of clothing, bedding, towels, etc. and cut tags out of clothing if requested. Slowly introduce messy play activities/new textures gradually.	Use touch to get child's attention before speaking to him/her. Provide many opportunities for messy play, plenty of different textures for hands, fidget toys etc.
Vestibular	Encourage 'heavy work' (proprioceptive) activities prior to and following movement activities. Provide opportunities for slow, regular linear movements (e.g. gentle back-and-forth motion, starting with feet on the ground first incl. rocking chair) rather than fast or jerky angular/rotatory movements.	Encourage regular movement breaks throughout the day, e.g. rough and tumble play, 'animal walks', playground, trampoline, swing (including rotary swings), self-spinning toys, slide, space hopper, exercise ball, 'move and sit' cushion, etc.

Auditory	Use quiet voices and try to minimize loud, unexpected noises as much as possible.	Vary tone of voice when speaking.
	Have quiet space for child to retreat to at home and school.	Lots of music, singing, nursery rhymes.
	Offer ear-defenders to block out noise when needed, e.g. shopping centre, vacuum, lawn mower etc.	Provide opportunities to experiment with noisy toys, e.g. musical instruments, drums, shakers, whistles etc.
	Carry laminated 'out of order' sign to stick on to hand dryers in public toilets if necessary.	
Visual	Uncluttered visual spaces, soft lighting, muted colours (turn off fluorescent lights).	Visually exciting environment, bright colours, posters/mobiles, light up/flashing toys etc.
	Allow child to wear sunglasses (even indoors).	Visual discrimination and hand-eye coordination games, e.g. batting at balloons, throwing bean bags into washing basket, popping bubbles, fishing games, visual treasure hunts/Where's Wally?, etc.
Olfactory	Avoid perfumes, scented body lotions, and strong laundry powder.	Use scented 'play dough' or pens.
	Turn on fan in kitchen to disperse cooking odours.	Encourage child to smell different foods during cooking activities.

(Continued)

Table 5.6 (Continued)

	Over-responsiveness	Under-responsiveness
Gustatory	Often oversensitivity is due to texture, i.e. touch rather than taste, commonly lumpy foods (mixed texture) are difficult to tolerate and child may gag	Offer crunchy/chewy foods and/or foods with strong flavours, e.g. grapefruit juice, peppers, adding herbs/spices
	Encourage oral motor skills, e.g. chewing, sucking, blowing etc.	Try an electric toothbrush
	Don't pressure child into eating foods that he/she finds uncomfortable	
	Have non-preferred foods available throughout day for child to experience on own terms (e.g. messy food play, involvement in cooking activities) rather than pressuring child to eat and increasing stress at mealtimes	
	Provide a wide range of foods, and offer a variety of different textures and temperatures of each food	
	Consider referral to dietician if there are concerns regarding nutritional intake or to speech and language therapist if there are concerns regarding drooling/chewing/swallowing	

- *Raising a Sensory Smart Child: The Definitive Handbook for Helping Your Child with Sensory Processing Issues* by Lindsey Biel and Nancy Peske (2009).
- SPD Foundation website: ⚘ http://spdfoundation.net/index.html

Speech and language therapy: aims, approaches, and conditions

Aims
- To promote comprehension and clear expression of language.
- To enable child to communicate with others.
- To develop oral feeding skills (see 🕮 p88).

Approach
- Work is carried out either 1:1, in groups and with parents, carers, and other professionals to help child develop their skills.
- Increasingly SLTs work through people who are in daily contact with the child, providing training and treatment programmes for them to carry out.
- Services are split into early years and school age:
  - Preschool SLTs work primarily in clinics, children's centres, and
  - early years settings.
  - School-age SLTs visit children at school and services are generally restricted to those children who have a SEN (see 🕮 p524).
  - Children with complex needs may have specialist staff who visit at home or in mainstream or special schools (see 🕮 p534).

Prevalence
- ~7% of 5-year-olds entering school have significant difficulties with speech and/or language. The majority of these children have expressive language delay.
- ~1% of 5-year-olds have the most severe and complex speech, language, and communication needs. These children have limited comprehension and expression.
- In socially disadvantaged areas, it's possible that up to 54% of children at nursery age have significant delays.

Descriptions of speech and language conditions
- *Language delay:* delayed development of comprehension or expressive skills (see 🕮 p52).
- *Language impairment:* atypical development, e.g. expressive skills appear in advance of comprehension, or severe delay of either or both.
- *Speech (phonological) delay:* pronunciation similar to that of a younger child, e.g. no use of consonant clusters ('poon' for 'spoon').
- *Speech (phonological) impairment:* atypical pattern of development or use of sounds; or severe speech delay.
- *Articulation disorder:* difficulty in moving tongue, lips to create sounds
  - Mild: lisp ('th' for 's'), difficulty with 'sh', 'ch', 'r', or 'l'.
  - Severe: dysarthric type oral motor difficulty affecting articulation, e.g. slow laboured speech.
- *Verbal dyspraxia:* difficulty in the motor planning of articulatory movements, leading to limited number of sounds and sound sequences produced or copied (see 🕮 p141).

- *Disorders of nasal resonance:* hypernasal quality to speech or at worst, inability to make oral consonants such as 'b/d' instead producing 'm/n'. This could be as a result of cleft palate, submucous cleft, or velo pharyngeal insufficiency (short soft palate, increased dimensions of nasopharynx post adenoidectomy, or poor motor control).
- *Dysfluency:* stammering 1% of population. Prevalence of ~5% in <6 years have been reported.
- *Voice disorders:* hoarse or breathy voice, generally due to vocal abuse such as excessive shouting or structural abnormalities/pathology, e.g. laryngeal webbing/vocal fold palsy or dysarthric type motor difficulty, e.g. in CP (see 📖 p67).
- *Social communication disorders:* ASDs or pragmatic disorders i.e. difficulty in use of language to communicate (see 📖 p107).

Speech and language therapy: assessment

The following areas are assessed to aid diagnosis:

Attention and listening skills
- Attention span and ability to switch attention from play to speaker is noted.
- Ability to attend to activities that are adult-directed are observed.

Play skills
- The ability to show functional use of objects (e.g. brush for hair, cup for drinking) is a precursor to pretending and develops by 12 months.
- The presence of pretend play is linked with early language development. It emerges from about 15 months.
- The ability to sequence play actions to create a story line is also observed (this develops by 3 years).

Social interaction skills
- The ability and desire to interact with others.
- Using appropriate eye contact.
- Facial expression.
- Gesture.
- Pointing.
- Use of language to request, comment, respond to questions, ask questions, direct, retell events.
- Conversational skills and joint play skills.

Verbal comprehension skills
- Verbal comprehension skills are assessed using increasingly complex instructions that require a motor response, i.e. selection of objects or pictures by pointing, or moving toys.
- This enables differentiation between children with purely expressive difficulties and those with comprehension and expressive problems.
- Tests start with single object label recognition, verb recognition, then testing 2–4 key word level instructions as well as concept and grammatical understanding.

Expressive language skills
- Counting number of words/signs/symbols used by child to communicate.
- Types of words, i.e. nouns, verbs, adjectives, prepositions, etc.
- Length of phrases. These phrases must be flexible and not rote learned as 'chunks', e.g. here-it-is.
- Grammatical complexity of sentences, e.g. use of pronouns he/she/they; use of verb tenses fell/washed. Use of sentences linked with and/because/that.
- Functional use of expressive language, e.g. to make requests, comment, ask and answer questions, describe, converse.

- Formal testing involves eliciting specific responses to pictures, toy materials or questions.
- Informal testing involves transcribing child's language during relaxed play or interaction. This often results in a more reliable sample of child's language but is more time consuming.

Speech/articulation skills

- Speech is assessed by presenting target pictures which contain all the sounds of speech in different word positions.
- The child's system of simplification (phonological system) can then be analysed.
- Typical patterns of error in development include:
  - *Stopping,* i.e. f s sh ch all substituted by b/d. Generally resolves by 3 years.
  - *Fronting,* i.e. k/g substituted by t/d. Can be as late as 4 years.
  - *Consonant blend deletion,* i.e. sp becomes p, bl becomes b. Generally correct by 4½ years.
- Child's ability to copy different speech sounds in isolation is also tested. This will show if any articulation difficulties with specific sounds exists.
- *Dyspraxic* children struggle to copy consonant vowel sequences. Many have limited range of vowels and consonants and would have made very slow progress with speech development (see 📖 p141).
- If *dysarthria* is suspected, DDK rates (diadochokinesis—the speed at which sounds such as p/t/k can be repeated) can also be tested and the difference between connected speech (longer strings of words) and single word naming compared. In dysarthria, there is often a tiring effect with worsening intelligibility as the sentence continues or over a longer word.

Resonance

Hypernasal speech may suggest some structural abnormality such as cleft or submucous cleft palate or some neuromuscular condition (see 📖 p257) affecting control of the velopharyngeal sphincter (The VP sphincter elevates soft palate to close nasopharynx so as to allow oral airflow.)

Voice

- Persistent hoarse or breathy voice needs ENT investigation and may require follow-up therapy to teach more effective and less damaging voice use.
- Dysphonia in children is often due to vocal abuse (i.e. shouting) but actual pathology is important to rule out, e.g. abnormalities such as webbing, unilateral cord palsy, nodules, or polyps.

Fluency

- Dysfluency (stammering) is an issue for a small percentage of children.
- For most it is a transient stage as linguistic output increases.
- If it persists for >6 months, referral to SLT is essential.

- Good outcomes exist for children <5 years using programmes such as *Lidcombe Therapy* which reinforces fluency in work with mother and child.
- Assessment includes type of dysfluency experienced, history of dysfluency, measures of amount of stammering in several minutes of speech and differences across different situations, and secondary behaviours associated with stammer, e.g. blinks, gestures, word switching, avoidance.

Assessment tools (Table 5.7)

Table 5.7 Common assessment tools used by SLTs

Area assessed	Name of test	Age range tested
Comprehension	Assessment of comp/expression	6–11 years
	Bracken test for concepts	3–7 years
	British Picture Vocab Scales	3–16 years
	CELF preschool	3–6 years
	CELF	5–17 years
	Derbyshire Language Scheme	1–4½ years
	Test of problem solving	6–11 years
	TROG	4–18 years
	Reynell Scales III	21 months–7 years
	Preschool Language Scale	Birth to 6:5 years
Expression	Derbyshire Language Scheme	1–4:6 years
	Renfrew Action Picture Test	3½ –8:5 years
	Renfrew Bus Story	3–8 years
	Renfrew Word Finding	3–9 years
	STASS	3–5 years
	CELF preschool	3–6 years
	CELF	5–17 years
Speech	STAP	Any
	DEAP	3–7 years
	Nuffield Dyspraxia assessment	3–6 years
Social interaction	Pragmatics profile	All ages
	Social communication profile	All ages
	Social use of language programme	All ages

Speech and language therapy: treatment strategies

For verbal comprehension

- Observe, watch, listen (OWL) and follow child's lead in play and conversation, reduce language complexity to child, and use descriptive commentary.
- Repetitive practice of target words/concepts in play and everyday situations.
- Use of photos, pictures, real objects.
- Practise listening to increasing amounts of information.
- Teach conceptual vocabulary such as size, position words, colours, numbers and grammatical items: pronouns, tenses, why, because, etc.
- Use of signs (e.g. Makaton) or photos/pictures to augment spoken communication.

For language expression

- OWL and follow child's lead in play and conversation.
- Repetitive input of target words in play and everyday situations.
- Use of a descriptive commentary, i.e. talk about what child is doing while he does it to input appropriate language models.
- Reduce number of questions to child as these produce limited response or are too stressful for some children.
- Add one word to what child says, i.e. expansion.
- Model phrase child needs to copy.
- Use signs and/or picture prompts to promote longer phrases.
- Teach noun, verb, adjective vocabulary, setting up games and activities for repetitive practice.
- Teach grammatical aspects, e.g. pronouns, tenses and use of linking words such as 'and', 'because', etc.

For speech

- Practice with target sounds, listening to meaning differences (minimal pair work, e.g. tea/key).
- Practice of target sounds in words, phrases and connected speech.
- Options are to target one process, e.g. fronting—making all sounds at the front of mouth, or to target one sound at a time.
- Use of visual representation of sounds (pictures, letters) to aid sequencing of sounds—particularly useful in dyspraxia.
- Work on improving intelligibility of highly motivating words.
- Cued articulation—use of hand gestures to prompt specific articulatory movements.
- In dysarthric children, practice with oral movements to increase range, speed, accuracy of tongue articulation and use of pacing to improve intelligibility.

For social interaction/pragmatic use of language

- Interactive play including turn taking, action songs, peek-a-boo, etc.
- Specific work to teach rules of conversation.

- Modify environment to promote requests and comments (e.g. stop automatic provision of items for child, use of waiting for child to respond, introduce novelty or bizarre events).
- Use of PECS to develop functional ability to request and comment.
- Use of AAC to support communication (see 🕮 p208).

For resonance

Practise producing oral consonants and use of visual feedback to encourage self-monitoring of nasality.

For dysfluency

- General advice to parents/carers regarding strategies to create a relaxed communication environment (e.g. reduce number of questions and demands for verbal responses).
- Practise relaxed ways of producing difficult words or sounds (methods generally use slowed articulation or use specific breath control techniques).
- Practice of these in increasingly difficult situations.
- Cognitive behavioural approaches to anxiety created by stammering (see 🕮 p373).
- *Lidcombe therapy* is widely used in younger children. This teaches children to approach difficult words in a more relaxed way and reinforces fluency in activities carried out with the parent and child together.
- In older children, the psychological impact of having a stammer is addressed in group therapy as well as tackling the stammering behaviour itself by using relaxed articulation, slowed speech, or breathing techniques.

For voice

- Therapy for vocal misuse involves teaching child to use better breath support for voice and less tension to produce volume (to 'yell well') as well as advocating lessening of shouting.
- Children with neurological conditions may need help to practise stronger voice or use better breath control to maintain voice during speech.

Autism Diagnostic Observation Schedule (ADOS)

- Semi-structured, standardized assessment of communication, social interaction and play/imaginative use of materials for individuals with possible autism (see 📖 p107).
- Used for whole range of developmental levels from children with no expressive language to those with fluent, full adult grammar.
- Designed to be a complimentary assessment to the Autism Diagnostic Interview (ADI).
- ADOS provides a measure of ASD that is minimally affected by language level.
- Assessment is carried out during play and conversation/verbal interaction during which there are 'social presses' (planned social situations), to stimulate a response from the child which is then recorded.
- There are 4 modules, each of which takes approx 30–45min to administer. Modules are chosen according to the child's expressive language ability.
- Social interaction is assessed in the ADOS under 2 headings:
  - Communication.
  - Reciprocal social interaction.
- Aspects of communication assessed are:
  - Frequency of vocalization directed to others.
  - Stereotyped/idiosyncratic use of words or phrases.
  - Use of other's body to communicate.
  - Pointing.
  - Gestures.
  - Amount of social overtures.
  - Conversation.
- Aspects of reciprocal social interaction assessed are:
  - Unusual eye contact.
  - Facial expressions directed to others.
  - Shared enjoyment in interaction.
  - Showing.
  - Spontaneous initiation of joint attention.
  - Response to joint attention.
  - Quality of social overtures.
  - Quality of social response.
  - Amount of reciprocal social interaction.
  - Overall quality of rapport.

Alternative and augmentative communication

This includes use of objects, pictures and signs to communicate (low-tech AAC) or computerized voice output communication aids (VOCAs— high-tech AAC).

Objects
- For children who do not recognize pictures or signs, and for those who are visually/dual sensory impaired, 'Objects of reference' can be used.
- An object is associated with an activity, e.g. spoon for mealtime, towel for swimming.
- Child is presented with object before the activity to help them understand what is happening.
- Children can learn to request by selecting an object of reference from a bag or box.

Signs
- Signs with speech (Makaton, Sign-a-long, Signed English) are commonly used to provide additional visual input to aid comprehension and development of expressive skills.
- Signing is used with children who have:
  - Hearing impairment (see 📖 p296).
  - Cognitive delay (see 📖 p117).
  - DS (see 📖 p387).
  - Severe language delay (see 📖 p52 and p57).
  - Poor speech intelligibility, e.g. dyspraxic children (see 📖 p141).
- Some children continue to use sign as a means of communication alone.
- Many go onto develop speech with their signing and it is used as a temporary aid until speech intelligibility and language structure develops.

Pictures
- Photos, pictures, and picture symbols (Mayer Johnson/Boardmaker, Widgit, Makaton, Rebus, PECS) can be used on their own or with signing.
- Picture communication is used with:
  - Children who are unable to sign due to coordination difficulties (see 📖 p136) or neurological conditions, e.g. CP (see 📖 p67).
  - Children on the autism spectrum (see 📖 p107 and p327) who have limited speech generally prefer this way of communication. Autistic children use pictures in two ways—one to communicate with others i.e. PECS and one to understand what is happening—picture schedules (showing a sequence of events).
- Pictures can be used in charts, individually, on key rings, in picture schedules (showing a sequence of events) or on VOCAs (see following section).

VOCAs/communication aids

- These are for children who are unable to speak or whose speech is unintelligible, e.g. children with motor speech disorders such as dysarthria (see 📖 p67), dyspraxia (see 📖 p141), etc. to give the child a 'voice'.
- Children first have to have picture recognition and some verbal comprehension of the items they are requesting.
- Most VOCAs are accessed by selection of a picture or photo either by eye pointing, pressing with a hand, fist or finger, head pointer, or selecting with a switch.
- Therapeutic intervention is required initially to ensure children understand use of pictures to communicate and can make use of a VOCA.
- Joint assessment with specialist SLT, OT (see 📖 p188), and advisory teacher is generally required for children with conditions such as CP to ascertain best type and position of switches/aids.
- VOCAs can be as simple as a single message or word, 4, 6, 9, 12 messages on a touch pad, up to computer type aids that contain extensive vocabulary with unlimited scope for development and customization.
- Recent development of iPhone and iPad apps to include communication aid software (also see 📖 p226) can enable children with reasonable hand function and EHC (see 📖 p46) to access VOCAs with these.

Useful contacts

- AFASIC supports parents and carers of children with Speech Language and Communication Needs (SLCN). Operates a parents' helpline: ✆ http://www.afasicengland.org.uk
- Communication Matters is a national organization providing information and symposia on AAC (Augmentative and Alternative Communication): ✆ http://www.communicationmatters.org.uk
- ICAN supports children with SLCN and provides information and training for parents and professionals: ✆ http://www.ican.org.uk and ✆ http://www.talkingpoint.org.uk
- Royal College of Speech and Language Therapists is the professional body of and for Speech and Language Therapists in the UK and Ireland: ✆ http://www.rsclt.org

Psychology: assessment and management of behavioural problems

Assessment of behavioural problems

Involves understanding the purpose and function of the behaviour by functional analysis (ABC analysis):

Antecedents
- What triggers it? Situation, timing, place, people present, environment.

Behaviour
- Detailed description of the behaviour. Nature, frequency, severity, duration.

Consequences
- What occurs after the behaviour? How is it managed? Child gets their immediate wants/attention, change in demands/expectation of child.
- Information gathering methods:
  - ABC diaries kept by parents.
  - Direct observation at home/school.
  - Videos of behaviour.

Treatment or behavioural modification

Is based on the idea that patterns of behaviour are reinforced by the response they elicit.

Desirable behaviours can be increased by:
- Positive reinforcement: rewards, praise, star charts, adult positive attention, privileges.
- To be most effective, rewards should be given as soon as possible after desired behaviour (unlike bribes which are offered in advance), consistently given, tangible, in proportion to achievement, readily achievable so child experiences early success.
- But threshold for receiving reward should increase with time until eventually desired behaviour is achieved and maintained without need for reward.

Undesirable behaviours decreased by:
- *Remove/change antecedent stimuli:*
  - E.g. taking hyperactive child to park rather than staying indoors all day.
- *Extinction:*
  - Removing unintended reward (e.g. attention) for undesirable behaviour, ignoring undesired behaviour (behaviour may temporarily escalate in attempt to elicit response).
  - Not appropriate for serious bad behaviour.
- *Time out:*
  - Child taken away from context where behaviour occurred to quiet place for agreed period of time, e.g. few minutes and child should be calm before coming out.

- Should be undertaken as part of behavioural programme.
- Rules must be clear, warning and alternative behaviour should be given to child before removing them.
- Time-out place should be free of stimulus/entertainment.
- Parent should supervise but not interact with child.
- *Punishment:*
  - E.g. telling off, withholding rewards, loss of privileges.
  - Must be immediate, time-limited, proportionate, and perceived as negative by child.
  - Child can habituate quickly to punishment and so use only sparingly if behaviour unacceptable/dangerous.
  - Must be coupled with explanation and lots of positive reinforcement of desirable behaviour.
  - Avoid trap of unwittingly giving child too much attention for negative behaviour.

Setting up behavioural programme

- It is easy to become overwhelmed so initially focus on one or two behaviours, that can be relatively easily be achieved—helps build confidence in child and parents.
- Specify target behaviour precisely and agree desired outcome in precise behavioural terms. Focus on formulating positive desired behaviours rather than stopping negative behaviours.
- Share understanding of the behaviour (ABC analysis) and impact on child/family with parent and child emphasizing possibility for change.
- Establish system of rewards, time out, etc. as previously described.
- Parents should minimize anger when enforcing rules.
- Once target behaviour has been established threshold for reward is increased and frequency of rewards decreased until target behaviour firmly established when rewards should cease.
- A new behaviour may then be targeted if necessary.

Clinical neuropsychology

Introduction
- Clinical neuropsychology is practised by clinical psychologists who require additional (Qualification in Clinical Neuropsychology) training in neuropsychology.
- The primary concern of clinical neuropsychology is to elucidate brain–behaviour relationships.
- Assessments may be diagnostic, therapeutic, or serve as a baseline against which to measure developmental trajectory, recovery, or change following treatment.
- Following a detailed clinical interview (with the child and family) and examination of relevant medical and educational records, age-appropriate tests are typically administered over a period from 1–4 hours, with breaks as necessary.
- Questionnaire measures designed to screen and/or quantify behaviour, psychological or physical symptoms and quality of life may also be given.
- A neuropsychology assessment should yield:
  - A formulation of whether the observed clinical presentation and cognitive profile are consistent with any known neuropsychological syndrome, developmental/congenital disorder, neurological illness/injury, or other medical/psychiatric condition.
  - Whether clarification of presenting difficulties are 'organic' and/or 'functional', and/or whether there are any social or mental health difficulties.
  - Detailed feedback of findings to parents and/or child and discussions/advice regarding implications for likely future developmental trajectory, education/training, social-emotional adjustment, behaviour management, etc.
  - Recommendations for education, therapy, further investigation or assessment (see 📖 p218).
  - If appropriate, short psychological interventions (see 📖 p373) for acute mental health issues (i.e. CBT, supportive counselling).
  - If appropriate, time-limited out-patient case management/monitoring.
  - Ongoing liaison with education (see 📖 Chapter 15: Educational Paediatrics) and any other relevant health professionals.

Rough guide to cognition

- All skills are dependent on age and environment (including education and familial factors, especially with verbal skills).
- All skills are mediated by arousal, disposition, effort, mood, and attention (see 📖 p36).
- Consider carefully if there is a general learning disability (GLD) (see 📖 p117); clues may include:
  - Indolent early development.
  - Features of medical history.
  - Pervasive school failure (see 📖 p519).
- If GLD, then most if not all more selective cognitive domains are likely, by definition, to be similarly delayed. GLD may present as 'poor memory/concentration', 'learning', or 'poor school attainment'; there may, however, also be islands of relative ability (i.e. rote memory, motor skills).

If GLD is unlikely, consider cognition in terms of 'domains' as an heuristic

Language expression and comprehension

(Dominant brain hemisphere.)

- Problems may present as:
  - Inability to understand what is said reliably (with no contextual clues).
  - Difficulty in naming objects/pictures, repeating sentence/word and/or expressing self.
  - Poor prosody, semantics, syntax, or articulation (also see 📖 p202).
- Try 'open-ended' questions (e.g. 'What do you enjoy doing when you are not at school?').

Spatial skills

(Non-dominant brain hemisphere.)

- Problems may present as:
  - Left–right disorientation.
  - Getting lost easily.
  - Inability to read analogue clock face.
  - Putting clothes on wrong way round.
  - Putting shoes on wrong feet.
  - Inability to tie shoe laces.
  - Inability write without guide lines.
  - Inability to read maps/graphs.
- Ask the child to copy simple shapes, i.e. most can draw a circle at 3 years, square at 4 years, triangle at 5 years, diamond at 7 years (also see 📖 p46).

Memory/new learning skills

(Medial temporal lobes, diencephalic.)

- Neuropsychologists generally refer to 'long-term' rather than 'short-term' memory. Broadly equivalent to storage of information on computer 'hard drive'; requires both adequate registration of material and retrieval skills. Fractionation may include:
  - 'Remote' memory is memory for events some years ago and/or memories that pre-date the index illness/injury.

- 'Prospective' memory refers to planning for/remembering future events.
- 'Semantic' memory refers to fact-based knowledge.
- 'Autobiographical' memory refers to personal memories.
- 'Episodic' memory refers to memory for events placed in time.
- The younger the child the less able to recall spontaneously; their recognition recall, or cued recall is better.
- Verbal recall is mediated by adequate language skills.
- Executive skills may mediate recall.
- GLD, word-finding, difficulties or certain executive deficits may present as 'problems with memory'.
- Problems with 'long-term memory' may present as:
  - Forgetting activities, conversations, or events day-to-day.
  - Losing the thread of meaning while reading a book or watching TV programme.
  - Inability to recount favoured TV episodes.
  - Repeating self or questions.
  - Getting lost.

Attention-executive skills
(Prefrontal and frontostriatal.)
- 'Meta-cognitive' (e.g. mediating the use of language, attention, spatial and memory skills) executive skills continue to develop up to, and through the adolescent years.
- They correlate highly with IQ till approximately 8 years (and remain weak in GLD).
- Until 7–8 years distractibility and disinhibition are hallmark features of a 'dysexecutive' syndrome.
- A dysexecutive' syndrome can be cognitive and/or behavioural (also see 🕮 p126):
- These skills are heterogeneous and difficult to assess in structured situations.
- They can include difficulties with organization, attention, and the self-regulation of behaviour (i.e. poor impulse/affect control).
- Disinhibition or 'inappropriate' behaviour is defined contextually; 'normal' adolescent adjustment may appear dysexecutive.
- Auditory attention span (i.e. digit span) is sometimes referred to as 'working' memory broadly equivalent to 'random access memory' (RAM) on a computer.
- Ask the child to repeat back a 2-, 3-, 4-, or 5-digit sequence (e.g. 6–7/4–3–7/5–7–3–2/ etc.), read at the rate of one per second. Then ask for same spans (but different digits) repeated back *in reverse* (i.e. 8–9–4 repeated back as 4–9–8). Backwards digit span should not normally be >1/2 than forwards.

Speed of information processing
- Problems with slowed mentation; sometimes confused with psychomotor speed.
- Can present as problems with divided attention or multitasking (e.g. keeping more than one 'ball in the air' cognitively).
- Broadly equivalent to the speed of the processor on a computer.

Dexterity
- Problems can present as clumsiness, poor writing (see 📖 p46).
- Consider handedness (note: switching preferred hand till 4 years is not uncommon; 70% of left-handers are left hemisphere dominant).
- Gross motor skills: cycling, swimming, catching, running, sports (see 📖 p44), etc.

Attainments
These are learned, not necessarily innate skills.
- Problems with literacy and/or numeracy; single word/sentence reading, reading comprehension, spelling, adding, subtracting, times tables, etc.
- Referred to as 'dyslexia' (see 📖 p147) and 'dyscalculia' (see 📖 p151).
- There are many reasons why children have difficulties in reading—for *dyslexic* diagnosis poor reading should normally be within a context of relatively well-preserved general intellectual skills.
- A *selective* dyscalculia is very rare.

Neuropsychology: referral considerations and indications

Indications from 1ˢᵗ- and 3ʳᵈ-party observations and reports

- Younger children may not complain of cognitive problems explicitly, especially if slow developing or chronic; it may need to be indirectly inferred from reliable 3ʳᵈ-party observation or concerns of maladaptive behaviour (i.e. aggression, withdrawal, disorientation).
- Parental perspective needs to be weighed carefully (consider: are there older sibs for comparison? the perspective of extended family? any relevant sociocultural factors? parental expectations, presentation, occupation, education and mental health). Seek/consider *both* parents and/or extended family's perspective on problem.
- Corroboration from school needs to be weighed carefully (consider: pedigree and specificity of school report, compliant children may be overlooked, ethnicity, language, literacy level, parental involvement). Consider whether major transitions at school (i.e. primary to secondary, exams) are unmasking underlying weaknesses. Seek continuity of opinion from school.
- What do reports from others in the health or educational sector say?
- Your own observations and consideration of all available evidence is crucial.

Medical indications

Any injury, illness or congenital condition that may have compromised normal brain function could be a potential referral to neuropsychologists. These conditions generally present with abnormal neurology or physical malaise. The following list is illustrative rather than exhaustive.

- Traumatic: acceleration–deceleration (RTAs, falls, NAI) (see 📖 p267), missile wound, birth trauma, CP (see 📖 p67).
- Cerebrovascular: stroke, haemorrhage, arteriovenous malformation (see 📖 p255).
- Seizure disorder (see 📖 p240): poorly controlled, absences, status epilepticus, nocturnal, subclinical activity, Rasmussen's.
- Space-occupying lesion: neoplasms, hydrocephalus (see 📖 p264).
- Infection: meningitis, encephalitis, abscess, herpes, HIV, syphilis.
- Neurotoxic: metals (lead, mercury), solvents/fuels (glues, paints) pesticides, carbon monoxide.
- Metabolic disorder (see 📖 p155): hypoxia, diabetes, PKU.
- Environmental/social: severe neglect/abuse (see 📖 p440), FAS.
- Pervasive developmental disorders: ASD, (see 📖 p107) Rett syndrome (see 📖 p405).
- Other neurodevelopmental disorders: e.g. ADHD (see 📖 p126), ADD Tourette (see 📖 p332) syndrome.
- Genetic (see 📖 p403): i.e. Williams, fragile X, Turner, Prader Willi, Angleman syndromes.
- Iatrogenic: radiotherapy, chemotherapy, medications (anticonvulsant; i.e. topiramate) postoperative cognitive disorder (cardiac surgery, kidney dialysis, chronic anaesthetic neurotoxicity)

Issues to consider before a referral to neuropsychology

General considerations

- Consider whether the service that is described in the introduction (📖 p212) above would in any way advance the care of the child/young adult. If in doubt seek guidance from the clinical neuropsychologist.
- Consider '1st-party/3rd-party and medical indications (see 📖 p216).
- Children with a GLD (typically defined as a child with global intellectual abilities at or below 2 sd below the mean i.e. IQ <70) should normally be referred to local Learning Disability Services. At the extremes of the normal distribution of ability (i.e. either very able or disabled), the efficacy and utility of neuropsychological assessment diminishes as the 'ceiling' or 'floor' of age-appropriate tests is reached.
- If there is no medical or psychiatric dimension, general difficulties at school are often best dealt with by educational psychology services (see 📖 p531).
- If there is no neurological dimension, then referral to CAMHS may be more appropriate in the event of general behavioural or social–emotional problems (see 📖 p319).

Age considerations

- The extent to which cognition can be usefully fractionated depends upon age.
- With infants less than ~3 years, general developmental scales (i.e. assessment of gross and fine motor skills, language, social, and adaptive skills as, e.g. in the BSID-III or GMDS-ER) need to be employed (see 📖 p36). The results of any cognitive assessment (other than some quasi-experimental paradigms) at this age will be a poor predictor of later intellectual skills.
- With preschool (3–6 years) children, assessment will generally be confined to verbal and non-verbal general intellectual skills, psychomotor/processing speed, attention and language skills; there are also measures of more selective skills (i.e. memory, attention-executive, spatial skills), though these are less commonly available outside specialist centres and may be less reliable.
- Until children first start to be exposed to school disciplines many are not familiar with or biddable to sitting down and completing tests over a period of time, which is required for successful neuropsychology assessments (also see 📖 p42).
- All raw scores on the neuropsychology tests administered to children are referenced against a normal population of same age peers, and reported in terms of sd from the mean scores for that age band. Scores may be expressed as:
  - Percentiles.
  - T-scores (where the mean = 50, sd 10).
  - Standard scores (mean = 100, sd 15).
  - Age-scaled scores (mean = 10, sd 3).
  - 'Mental-age' equivalents.

Neuropsychology: advice to parents and school

- If a program of 'cognitive rehabilitation' is offered consider carefully:
  - Has there been a proper neuropsychological formulation of the quality and distribution of any cognitive impairment?
  - Is there a sound, peer-reviewed evidence base for the intervention?
  - Is it costly?
  - Is it onerous for the child?
  - Is there a sport or activity which the child could engage in pleasurably which might be of equal benefit and have incidental social value?
  - Does it purport to 'retrain', 're-organize', or 'recover' lost brain function? If so treat with caution.
  - Does it purport to educate (i.e. understanding distribution of strengths and weaknesses correctly), support (i.e. re-establish self-confidence and insight) and/or maximize external and organizational aids (i.e. calendars, mobile phones, mechanical/electronic aids to recall, organization of function)? If so, it may be helpful.
  - COGMED Working Memory Training is one computerized cognitive training program of working memory for which there is a reasonable, independent evidence base. The program is suitable for children aged 4 years and older. There are peer-reviewed studies available, which suggest that COGMED training might improve some features of 'working memory', with some sustained and generalizing benefit. It is, however, a commercial program which requires considerable commitment from parents and children over a number of weeks
- Recovery or rehabilitation (see 📖 p183, p186, p191, p208, p225) is often more about maximizing adaption, accommodation, and insight than restoration of lost function.
- Restore normal daily routines as far and as quickly as possible given the nature and severity of illness/injury.
- Encourage age-peer social activities whenever possible and/or appropriate.
- Consider carefully whether it is better to 'work' on lost skills which may never fully recover or focus instead on residual strengths (NB the importance of self-confidence and self-esteem in adaption and recovery).
- Be aware of recovery gradients:
  - Following acute injury/illness recovery takes for up to 2–3 years with the rate of recovery diminishing over time; recovery in year 1 is much more marked than years 2–3.
  - Cognitive development can 'plateau' with new skills still being acquired but not at the same rate as age-peers. For example, following radiotherapy the younger the child the greater and more quickly apparent any deleterious effects. Older than 7/8 years effects are more subtle and take longer to be expressed—often in speed of information processing and/or attention.

- Recovery can be 'stepwise' when interrupted by treatment or complications.
- The evidence for delayed emergence of cognitive or behavioural deficits (i.e. 'executive' deficits in adolescence following a frontal injury/illness in infancy) is very weak if there has been no manifestation of the deficit in intervening years. Pre-existing deficits can, however, be *exacerbated* or exaggerated by adolescent adjustment.
- Extent of impaired awareness/cognition acutely does not always correlate with longer-term neuropsychological outcome.
- Age related vulnerability-plasticity. There is some evidence to suggest that approximately:
  - 0–12 months: confers increased vulnerability to brain insult (which outweighs beneficial effects of potential plasticity).
  - 1–6 years: vulnerability is less but there is still plasticity, which may lead to greater recovery potential.
  - 6–7 years: the evidence for true brain plasticity (i.e. ability to spontaneously reorganize or recommit skills to non-damaged brain area) is limited (also see 📖 p59 and p60).
- In adolescence, maladaption to chronic or serious acute illness/injury (see 📖 p363) is more common that in the younger or middle years of childhood.

Orthotic management of neurodisability

- *Orthoses*, often referred to as splints or braces, are externally applied medical devices that compensate for impairments in the musculoskeletal (see 📖 Chapter 11: Orthopaedics) or neurological systems (see 📖 Chapter 6: Neurology).
- *Orthotists* are the allied health professionals specifically trained to advise on whether and how an orthosis can be designed and made.
- Orthoses are prescribed to achieve clinical objectives such as to prevent deformity or to improve functioning (see 📖 p67).
- Orthoses are usually custom-moulded from plastics, such as polypropylene, and incorporate judiciously placed straps and padding in order to achieve their goals.

Biomechanical principles

- The means by which orthoses work is biomechanical, through the application of force and lever systems.
- Typically the forces that orthoses apply are 'reaction' forces generated in response to gravity, where muscles are weak, and/or to counter forces of muscle imbalance, as in the case of spasticity.
- Key biomechanical principles underpinning orthotic management are that using longer lever arms means less force is required; and that applying forces over large surface areas means less pressure is applied to the body. For stability, the centre of mass of the body must be within the base of support.
- An appreciation of gait analysis (see 📖 p433) is necessary to understand how orthoses can improve the efficiency of walking.

Terminology

- Terminology for orthoses can be confusing. The standard system is to describe an orthosis by the joints that are encompassed in the device. For example, an orthosis enclosing the ankle and foot but finishing below the knee is an ankle–foot orthosis, with the acronym AFO. Similarly, a spinal orthosis encompassing the thoraco-lumbar and sacral spine is referred to as a TLSO.
- Sometimes the aim of the orthosis is included in the name, such as hip abduction orthosis.
- Confusion can occur when orthoses are named after people or places or referred to by trade names. Terms such as dynamic are vague and should be avoided.

Foot orthoses

- Insoles, supportive footwear, and shoe modifications can all be used to increase stability during standing and walking.
- Mild plano-valgus or varus deformities (see 📖 p422) can be controlled by foot orthoses that are designed to encourage better skeletal alignment.
- Foot orthoses occasionally extend just above the ankle to gain greater control, and these designs are termed supra-malleolar orthoses (SMOs).
- Insoles can also be moulded to redistribute plantar pressure under the foot.

Ankle–foot orthoses (AFOs)

- To control equinus (see 📖 p422) or calcaneus deformity, or moderate to severe valgus or varus deformities, an orthosis need to encompass the ankle and foot and extend to just below the knee.
- AFOs provide longer leverage and control in the sagittal plane. AFOs may be trimmed to be flexible or incorporate hinges to allow dorsiflexion, or made rigid to provide maximum control.
- AFOs are widely prescribed for children with CP (see 📖 p67), spina bifida (see 📖 p261), and other neuromuscular conditions (see 📖 p257) to improve gait efficiency.
- AFOs are also used to control foot position and prevent deformity in non-ambulant children.
- Sometimes AFOs are used at night, although this should not be pursued if this interferes with sleeping.

Knee–ankle–foot orthoses (KAFOs)

- A KAFO extends from the thigh and includes the ankle and foot; a hinge is usually included at the knee to enable flexion during sitting but these are often designed to be locked in extension for standing and walking.
- Children with neuromuscular conditions such as muscular dystrophy (see 📖 p257) or spinal muscular atrophy (see 📖 p258) may find that KAFOs enable them to stand and walk; however, KAFOs are rarely used with children with CP.

Hip–knee–ankle–foot orthoses (HKAFOs)

- HKAFOs can enable children who are unable to maintain standing unaided to stand and become mobile.
- HKAFOs extend from the trunk and control the whole lower limb. Children with spina bifida or paraplegia can learn to use custom-fitted modular orthoses such as the Swivel Walker or ParaWalker.

Thoraco-lumbar sacral orthoses (TLSOs)

- Spinal orthoses (TLSOs) are used to control scoliosis (see 📖 p416) in children with a variety of neuromuscular conditions.
- Although orthoses may not prevent progressive scoliosis, TLSOs are often used to reduce the rate of progression and delay the need for surgical stabilization, or when surgery is not possible.

Upper limb orthoses

- Orthoses are used to position the arm, wrist and hand to improve upper limb functioning and/or manual ability (see 📖 p193).
- Wrist–hand orthoses (WHOs) usually hold the wrist in extension, and may extend to control thumb posture to promote a functional position.
- 'Paddle' type designs of WHOs may be used to resist flexion deformities in the wrist and fingers.

Head orthoses

- A protective helmet may be indicated when a child is prone to falling, for instance during seizures (see 📖 p240), or injuring themselves.
- Helmets vary in design; some are constructed from dense foams whilst other designs have hard exteriors.

Lycra-based orthoses

- There has been increasing interest in fabric orthoses that use Lycra-based materials to control body postures.
- These types of orthosis can be designed to fit different parts of the body.
- However, there is limited evidence that Lycra-based orthoses are effective, or to inform patient selection.

Summary

- Orthoses can be very useful to improve functioning in children with neurodisability, and may reduce the rate of progressive deformity.
- However, orthoses can occasionally create skin problems due to pressure or friction; and repairs may be required. Therefore families should be able to easily access an orthotist directly, and the fit of an orthosis should be checked by an orthotist as necessary.
- Typically a child grows out of their orthosis between 6–14 months, reassessment and replacement of the orthosis needs to be considered.
- There can be stigma associated with using equipment that identifies children as different to their peers. Therefore the benefits of orthoses for individual children should be carefully assessed and re-evaluated over time.
- An orthotist with an understanding of the nuances of neurodisability should be an integral member of the multidisciplinary team (see 📖 pp20–3).

Prosthetics

What is a prosthesis?

A prosthesis replaces a part of the body, e.g. a missing limb. It should be distinguished from an orthosis, which is a device to hold part of the body in a more correct or desirable position (see 📖 p220).

What is a prosthetist?

Prosthetists and orthotists are the health professionals trained to design and manufacture these devices. They are dual trained in the two roles but generally specialize in one or the other later on.

Prosthetics in childhood and adult life

- The requirement for a prosthesis is rare in early childhood and is usually the consequence of a congenital abnormality, often, for example, a trans-radial deficiency resulting in an absent hand.
- In childhood other causes of limb deficiency accumulate: trauma, cancer, and increasingly frequently as a result of a child surviving sepsis.
- This contrasts dramatically with adult-onset limb deficiency which is overwhelmingly the result of vascular problems due to diabetes, smoking, and atherosclerosis.

Some key principles

- Use play to help the child to want to wear the prosthesis, e.g. encourage them to wear it while a story is being read aloud or particular toys are being played with.
- Enable the child to reach their developmental milestones on time, e.g. have the prosthetic leg ready for learning to walk.
- Children are infinitely adaptable; they find ways round limb deficiencies very often, e.g. using the elbow flexion of an arm with no hand, to replace the hand. This can make encouraging them to use the artificial hand very difficult. The residual limb has good sensation, the prosthesis none at all.
- Make sure the prosthesis is functionally useful at that time for the child. An upper limb device is more of a tool than a hand, e.g. to hold a bicycle handlebar, or play with a particular toy.
- Involve the child's carers or parents in the process of learning to use a device.
- Parents of children who lose a limb through trauma are often overwhelmed by feelings of guilt, and may themselves need a chance to spend time with a counsellor.
- For parents of a child with a congenital limb deficiency the major impact comes at a much earlier stage in the child's life, even before they are born if the deficiency has been identified on a scan.
- Making a decision to remove parts of a residual limb that get in the way of making prosthetic progress is an agonizing and protracted process, e.g. removing a deformed and inappropriately placed foot in proximal femoral deficiency.
- Using other body parts to replace a missing hand, e.g. using the mouth and teeth as a surrogate hand, can have significant consequences for

the part that is used later in life—such as wear and tear on teeth, painful joints if feet are used as hands.
- The prosthetic user will have lifelong contact with a prosthetic service, with differing needs at different stages of life.
- Children with limb deficiencies will benefit greatly if there is close liaison with the school or nursery, to educate staff and other children, ensure appropriate adaptations are made. Points of transition (see 📖 p171) are particularly important, e.g. starting science laboratory lessons, going on school trips away from home.

About prostheses
- The first prosthesis tends to be very simple mechanically.
- As the child grows there is space for a more sophisticated component.
- As the child ages different priorities apply, e.g. cosmesis over functioning at a stage in the early years of adolescence onwards, the need to ride a bike at an earlier stage.
- An upper limb prosthesis is really a tool to do tasks and children may need several devices to carry out different tasks.

Clinical engineering

Clinical engineers work across a wide spectrum of areas to provide a technical solution to clinical problems. They also work as part of the clinical team in elucidating the nature of the problem and in planning technical solutions.

Diagnostics

Gait lab (🕮 p433)
- The gait lab is used to analyse a client's gait pattern and posture.
- Engineers work on analysing the gait and collaborate with orthopaedic surgeons (see 🕮 p410 and p411), orthotists, (see 🕮 p220) and PTs (see 🕮 p176) in planning surgical and therapy interventions to improve gait and posture.

Clinical measurement
Examples of this include:
- Interface pressure mapping, e.g. for wheelchair seating (see 🕮 p186).
- Monitoring of sensory and motor signals along the spinal cord during spinal surgery.

Technical solutions for clinical problems

Wheelchairs and special seating (see 🕮 p186)
Clinical engineers work with PTs and OTs (see 🕮 p191) in assessing posture and pressure areas to provide seating which maximizes functioning and minimizes the risk of pressure sores.

Environmental control units (ECU)
- A child with complex impairments (see 🕮 p67, p267, and p268) that severely restricts his/her independence can be helped to achieve a much higher degree of independence by the provision of an ECU system.
- The fundamental requirement is for the client to have one reliable means of signalling—this can be as little as a reliable head or mouth movement.
- The ECU is designed by the engineers around the client's abilities and wishes, enabling them to do things independently such as:
  - Open a door which has been set up to respond.
  - Turn on lights.
  - Turn on or off other electronic devices.
  - Drive electronic wheelchairs.
- A system setting up a single room can cost in the region of £3000.
- Specialist centres are located in Bristol at the Frenchay Hospital, Birmingham at the Regional Rehabilitation Unit, Oxford at The Oxford Centre for Enablement.

Computer access
- There is a wide variety of both hardware and software which enables the client to make use of computers.
- Hardware examples include:
  - Keyboards having guards to avoid pressing multiple buttons at once.

- Alternative mouse to match limited hand function, e.g. to cope with tremor.
- Screens which respond to eye gaze as a means of control.
- Software can be provided to allow improved speed and response where limited movement and limited cognition are in evidence.
- Increasing use is being made of commonly available equipment such as smart phones, tablet PCs, and 'apps'.

Communication aids (Also see 📖 p208)
- There is a huge range of equipment. Examples include:
  - Touch pads with letters that can spell out words or phrases using an electronic voice.
  - Letter boards (ETRAN) to spell out words using eye movements.
  - 'Litewriter' which has a keyboard input and displays the output visually or audibly.
- Clinicians seeking a technical solution are advised to contact a specialist centre as the range of technology is huge.

Functional electronic stimulation (FES)
- If a client has a foot drop, causing a tendency to catch the toes against the ground resulting in a trip, the FES can be set up to follow the gait cycle and trigger the foot dorsiflexors to act, reducing the trip risk.
- FES devices cost in the region of £700–£5000 according to the degree of sophistication.

Contacting a clinical engineering department
Specialist services can be contacted at: Oxford University Hospitals (The Oxford Centre for Enablement 01865 227 447), Kings College Hospital in London, Birmingham, Manchester, Leeds.

Neurology

Above the clouds, the sky is always blue.

Scandinavian proverb

Evaluating a child with a neurological disorder

The key to neurological diagnosis is a meticulous history, careful examination, and good observation. One needs to keep an open mind and avoid bias.

▶ Always listen to the parent and child. They are trying to tell you the diagnosis.

Important components of a neurological history

1. *Birth history:* history through pregnancy—drug use, illnesses, trauma, fetal movements, ultrasound findings (polyhydramnios), and antenatal bleeds, etc. Resuscitation history—significant oxygen requirement, ventilatory support, instrumentation, dysmorphism noted at birth, joint contractures/hip dysplasia noted at birth. Apgar scores.

2. *Neonatal history:* birth records must be checked. Gestational age, head circumference, and weight at birth. Feeding difficulty, oxygen requirements, special care, hypoglycaemia, jaundice, seizures.

3. *Family history:* meticulous FHx going back 3 generations and including half siblings etc. Common conditions such as heart disease, diabetes, hearing difficulties, thyroid problems, any autoimmune diseases, etc. may seem irrelevant but can be very important. Keep in mind inheritance patterns, particularly recessive and maternal when asking Hx. Always examine parents if considering dominant or maternally inherited conditions. Unexpected sudden deaths must be probed.

4. *Medication history and toxins:* regular medications, substance abuse, accidental ingestion, allergic reactions, side effects must all be borne in mind especially in acute presentations. Pets, foreign travel, etc. which seem unimportant can become very relevant (TB, Lyme disease, tick paralysis).

5. *Immunisation history* (see 🕮 p620).

6. *All recent and past medical history:* must be sought and all associations of that history with the current problem must be thought of. Previous head injuries, seizures, any faints or funny turns must be asked for.

7. *Social and developmental history:* this is of course critical. Plotting the head circumference and growth (see 🕮 p602 and p616) are very important. The child's schooling (see 🕮 p520), participation in sport and peer group activities, family circumstances, learning difficulties (see 🕮 p117), bullying (see 🕮 p342), work pressures, all need to be explored.

The child should always be part of the history-taking process and should be given the opportunity to say what is bothering them. Drawing pictures can be an excellent alternative to a narrative story.

A timeline for the history should be sought and will give clues as to whether the problem is static, progressive (acute or chronic), or paroxysmal. Loss of acquired skills always has a sinister connotation and needs to be actively teased out from history.

Examination

There is an enormous emphasis on meticulous examination and trying to localize the pathology in adult neurology. Whilst there is no substitute to meticulous examination where possible, in children observation plays an equally if not more important part. Watching them ambulate, talk, interact with friends, siblings, and family gives a lot of information. Even before starting formal examination certain observations are very useful.

Gait and posture

- The way a child walks into the clinic should never be missed. Watching the child's standing, sitting and lying down posture often suggests the diagnosis in neuromuscular disorders (see ☐ p257). Their gait (see ☐ p433) gives clues to the identity of motor disorders.
- Formal testing of power is often impossible and observing the child walk and get up from sitting or lying down will clearly indicate the degree of weakness.
- Hemiplegic and ataxic gaits can be noticed.
- Facial asymmetry when talking or smiling and expressionless myopathic facies are worth noting.
- Examining parents particularly eliciting maternal myotonia in a weak child should be part of routine examination.
- Subtle asymmetries and motor weakness can be uncovered by performing a Fog test.

Dysmorphism

- One can't make much of dysmorphic features until you have seen the parents but gross dysmorphism such as hypertelorism, sutural prominence, and facial dysmorphism (see ☐ p384) can be noted easily. Micro- and macrocephaly can sometimes be easily identified.
- Some syndromes are recognizable to trained eyes, e.g. fragile X (see ☐ p403), Angelman syndrome (see ☐ p404), Rett syndrome (see ☐ p405), and of course more familiar chromosomal abnormalities such as Down syndrome (see ☐ p387).

Neurocutaneous markers

Should be looked for, e.g. port wine stains (Sturge Weber syndrome) (see ☐ p251)), ash leaf macules (tuberous sclerosis—may need Wood's lamp exam (see ☐ p251)), café au lait (neurofibromatosis (see ☐ p250)).

Other suggestive signs

For example, telangiectasia, jaundice, stiff wiry hair (Menkes disease), hirsutism and coarse facial features (mucopolysaccharidosis), hyperventilation and hand stereotypes (Rett syndrome), fatigable ptosis (myasthenia), frog leg posture and tongue fasciculation (spinal muscular atrophy (see ☐ p257)), etc.

Behaviour and interaction

- May suggest hyperactivity, attention deficit (see ☐ p126), or autism (see ☐ p107).
- There is nothing different from adult examination in the formal neurological examination of a child. By age 7 most children can be fully examined as an adult and sometimes as young as 3. This depends on their cognitive ability and cooperation.

Additional examination points in newborn and infant neurological examination

- Chart their head circumference, body growth, and weight gain.
- Neonatal reflexes should be examined and their persistence beyond a certain age documented as abnormal. These include Moro (noting the persistence and asymmetry, if any), asymmetric tonic neck reflex, palmar and plantar grasp reflexes, stepping and placing reflexes and parachute reflex.
- A weak floppy neonate or infant lying in a frog leg posture (see 📖 p233) with poor antigravity movements, weak cry, laboured breathing, tongue fasciculation, and absent deep tendon reflexes suggests spinal muscular atrophy or a severe congenital myopathy.
- An exaggerated startle to nose tap especially in a stiff neonate with or without cyanotic spells suggests hyperekplexia.
- Neonatal seizures can be subtle especially in preterm babies and may be easily missed. Jitteriness can be seen in hypoglycaemia and hypocalcaemia. Persistent hiccups are sometimes seen in non-ketotic hyperglycinemia.
- Nerve root injuries (Erb and Klumpke) as well as more traumatic cervical cord injuries may occur during the process of delivery and can present initially with flail limbs, areflexia, and swallowing and breathing difficulties. Hip dysplasias (see 📖 p419) and joint contractures should be noted.

Signs and symptoms

Abnormal head size

- It is important to measure the OFC at its widest point accurately accounting for gestational age.
- A sequential plot is more valuable than a single measurement.
- Parental head circumference must be measured and mid parental head circumference centile worked out.
- Appropriate charts must be used. OFC has to be interpreted in the context of the child's neurodevelopmental assessment, intracranial pressure and story of regression if any.

Causes of large head (> 2 sd above mean for age)

- Familial large head (most likely)
- Hydrocephalus (see 🕮 p264) (true obstructive as in aqueduct stenosis, tumours, Chiari malformation, or poor absorption as in post meningitis or post haemorrhagic)
- Increased extra-axial fluid spaces: This has to be excessive and progressive as it is a common finding on imaging (achondroplasia, Menkes disease, glutaric aciduria type 1).
- Hydranencephaly: very rare, may be part of holoprosencephaly sequence.
- Megalencephaly: genetic or associated with neurocutaneous syndromes such as NF, tuberous sclerosis, gigantism as in Soto syndrome.
- Metabolic disorders (see 🕮 p155): Alexander and Canavan disease, galactosaemia, glutaric aciduria type1, MPS, gangliosidoses.
- Subdural effusions/haemorrhages.
- Thickened skull causing large head: rickets, osteogenesis imperfecta, cleidocranial dysostosis, epiphyseal dysplasia, osteopetrosis, etc.

Causes of microcephaly (OFC < 2 sd below normal for age)

- Primary microcephaly.
- Genetic.
- Chromosomal abnormality.
- Anencephaly and encephalocoeles.
- Agenesis of corpus callosum.
- Lissencephaly or pachygyria.
- Holoprosencephaly.
- Secondary microcephaly.
- Intrauterine infection/toxin exposure.
- Hypoxic ischaemic injury.
- Intracranial haemorrhage or perinatal stroke.
- Post meningitis/encephalitis.
- Chronic renal/cardiac disease.
- Chronic malnutrition.

Abnormal head shape

Postural plagiocephaly is the most common. In the absence of developmental concerns or abnormal examination findings, no further investigation is required.

Causes of abnormal head shape
- Intracranial causes, e.g. cerebellar agenesis, temporal lobe agenesis, hydrocephalus, Dandy–Walker malformation, chronic subdural effusions.
- Extracranial causes, e.g. plagiocephaly, craniosynostosis which may be syndromal, genetic, or associated with other conditions such as MPS, polycythaemia, hyperthyroidism, hypercalcaemia, rickets, and ataxia telangiectasia.
- Some well recognized craniosynostosis need mention which can be diagnosed readily on the basis of head shape. Examples are clover leaf skull of Pfeiffer syndrome, brachycephaly and synostosis of Apert syndrome and generalized synostosis of Crouzon or Carpenter syndrome with associated facial malformation in Crouzon and obesity and hypogonadism in Carpenter.

Further resource
Microcephaly Support Group: ☎ 01638 552689 🖰 http://www.micro-cephaly.co.uk

Floppy infant

- Floppiness can be due to hypotonia, weakness, or ligamentous laxity and all 3 may coexist.
- Benign hypotonia in the absence of weakness and normal cognitive development is very common and one should avoid over-investigating a floppy infant in the absence of specific concerns other than just hypotonia.
- Ligamentous laxity is also very common and often familial and can cause significant motor developmental delay.
- GDD (see 🕮 p117) is unlikely in a pure neuromuscular disorder although there are exceptions with autism (see 🕮 p107) and learning difficulty (see 🕮 p117) in association with Xp21 muscular dystrophies and seizures (see 🕮 p240) and learning difficulties in congenital muscular dystrophies.
- Hypothyroidism (Semelaigne syndrome) can present with weakness, calf hypertrophy, and raised muscle CK enzyme levels akin to muscular dystrophies and must always be actively excluded.

As a general approach one needs to determine whether hypotonia or weakness is the predominant feature.

If hypotonia is predominant, the causes are more likely to be central

For example:
- Hypoxic ischaemic damage.
- Cerebral dysgenesis.
- Metabolic disorders (see 🕮 p155), e.g. Menkes disease, glutaric aciduria type 1, MPS, gangliosidoses, glycosylation defects, etc.
- Hypothyroidism, rickets, hypocalcaemia, hypophosphataemia
- Recognizable syndromes, e.g. PWS, Worster-Drought syndrome, Moebius syndrome, Angelman syndrome (see 🕮 p404), Rett syndrome (see 🕮 p405), etc.
- Chromosomal abnormality, e.g. 22q11 deletion, trisomies (see 🕮 p387), fragile X (see 🕮 p403), etc.

Examination will usually reveal normal to brisk deep tendon reflexes, no weakness, global developmental concerns, dysmorphism (see 🕮 p384).

Investigations most likely to help are chromosome analysis, genetic opinion, metabolic investigations, and imaging.

If weakness is predominant, it is likely to be a peripheral neuromuscular problem

For example:
- Spinal muscular atrophy (SMA): characterized by normal cognition but profound weakness, flopped posture, tongue fasciculation, and absent deep tendon reflexes.
- Peripheral neuropathies. Most neuropathies do not present in infancy.
- Myasthenia: if presenting in infancy it is more likely to be a congenital myasthenia and early history is very important. Autoimmune myasthenia can sometimes present as early as second year of life.

Transient neonatal myasthenia can carry on into the first few months of life in infants born to mothers with myasthenia gravis. Eliciting a history of or demonstrating fatigue is critical.
- Congenital myopathies.
- Congenital myotonic dystrophy (DM1). This is very important to consider and the examination repertoire should include a parental examination to exclude myotonia.
- Congenital muscular dystrophies.
- Other muscular dystrophies that rarely present in infancy—Xp21 muscular dystrophies, limb girdle muscular dystrophies, facioscapulohumeral muscular dystrophy.
- Collagen-related myopathies—Ullrich and Bethlem myopathies.
- Metabolic myopathies—in particular Pompe disease can present with early cardiomyopathy and McArdle disease.
- Mitochondrial myopathies.

Examination will usually reveal significant weakness, depressed or absent deep tendon reflexes, and normal cognitive development (see 📖 p36) in general. It is important to include a cardiac and respiratory system examination and inquire for symptoms of cardiac and respiratory failure.

Investigations most likely to be useful are thyroid functions, CK, lactate, blood film for vacuolated lymphocytes (if metabolic myopathy suspected), ECG, EMG, nerve conduction studies, and a muscle biopsy. DNA analysis can give rapid diagnosis in SMA and DM1.

Headache

Headache is very common in school-age children and may be present from infancy in some cases. Distinction must be made between acute and chronic headache causes of which differ. Further distinction is between symptomatic and idiopathic headaches. Chronic idiopathic headaches are the ones most likely to be encountered in the office setting.

Causes of symptomatic headaches

- Raised intracranial pressure: secondary to acute hydrocephalus, cerebral oedema, benign intracranial hypertension, venous sinus thrombosis, etc. The characteristics symptoms of headache, vomiting, deteriorating cognitive function, cranial nerve palsies, and papilloedema are seen in established cases.
- Ear, nose, throat, and sinus disease.
- Dental disease (see 📖 p165).
- Visual acuity problems (see 📖 p271).
- Vascular—subarachnoid or intracranial haemorrhage from aneurysms, arteriovenous malformations (rare and usually catastrophic).
- Post-traumatic, e.g. concussion acutely and chronic headaches.
- Infections, e.g. meningitis, encephalitis.
- Toxins, e.g. substance abuse, analgesic overuse, carbon monoxide poisoning.
- Metabolic causes, e.g. hypothyroidism.
- Miscellaneous, e.g. OSA (see 📖 p90), hypoventilation (neuromuscular disorders), hypertension (rare).

Common causes of chronic and paroxysmal idiopathic headaches

- Migraine (with and without aura).
- Variants of migraine, e.g. abdominal migraine and cyclical vomiting, paroxysmal vertigo, and torticollis.
- Complicated migraines, e.g. hemiplegic migraine, basilar migraine, ophthalmoplegic migraines, confusional migraine.
- Chronic daily headaches (episodic and chronic tension type).
- Cluster headaches (rare).
- Chronic depression (often under-recognized in children, (see 📖 p350)).

Migraine

- The common characteristics are as follows:
  - Unilateral (sometimes bilateral).
  - Throbbing character.
  - Lasts 3–72 hours.
  - Associated photo and or phono phobia.
  - Associated nausea and or vomiting.
  - Often positive FHx.
  - Relieved by rest.
  - Sometimes precipitated by menses, stress, dehydration, sleep deprivation, long periods of starvation.

- Aggravated by movement and continued activity.
- Perhaps the most important feature is the disabling nature of migraine which has to be a feature in the history.
- Auras are uncommon in younger children. They take the form of visual auras (positive—scintillation, wavy or crisscross lines, dots, spectral, distortion of imagery, macropsia; negative—scotomas, micropsia, hemianopias, etc.), auditory, gustatory, olfactory, etc.
- Once the headaches are recurrent and fairly stereotypic with consistent features, a confident diagnosis of migraine will save unnecessary investigations. EEG will show slowing of background during an attack and is unhelpful. Imaging is normal or may show incidental abnormalities which complicate the issue and increase anxiety. Very rarely an atrial septal defect or patent foramen ovale is present and closure of these can lead to a resolution of migraines.
- Treatment is symptomatic in the form of simple analgesia often in combination with an antiemetic, plenty of fluids (once vomiting has resolved), oral or intranasal triptans. Prophylaxis in frequent attacks is in the form of avoidance of triggers where identifiable, sanomigran and various other drugs such as propranolol, topiramate, and sodium valproate.

Episodic and chronic tension-type headaches

- Are commonly experienced by everyone due to life stresses, fatigue, and exertion. Headache is dull, constricting in character and lasts up to a day sometimes a little longer.
- Chronicity should raise the suspicion of chronic anxiety (see 🕮 p354) and depression. Headache is present at all times and for days or weeks with none of the typical migraine characteristics and is not disabling in the same way as an acute migraine attack.
- Amitriptyline and psychotherapy (see 🕮 p373) may be required.

Unsteadiness and falls

There are many reasons for being unsteady and its presence does not equate to a diagnosis of ataxia. Careful history and examination is the key.

Important questions in the history

- Duration and time course: is it a new symptom or has it been since the child started walking and is just more noticeable? Is it episodic and paroxysmal or persistent?
- Are there any associated concerns, e.g. weakness, speech and articulation problems, vision or hearing difficulties, feeding and swallowing difficulties. Are the problems restricted to gait alone or is it upper limb function as well? Is there associated nausea, vomiting, vertiginous sensation etc.?
- What are the fine motor skills like? Ask questions about all aspects of praxis, e.g. articulation of words, dressing, fine motor skills, sequencing tasks.

Examination

When examining, one needs to focus on certain points such as:

- Presence of true ataxia: is there gait, trunk, and limb ataxia? Are there cerebellar signs, e.g. nystagmus, difficulty with tandem walking, dysmetria?
- Is there any weakness: is it fatigable (myopathy, myasthenia)?
- Is the proprioception intact? Romberg test and finger nose test with eyes closed, drift of outstretched arm (may be due to weakness).
- Is the coordination appropriate? Sequential finger thumb opposition, Berges and Lezine repertoire, copying a sentence in sequence, performing sequential tasks.
- How is the fine motor coordination, e.g. stringing beads, cutting or folding paper, handwriting?
- Are there any vestibular features, e.g. nystagmus, tinnitus, vertigo?
- Is there any evidence of a neuropathy? Check reflexes. Are there any neurocutaneous markers, e.g. telangiectasia?
- Any other unusual examination findings, e.g. opsoclonus, altered conscious state (non-convulsive status), pupillary abnormalities (toxins), papilloedema (raised ICP), pyramidal tract signs, Achilles tendon or hamstring contractures, movement disorders, e.g. tremors, dystonia, chorea?

Unsteadiness thus can result from various causes

- Vestibular.
- Peripheral neuromuscular problems, e.g. myopathies and neuropathies.
- Weakness (often weakness in Guillain-Barré syndrome is interpreted as ataxia).
- Ataxia (see 🔲 p247).
- Developmental coordination disorder (definitions vary between therapists and clinicians) (🔲 p136). This is essentially 'clumsiness' in the absence of any weakness, ataxia, or other neurological dysfunction. Degrees of functional impairment vary. It affects fine and gross motor function and most markedly sequencing. There are no alarming examination findings and no cerebellar signs. It is static but may become more obvious as more demands on co-ordinated functioning are placed on a growing school-age child.

Abnormal movements

Common movement abnormalities seen are:

Tremor
- Rhythmic oscillation of a part of or whole body.
- Amplitudes can vary.
- It can be postural when trying to maintain a posture, action or intentional when precipitated by voluntary action (usually cerebellar pathology), and extrapyramidal which is high amplitude tremor present at rest and gets worse with posture and movement (pathology in superior cerebellar peduncle or substantia nigra).

Chorea and ballismus
- A sudden jerky trunk or limb movement which is purposeless.
- Ballismus is a more severe form with violent high amplitude proximal limb movements.
- Typically seen in rheumatic fever and lupus when acute and in CP (see 📖 p67) alongside athetosis and dystonia. May also be seen in metabolic conditions such as Wilson disease.

Athetosis and dystonia
- Sustained abnormal contractions of agonist and antagonist muscles with cramp like pain and postures.
- Slow writhing distal movements that accompany dystonia are termed athetosis. Often coexists with chorea.
- Dystonias may be generalized due to genetic/metabolic conditions such as PKAN, Wilson disease, DYT1, and focal such as in blepharospasm, torticollis, writer's cramp.

Myoclonus
- Sudden involuntary muscle contraction lasting <250ms.
- May be focal, multifocal, or generalized.
- May be spinal or cortical.
- May be spontaneous as in epilepsy or triggered by noise or touch.

Rigidity and bradykinesia
- These are features of Parkinsonism and are rare in children.
- There is paucity of spontaneous movement and initiation of action.
- There is a persistent abnormal increased tone with increased resistance to passive movement (lead pipe rigidity). There is often superimposed tremor causing the 'cog wheeling' phenomenon.

Tics and other stereotypes
- Various behavioural stereotypes like arm flinging, hand wringing, head nodding, body rocking are seen in children with learning difficulties but sometimes in developmentally normal children as well.
- Tics are the commonest movement stereotypes (see 📖 p332).
- They often involve face and limbs and can change from one body part to another over time.
- There are quiescent periods with exacerbations at times of stress.

- They may take the form of simple or complex motor phenomena. Ocular tics may be mistaken for opsoclonus or nystagmus.
- If they persist without remission over more than 6 months in a 12-month period and are accompanied by distressing vocal tics a diagnosis of Tourette syndrome needs to be considered.
- They can be voluntarily suppressed and extinguish in sleep.
- Simple motor tics do not need treatment other than reassurance.
- Psychological input and medication such as sulpiride, pimozide, haloperidol, and clonidine may be needed in more intrusive intractable tics and Tourette syndrome.

Other rare paroxysmal abnormal movements

Tonic upgaze of infancy, torticollis of infancy, cataplexy, paroxysmal kinesogenic, and non-kinesogenic choreoathetosis.

Epilepsy and non-epileptic paroxysmal events

- When considering paroxysmal events and diagnosing epilepsy a meticulous history is required.
- Ample time needs to be spent in taking a careful history and eliciting a FHx. History taking needs to be aided by eye witness accounts, diaries, school accounts and where possible video footage even from a cell phone camera.
- Where unsure it is better not to make a diagnosis of epilepsy and keep an open mind than to hastily commit to a diagnosis and worse still treatment.

Five primary questions need to be answered when considering epilepsy as a diagnosis

1. Is it epilepsy?
- Exclude other paroxysmal non-epileptic phenomena.

2. What are the seizure types?
- Tonic, clonic, tonic–clonic, myocyclonic, atonic, absences, etc.

3. What is the cause of the epilepsy?
- E.g. idiopathic (genetic predisposition) or symptomatic (structural malformation, metabolic defect), etc.

4. What is the epilepsy syndrome?
- Based on the seizure types, age of onset, and EEG characteristics can we fit the child into a known epilepsy syndrome? This is not always possible.

5. Are there associated behavioural or cognitive difficulties?
- Are there any psychosocial factors that need addressing?

A suggested helpful approach

D—Describe the observed event in simple terms
E—Is it epilepsy based on the history?
S—Is there an epilepsy syndrome that fits the description?
C—What is the cause?
RIBE—Any Relevant Impairment of Behaviour or Educational abilities. These are often ignored but are probably the most relevant in terms of overall management of the child.

Epilepsy is by definition recurrent, stereotypic unprovoked seizures. When answering the first question one needs to consider the other *non-epileptic paroxysmal events* some of which are listed as follows.

Syncope
- Could be secondary to cardiac arrhythmias such as prolonged QT, breath holding, reflex asystolic syncope (RAS).
- Every child being investigated for epilepsy must have an ECG.
- RAS typically presents with episodes of pallor and loss of consciousness precipitated by a painful stimulus. ECG shows a brief asystole.

- Breath holding is a voluntary apnoea induced by holding one's breath against a closed glottis causing cyanosis. In both the secondary hypoxia can induce a seizure but it is not epileptic as it is not unprovoked.

Febrile seizures
- Occurs in 6 months to 6 years age group.
- Associated with fever but not necessarily high pyrexia.
- Developmentally normal child.
- FHx may be present.
- Frequency tails off beyond 2 years.
- If developmental concerns and increasing frequency of seizures followed by afebrile seizures and myoclonus consider severe myoclonic epilepsy of infancy (SMEI).

Gastro-oesophageal reflux (Sandifer syndrome)
Feed related (see 🕮 p83). Very painful dystonic posturing.

Shuddering attacks
Looks like shivering, usually in the context of excitement.

Sleep myoclonus
- Occurs at few weeks of age.
- Only in sleep.
- Synchronous or asynchronous limb jerks which may be quite violent and may occur in clusters.
- Does not involve the face and does not wake the child.
- Normal development

Self gratification
- Leg adduction and rubbing, flushed, vacant expression, irritable if disturbed.
- Common and self-limiting.

Behavioural stereotypes
Common in children with learning difficulty but sometimes in developmentally normal children.

Tics and mannerisms
Paroxysmal kinesogenic dyskinesias—precipitated by movement, several times a day, can take form of dystonia or choreoatheoid movements, treated with carbamazepine or phenytoin.

Cataplexy
- Can occur in isolation, as part of narcolepsy complex or in some storage disorders.
- Sudden loss of posture induced by surprise or laughter or loud noise.

Preoccupation (daydreaming)
Common especially where child is struggling at school.

Parasomnias
- Night terrors often confused with frontal lobe seizures.
- Frontal seizures are many/night at any time of sleep cycle and brief.
- Night terrors usually occur in the early part of sleep, are isolated events and quite long.

Benign myoclonus of infancy
- Normal EEG.
- Often difficult to distinguish from epileptic myoclonus.
- Normal development.

Hyperekplexia
- This is caused by a mutation in the gene encoding strychnine responsive glycine receptors.
- Can be dominantly inherited.
- Causes stiffness and exaggerated startle diagnosed by nose tapping to induce opisthotonic posture.
- Can be severe enough to cause cyanosis.
- Treated with benzodiazepines.

Non-epileptic attack disorder (pseudoseizures)
- Seizures are asynchronous limb jerks with pelvic thrusting movements with quick offset and no post-ictal phase.
- Can coexist with genuine epilepsy and may require video telemetry to untangle epileptic from non-epileptic events.

Early-onset epilepsies

Some common epilepsy syndromes are briefly covered here.

Benign neonatal convulsions (non-familial)
- Day 1–7.
- Focal clonic or subtle seizures.
- Ictal spikes or slow waves, interictal asynchronous theta rhythm.
- Treatment phenobarbitone/phenytoin.
- Excellent prognosis. Seizures remit when medication withdrawn.

Benign neonatal convulsions (familial)
- Autosomal dominant (ask grandparents a careful history).
- Can occur up to 3 months.
- Generalized clonic seizures, occasionally tonic with cyanosis.
- No specific EEG features.
- Treatment phenobarbitone/carbamazepine.
- Good prognosis—most stop seizing by 6–12 months.

Pyridoxine-dependent seizures
- Neonatal to 18 months (some may present with later onset intractable epilepsy).
- Very important to try pyridoxine in any intractable infantile epilepsy.
- Multifocal or generalized seizures/infantile spasms.
- Suppression burst or hypsarrhythmic EEG.
- Treatment with high dose pyridoxine 50–100mg.
- Urine analysis for alpha amino adipic semi-aldehyde (AASA) shows excess secretion.
- Recessive inheritance (antiquitin gene).

Early infantile epileptic encephalopathy (Ohtahara syndrome)
- 3–6 months of life.
- Tonic spasms.

- Suppression burst EEG.
- Brain malformations common, e.g. agenesis of corpus callosum.
- Intractable seizures.
- Poor prognosis—may evolve to West syndrome.

West syndrome
- 3–12 months (peak 3–7 months) as opposed to infantile colic which is very rare after 3 months of age.
- Infantile spasms in clusters at sleep–wake interface.
- Developmental plateau or regression (may occur before or after onset of spasms).
- Hypsarrhythmic EEG with attenuation following spasm (initially wake EEG may be normal, always ask for sleep EEG).
- Idiopathic (better outcome) or symptomatic, e.g. HIE, tuberous sclerosis (TS), DS.
- Treatment: vigabatrin for TS; steroids (ACTH or prednisolone) for other aetiology.
- Outcome better if spasms controlled quickly with normalization of EEG. Generally outcome is not good. About 70% will have learning difficulties (see 🕮 p117) and may evolve to Lennox–Gastaut syndrome.

Lennox–Gastaut syndrome
- 1–8 years.
- Tonic, atonic, myoclonic seizures, atypical absences.
- Slow spike waves in wake and fast spike bursts in sleep.
- Treatment valproate, lamotrigine.
- Poor prognosis for developmental outcome. Seizures initially intractable but improve with age.

Severe myoclonic epilepsy of infancy (Dravet syndrome)
- Febrile then afebrile hemiclonic or generalized seizures.
- Developmental plateau or regression.
- Myoclonus appears later.
- Spike-wave, polyspike waves on EEG, early photosensitivity.
- Seizures often intractable, ataxia develops with age, developmental outcome poor.
- Treatment: stiripentol, ketogenic diet.

Childhood absence epilepsy
- 3–12 years.
- Typical absences (can be induced by hyperventilating for 3min).
- 3Hz spike wave discharges on EEG.
- Treatment: ethosuximide, valproate.
- Seizures remit in 75%.
- May show subtle cognitive impairment especially if intractable.
- Consider GLUT-1 (glucose transporter defect) if intractable absences.
- Ketogenic diet may be useful.

Benign epilepsy of childhood with centrotemporal spikes (BCECT)
- 3–13 years.
- Focal or generalized motor seizures—orofacial muscles often involved.
- Centrotemporal spikes.

- Treatment none or carbamazepine.
- Outcome excellent with seizure remission by puberty.

Landau–Klefner syndrome (acquired epileptic aphasia)
- 2–10 years.
- Infrequent generalized tonic–clonic or focal clonic seizures (may precede or follow language regression in 60–80% cases).
- Language regression with normal hearing and audiometry.
- Multifocal spike waves in temporal or parieto-occipital regions. Continuous slow spike waves in slow sleep (CSWS).
- Treatment steroids.
- Outcome good for seizure control but not so good for language recovery.

Juvenile myoclonic epilepsy (JME)
- 10–18 years.
- Bilateral symmetrical myoclonus predominantly in arms; generalized tonic–clonic seizures, absences.
- Generalized spike or polyspike waves (>3Hz).
- Photosensitivity common.
- Treatment: valproate, lamotrigine.
- Needs treatment to continue into adult life. Good response to treatment.
- FHx of epilepsy common.

Progressive myoclonic epilepsies
- Generalized or fragmentary myoclonus, generalized seizures, atonic seizures.
- Associated cognitive decline, regression, ataxia.
- Conditions to consider include neuronal ceroid lipofuscinosis (NCL), lysosomal storage disorders like sialidosis, Gaucher disease and neuroaxonal dystrophy, mitochondrial disorders like MERRF (myoclonic epilepsy with ragged red fibres), Huntington disease, Wilson disease, neurodegeneration with brain iron accumulation including pantothenate kinase (PKAN).
- These need specialist opinions and extensive neurometabolic and physiological investigations.

Investigating epilepsies
- The investigation of epilepsies is determined by attempting to classify them into epilepsy syndromes. Doing so would give an idea as to whether they are idiopathic or symptomatic.
- Once they are thought to be symptomatic investigations can be directed accordingly. Progressive and degenerative epilepsies need extensive neurophysiological and neurometabolic investigations.
- First as an aid to classification of the epilepsies into syndromes an EEG is required. If a wake EEG is normal it is important to ask for a sleep EEG. This may be a natural sleep or sleep-deprived EEG or induced sleep with sedation or melatonin.

- If there is doubt about the paroxysmal events been described it is important to get more information. There are various methods that can be employed to get additional information such as:
  - More meticulous history taking.
  - Asking for description from carers, friends, school, etc.
  - Parental video recording with a cell phone camera, digital camera, or video camera.
  - Arranging an inpatient stay to observe and document seizures.
  - An ambulatory EEG recording over 48–72 hours. This can be complemented by parental records or video footage.
  - Video telemetry (simultaneous video and EEG recording).

It is not possible to have a standard set of investigations to fit all patients. Nevertheless some important investigations to consider include:
- Chromosome analysis: including fragile X (see 🕮 p403), ring chromosome 20.
- DNA analysis: where specific conditions need confirmation, e.g. *SCN1A* mutations in SMEI, *GLUT-1* mutations, etc.
- Neuroimaging: this should be a good quality MRI scan. Some centres can do thin sections and volume sequences (epilepsy protocol) especially where surgery is being considered.
- Specialized neurophysiology: this includes VEPs, video telemetry, ambulatory EEG recording, ictal SPECT scanning, MEG or fMRI scans for functional localization of ictal focus, intracranial grid mats. Most of these investigations are only available in centres that perform epilepsy surgery procedures.
- Metabolic investigations: including urine AASA (pyridoxine dependant seizures), CSF glucose paired with blood glucose (GLUT-1), biotinidase, lactate, copper, long chain fatty acids, white cell enzymes, etc.
- Other investigations, e.g. retinal examination, muscle biopsy, etc. may add further information.

Management of epilepsy

The mainstay of management is with AEDs. There is very little data on use of drugs specific to certain syndromes. NICE guidelines are available on choice of medication in seizure types (🕮 pp624–31).

AEDs (see 🕮 p624 and p629)
The following is only a suggested guide:
- Generalized seizures: valproate, lamotrigine, leviteracetam.
- Focal seizures: carbamazepine, topiramate, clobazam, lamotrigine.
- Myoclonic seizures: valproate, leviteracetam, clonazepam, topiramate, stiripentol (SMEI).
- Atonic seizures: valproate, topiramate, leviteracetam.
- Absences: ethosuximide, valproate.

It is not essential but prudent to check blood count and liver functions prior to starting AEDs. Routine blood tests subsequently are not recommended.

Drug levels are indicated only for toxicity or compliance monitoring.

Non-drug treatments
- Vagal nerve stimulation:
  - Implantable device which sends regular electrical stimuli to vagus nerve in the neck. Swiping a magnet over the device can deliver immediate impulse in acute situation.
  - Mechanism of action unknown.
- Ketogenic diet:
  - A high fat, low carbohydrate diet to induce ketosis.
  - Helpful in myoclonic epilepsies and intractable seizures.
- Epilepsy surgery:
  - Hemisherectomy, lesional and focal resections, corpus callosotomy, multiple subpial transection

Further resources

Epilepsy Action ☎ 0808 800 5050 🖰 http://www.epilepsy.org.uk
National Centre for Young People with Epilepsy (NCYPE) ☎ 01342 831342 🖰 http://www.ncype.org.uk
West Syndrome Support Group ☎ 01252 654 057
The Epilepsies: the diagnosis and management of the epilepsies in adults and children in primary and secondary care. Clinical Guidelines, CG 137. Jan 2012
Dietary Treatment for Epilepsy. 🖰 http://www.matthewsfriends.org

Chronic ataxia

- Acute to subacute ataxia result from:
  - Post-infectious cerebellitis (particularly 7–14 days post varicella).
  - Acute disseminated encephalomyelitis (ADEM).
  - Toxins.
  - Posterior fossa tumours.
  - Pseudo ataxia from weakness in Guillain–Barré syndrome.
  - Posterior circulation vascular events etc.
- Chronic ataxia may be:
  - Cerebellar.
  - Spinocerebellar.
  - Neuropathic.
  - Mixed.

Some causes of chronic ataxia are:

Opsoclonus–myoclonus syndrome

- Presumed parainfectious or paraneoplastic (neuroblastoma) condition.
- Often presents with altered behaviour and irritability, rapid chaotic synchronous eye movements in all directions of gaze (opsoclonus), and later myoclonus. Ataxia can be an important early component.
- Treatment is with steroids and intravenous immunoglobulin. Steroid sparing and other immunomodulating agents may be required.

Mitochondrial cytopathy

- Ataxia is just one component of the myriad symptoms that result from mitochondrial mutations.
- Retinopathy may accompany especially in the condition NARP (neuropathy, ataxia, retinitis pigmentosa with the typical 8993 mitochondrial DNA mutation).

Metabolic and degenerative disorders

Several metabolic disorders present with chronic ataxias. Some examples are:

- HARP (hypobetalipoproteinemia, ataxia, retinitis pigmentosa).
- Hartnup disease.
- Maple syrup urine disease.
- Pyruvate dehydrogenase deficiency.
- Vitamin E deficiency.
- Refsum disease.
- Adrenoleucodystrophy.
- GM2 gangliosidoses (hexosaminidase deficiency).

Genetic ataxias

Some examples are:

Episodic ataxia type 1

- Results from a potassium channelopathy (KCN1A mutation).
- Attacks begin at 5–7 years of age.
- Sensation of spreading weakness and stiffness accompanies the ataxia which lasts for about 10min but can last a few hours.

- Myokimia is seen and an EMG shows continuous spontaneous activity at rest.
- Treatment is with phenytoin or carbamazepine.

Episodic ataxia type 2

- Is a calcium channelopathy and has its onset in school aged children with accompanying vertigo and vomiting as well as a migraine.
- Attacks last from 1 hour to 1 day.
- Treatment is with acetazolamide or flunarizine.

Spinocerebellar ataxias (SCA)

- There are an ever increasing number of progressive dominantly inherited ataxias (SCA 1, 2, 3, 6, and 7 have onset in childhood as also dentatorubral-pallidolysian atrophy, DRPLA).
- They show a mixture of pyramidal, extrapyramidal, and cerebellar features as well as sensory neuropathies.
- The genetic defect is often a trinucleotide repeat.
- Diagnosis is largely based on DNA testing and no specific treatments are available.

Ataxia telangiectasia (AT)

- Several mutations in the AT gene have been identified in this recessive disorder.
- It causes a progressive ataxia, telangiectasiae in skin and conjunctivae and immune dysfunction causing frequent sino-pulmonary infections.
- Alphafetoprotein is elevated. Immunoglobulin (Ig) A and IgE are often significantly reduced.
- It is often life limiting because of infections and increased risk of lymphoma and leukaemia.

Ataxia and oculomotor apraxia

- Ataxia precedes the characteristic feature of oculomotor apraxia. Eventually a motor neuropathy develops.
- Also recessively inherited.

Friedrich ataxia

- Most common recessively inherited ataxia. Triplet repeats of frataxin gene.
- Onset between 2–16 years.
- Associated features include scoliosis, dysarthria, diabetes mellitus, and a hypertrophic cardiomyopathy.
- Typically tendon reflexes are absent.
- Genetic treatment trials are in progress and the drug idebenone has shown some encouraging results.

Investigations

- Are based on the clinical picture.
- DNA analysis is the mainstay in genetic ataxias.
- Metabolic investigations should include:
  - Vitamin E levels.
  - Alphafetoprotein.
  - Immunoglobulins.

- Cholesterol and triglycerides.
- Transferrins.
- Phytanic acid.
- White cell enzymes.
- Plasma amino acids.
- Urine organic acids.
- Carnitine profile.
- Lactate (blood and CSF).
- Bone marrow.
- Nerve conduction studies and EMG.
- Eye examination.

Further resource

Ataxia UK: ☎ 0845 644 0606 🖰 http://www.ataxia.org.uk

Neurocutaneous disorders

- The skin and nervous system have common embryonic origins.
- Skin malformations and markers are a useful clue in the diagnosis of neurocutaneous malformation sequences.

Well-recognized neurocutaneous syndromes include:

Neurofibromatosis type 1

- Both syndromes are dominantly inherited.
- Incidence is about 1:4000 live births.
- >50% are new mutations. Incidence1:3000 live births.
- NF1 gene lies on chromosome 17q.
- It is a progressive condition with onset in infancy.
- Cutaneous features increase through the first decade of life.

Clinical criteria for diagnosis are at least 2 of the following:

- 6 or more café au lait spots (>5mm pre-pubertal/>15mm post-pubertal).
- >2 neurofibromas or 1 plexiform neurofibroma.
- Axillary or inguinal freckling.
- Optic gliomas.
- >2 iris hamartomas.
- Characteristic bone lesions such as sphenoid wing dysplasia or bone cortex thinning with or without pseudoarthrosis.
- 1st-degree relative with NF1 diagnosed by the above listed criteria.

Minor features:

- Include microcephaly, short stature, learning difficulties in 60% of cases, epilepsy, hypertension resulting from aortic coarctation, renal artery stenosis, or phaeochromocytoma. Scoliosis is present in 10–40% of cases. Optic gliomas occur in 20% of cases.
- Other neoplasms associated are brainstem gliomas, malignant transformation of neurofibromas, ependymomas, meningiomas, and medulloblastomas. There is an increased risk of Wilms tumour, rhabdomyosarcomas, medullary thyroid carcinoma, melanomas, leukaemia, and phaeochromocytoma.

Principles of management include:

- Monitoring growth
- Monitoring blood pressure
- Monitoring visual fields and/or serial visual evoked potentials
- Treating hydrocephalus and spinal lesions causing cord compression

Neurofibromatosis type 2

- The gene for NF2 lies on chromosome 22.
- Is less common with an incidence of 1:40,000 live births.
- It is also dominantly inherited and a progressive condition.

Diagnostic criteria
- Bilateral vestibular schwannomas (90% cases).
- A 1st-degree relative with NF2 and either of the following in the index case:
  - Unilateral vestibular schwannoma or
  - 2 of the following: neurofibroma, meningioma, glioma, schwannomas or juvenile posterior subcapsular cataract (60% of children).

Or
- 2 of the following criteria:
  - Multiple meningiomas.
  - Unilateral vestibular schwannoma.
  - Neurofibroma, gliomas, schwannomas, cerebral calcification or juvenile posterior subcapsular cataract.
- Schwannomas are slowly progressive and may need surgical resection.
- Genetic counselling for family members is important in both conditions.

Tuberous sclerosis
- Incidence 1:20,000 live births.
- Dominantly inherited.
- Genes responsible for the syndrome are *TSC1* (chromosome 9q) and *TSC2* (chromosome 16p).
- 2/3 of cases are *de novo* mutations.
- The usual presentation is with infantile spasms.
- Skin associations are ash leaf macules (may need Wood's lamp examination to detect), shagreen patch, periungual fibromas, and adenoma sebaceum.
- TS results in multiple hamartomas (tubers) in the brain. Subependymal giant cell astrocytomas (SEGA) occur at the foramina of Munro and may cause obstructive hydrocephalus typically in or beyond the 2nd decade of life.
- Seizures are very difficult to control and cause severe learning difficulties (see 📖 p117). If a prominent tuber is the focus of most of the abnormal electrical activity removal of this area may be considered in intractable cases.
- Other associations are retinal phakomas, renal angiomyolipomas or hamartomas, cysts of the kidneys, bones, and lung, cardiac rhabdomyomas.
- Children usually have severe learning difficulties and autism (see 📖 p107).
- Other than seizure management it is important to monitor renal function, vision, and BP.

Sturge–Weber syndrome
- An association of a ipsilateral port wine stain in the first division of the trigeminal nerve dermatomal distribution and leptomeningeal angiomatous malformation causing focal epilepsy, progressive hemiatrophy of the brain, and contralateral hemiparesis.
- It is important to bear in mind that only about 15% children with port wine stain will have Sturge–Weber syndrome.
- Other associations are learning difficulties (90% cases), glaucoma (30% cases), and homonymous hemianopia.

- Seizures (see 📖 p240) may be difficult to control. Intractable seizures may warrant a hemispherectomy.
- Low-dose aspirin prophylaxis aiming to reduce stroke like episodes is recommended by some.
- Laser therapy is used to treat the cutaneous angioma.
- Regular ophthalmology follow-up for glaucoma is needed.

Ataxia telangiectasia
- Rare disorder with incidence of 1:40000.
- Autosomal recessive inheritance or *de novo* mutation in gene on Chromosome 11q.
- Clinical features consist of:
  - Slowly progressive cerebellar ataxia, dystonia, and dysarthria.
  - Nystagmus and oculomotor apraxia.
  - Telangiectasia of skin and conjunctiva.
  - Increased susceptibility to bronchopulmonary infections (70% cases) due to IgA and IgE deficiency.
  - Absence of lymphoid tissue—tonsils, adenoids, thymus.
  - Raised alphafetoprotein (AFP) and carcinoembryonic antigen (CEA).
  - Chromosome fragility which can be tested for.
  - Diabetes.
  - Short stature and progeric changes.
- There is increased risk of leukaemia, lymphoma, and skin malignancy.
- Heterozygotes also have increased risk of malignancy especially breast cancer.

Other neurocutaneous syndromes
Mainly present with seizures and learning difficulty, e.g.
- Epidermal naevus syndrome.
- Cutis marmorata telangiectatica.
- Hypomelanosis of Ito.

Further resources
Ataxia UK: ☎ 0845 644 0606 🖱 http://www.ataxia.org.uk
Sturge–Weber Foundation: ☎ 01392 464675 🖱 http://www.sturgeweber.org.uk
The Neurofibromatosis Association: ☎ 0845 602 4173 🖱 http://www.nfauk.org
Tuberous Sclerosis Association UK: ☎ 05602 420809 🖱 http://www.tuberous-sclerosis.org

Neurodegenerative disorders

This is a rare group of conditions resulting in progressive loss of skills (progressive intellectual and neurological deterioration). Initial development may be normal but as the disorder progresses there is evidence of global brain dysfunction.

The list is exhaustive but the most common conditions are:

Mucopolysaccharidoses (type 3 Sanfilippo in particular)

- Initial developmental delay, then a hyperactive, aggressive behaviour (see 📖 p369) change with insomnia (see 📖 p168).
- By 10–15 years rapid degeneration resulting in death by 15–25 years.
- Associated deafness (see 📖 p296) and diarrhoea.
- Diagnosed by excess urinary heparan sulphate excretion and white cell enzymes.

Adrenoleucodystrophy

- X-linked peroxisomal disorder.
- Presents 4–10 years with significant behavioural change—aggression, hyperactivity, irritability.
- There is a rapid cognitive decline with deafness, optic atrophy (see 📖 p275), and seizures (see 📖 p240).
- There may be adrenal failure in the late stages. Within 2–4 years the child becomes decerebrate.
- Biochemical testing shows elevated long-chain fatty acids.
- Bone marrow transplant may be beneficial in selected cases.

Metachromatic leucodystrophy

- Presents at about 18 months with regression, flaccid paralysis and absent reflexes, with decerebrate posturing and optic atrophy within 3–6 months and death by 8–10 years.
- MRI shows a tigroid appearance of the white matter.
- Urine exam shows the typical metachromatic granules and nerve conductions show a neuropathy.
- White cell enzymes confirm diagnosis.
- There is no treatment available.

Neuronal ceroid lipofuscinosis

- Late infantile variety caused by mutation of gene *CLN2* is the commonest.
- Presents with seizures at 2–4 years.
- Progressive myoclonic epilepsy results and causes ataxia (see 📖 p247), eventually blindness and death within 3–10 years.
- VEPs are abnormally enlarged in the face of an extinguished ERG.
- Inclusion bodies may be seen on skin and conjunctival biopsy.

Alper's disease

- Mitochondrial disorder presenting with hypotonia, developmental delay (see 📖 p36), failure to thrive, seizures and hepatic dysfunction.
- Status epilepticus and hepatic failure results in death.
- Valproate should never be used to treat the seizures.
- Mutations have been identified in POLG (polymerase gamma) needed for mitochondrial replication.
- VEPs are abnormal with normal ERGs.

Infantile neuroaxonal dystrophy

- Recessive disorder due to mutation in *PLA2G6*.
- Presents in infancy with hypotonia and areflexia.
- Eventually spasticity, opisthotonus and optic atrophy ensues with death by 5 years.
- MRI shows cerebellar atrophy. EMG shows denervation with normal nerve conduction.

Juvenile Huntington disease

- Dominantly inherited.
- Triplet repeat disorder showing anticipation.
- Rigidity, dystonia, myoclonic seizures develop. Adults present more with tremor, chorea, and dementia.
- MRI may show caudate atrophy.

Wilson disease

- Recessively inherited disorder of copper transport resulting in deposition of copper in brain, liver, and cornea.
- Presents with liver dysfunction in the younger child but extrapyramidal features in the older child.
- Slit lamp exam shows a Kayser–Fleischer ring.
- Chelation with penicillamine or zinc slows disease progression.
- Low plasma caeruloplasmin and low serum copper is seen and MRI shows low signal in lentiform nuclei and brainstem.

Neurodegeneration with brain iron accumulation

- Most cases result from *PANK2* gene mutation resulting in pantothenate kinase associated neurodegeneration (PKAN).
- Presents in first two decades of life with progressive dystonia, rigidity and choreoathetosis with cognitive decline.
- Retinitis pigmentosa and optic atrophy may be seen.
- MRI shows characteristic 'eye of the tiger' appearance.

Subacute sclerosing panencephalitis

- Late presentation due to measles virus reactivation in nervous tissue.
- Increasing incidence due to drop in measles vaccine uptake.
- Presents between 5–15 years with gradual deterioration in behaviour and school performance and myoclonus, tremor and seizures eventually appearing.
- A retinopathy is associated and EEG shows suppression burst pattern. There is rapid motor and cognitive deterioration leading to a coma and death.

Other neurodegenerative conditions

- Rett syndrome (see 📖 p405).
- Krabbe leucodystrophy.
- Vanishing white matter disease.
- HIV encephalopathy.
- Lafora body disease.
- Unverricht–Lundborg disease.
- Pelizaeus–Merzbacher disease.
- Niemann–Pick disease type C.
- Gaucher disease.
- Variant Creutzfeldt–Jacob disease (vCJD).

Stroke

- A focal neurological deficit lasting >24 hours due to a vascular event.
- A transient ischaemic attack lasts <24 hours.
- A stroke like event is a stroke of non-vascular aetiology.
- Stroke in children presents as an acute onset of focal neurological deficit.
- Associated symptoms are visual deficits, seizures particularly in neonatal strokes, headaches, and neck pain particularly where arterial dissection is aetiology.
- Fever, preceding neck trauma, pre-existing cardiac disease, sickle cell disease, and FHx of strokes or stroke like episodes should be sought.

Causes
- Arterial.
- Venous.
- Haemorrhagic.

Arterial stroke
May result from:

Embolic event
- Paradoxical embolus from the heart in a child with congenital heart disease (right-to-left shunt) or proximal vessels.
- An arterial dissection following a trivial trauma can cause a thrombus to form which later embolizes.

Thrombotic event
These are rare in children but include prothrombotic deficiencies such as:
- Protein C.
- Protein S.
- Antithrombin 3 deficiency.
- Mutations in methyltetrahydrofolate gene (*MTHFR*).
- Factor V Leiden.

Vasculopathy
- This is seen in small vessels in post-varicella vasculopathy and large vessels in Moya Moya syndrome, fibromuscular dysplasia, Lyme disease, Mycoplasma arteritis.
- In Moya Moya collateral circulation develops due to large vessel occlusion.
- It is also seen in neurofibromatosis (see p250), DS (see p387), and sickle cell disease.

Venous infarction
Polycythaemia
True or as a result of dehydration especially in newborn babies, congenital heart disease, sickle cell disease, etc.

Venous sinus thrombosis
- From infection or hypercoagulable state—in particular homocysteinuria needs to be considered.
- It may be precipitated by oral contraceptive use.

Haemorrhagic stroke
- Cerebral aneurysm rupture: catastrophic with headache, seizures and altered conscious level.
- Arteriovenous malformation
- Cavernomas: dominantly inherited, usually causes slow bleeds and seizures

Investigations
For a stroke include:
- Thrombophilia screen.
- Plasma homocysteine.
- Transthoracic echocardiogram.
- Carotid Dopplers.
- MRI and MR angiogram.
- Vitamin B12 and folate levels.
- Viral serology.
- Lactate, lipid profile, autoantibody screen, ESR.

Acute management
- Maintain airway, breathing, and circulation.
- Adequate oxygenation and hydration.
- Monitoring BP.
- Treatment of seizures.
- Neurosurgical intervention—evacuation of haematoma , intracranial pressure monitoring and craniectomy in the event of raised intracranial pressure.
- Thrombolysis: heparinization followed by warfarin should be considered where there is an underlying congenital heart defect, procoagulant defect or a definite arterial dissection and in sinovenous thrombosis.
- Treatment dose of aspirin is followed by low-dose aspirin for secondary prevention.

Neuromuscular disorders

These present with:
- Hypotonia (most children with hypotonia without weakness have a central cause for the hypotonia (see 📖 p233)).
- Weakness.
- Delayed motor milestones (see 📖 p44).
- Rarely with learning difficulties (see 📖 p117) and seizures (Xp21 muscular dystrophy and congenital muscular dystrophy).
- Absent, deep tendon reflexes.
- Cardiomyopathy.
- Respiratory failure and recurrent chest infections (see 📖 p91).

An anatomical approach to neuromuscular disorders is helpful in achieving a diagnosis.
- Anterior horn cell: SMA types 1, 2, and 3.
- Peripheral neuropathies: inherited (CMT) and acquired.
- Neuromuscular transmission defects: congenital and autoimmune myasthenia.
- Muscle disease:
  - Congenital myopathies.
  - Muscular dystrophies: Xp21, congenital muscular dystrophies, limb girdle, facioscapulohumeral, Emery–Dreifuss syndrome, etc.
  - Congenital myotonic dystrophy.
  - Myotonia congenita.
- Connective tissue disorders: Ehlers–Danlos syndrome, collagen related myopathy (Bethlem and Ullrich myopathies).
- Metabolic myopathies: acid maltase deficiency, muscle phosphorylase deficiency, mitochondrial myopathy.
- Inflammatory myopathies: dermatomyositis.

Congenital hypothyroidism can cause a severe myopathy with raised CK levels and must always be excluded

Salient features of the common neuromuscular problems

Xp21 muscular dystrophies
- X linked recessive inheritance.
- About 30% *de novo* mutations.
- Present with delayed motor milestones, raised CK levels in thousands (Becker) and tens of thousands (Duchenne), calf hypertrophy, sometimes calf pain and cramps.
- Progressive weakness causes loss of independent ambulation by about 13 years in Duchenne muscular dystrophy.
- Diagnosis is by raised CK, DNA analysis identifying a deletion, duplication or point mutation in the DMD gene and muscle biopsy showing absence of dystrophin staining.
- Learning difficulties are associated in a significant proportion with autistic spectrum features (see 📖 p107) in some.
- Cardiomyopathy and respiratory failure are late complications as are scoliosis and contractures of tendons.

Congenital myotonic dystrophy

- Autosomal dominant inheritance.
- Trinucleotide CTG repeat. Severity depends on length of repeats.
- Anticipation down generations.
- Polyhydramnios, reduced fetal movements, profound weakness and hypotonia at birth often requiring ventilatory assistance, congenital talipes and arthrogryposis are important features.
- Maternal grip myotonia and expressionless facies may offer diagnostic clues.
- Moderate to severe learning difficulties (see 📖 p117) accompany and late complications include cataracts, cardiac rhythm disturbances, and chest infections.
- Diagnosis is by DNA analysis of mutations in *DM1* gene.

Spinal muscular atrophy

- Autosomal recessive disorder due to deletion of exons 7 and 8 of the *SMN* gene.
- Classified clinically into:
  - Type 1 (never able to sit independently).
  - Type 2 (never able to stand independently).
  - Type 3 (achieve independent ambulation but get progressively weaker).
- Life expectancy in type 1 is less than 2 years.
- Recurrent chest infections (see 📖 p91) and respiratory failure are main causes of morbidity and mortality.
- Clinical features include profound weakness, absent deep tendon reflexes, and tongue fasciculation with intercostal weakness.
- Extreme weakness and hypotonia in type 1 is evident in the form of a frog leg posture of the legs and a jug handle posture of the arms with intercostal recession.
- Variants of SMA are SMA with respiratory distress (due to mutation in *SMARD1* gene) where there is predominant diaphragm weakness and paradoxical breathing and SMA with pontocerebellar hypoplasia. EMG shows denervation.

Congenital myopathies

- Various types such as core myopathy, nemaline myopathy, myotubular myopathy, etc.
- Common clinical features are arthrogryposis at birth, myopathic facies (marked facial weakness), sometimes ophthalmoplegia, feeding difficulties (see 📖 p81 and p88), recurrent chest infections, early onset of scoliosis (see 📖 p416), joint contractures, hypotonia and weakness which is relatively non-progressive or slowly progressive.
- Diagnosis largely rests on muscle biopsy and immunohistochemistry and genetic confirmation by DNA analysis for specific mutations.
- Muscle MRI showing patterns of differential muscle group involvement may add a piece to the diagnostic jigsaw.
- EMG reveals myopathic features with reduced amplitude of compound motor action potential (CMAP)

Congenital muscular dystrophies

- Inherited muscle diseases with or without CNS involvement and eye involvement in varying degree.
- Present with hypotonia and weakness as well as contractures at birth. Weakness is progressive although not very rapid.
- CK may be elevated.
- Learning difficulties, seizures (see 📖 p240) and visual impairment (see 📖 p275) may be associated particularly in those due to glycosyltransferase mutations.
- Diagnosis is based on muscle biopsy showing dystrophic features, neuroimaging abnormalities such as white matter abnormalities, structural brain defects and cerebellar cysts, confirmed by identifying mutations in genes responsible (*FKRP, POMT1, POMGnT1, Fukutin, LARGE*, etc.).

Congenital peripheral neuropathies (Chariot–Marie–Tooth)

- These are inherited neuropathies all genetically labelled as CMTs.
- Most common form is Type 1A (autosomal dominant).
- This presents with delayed motor development (see 📖 p44), foot drop, weakness of ankle eversion and dorsiflexion, absent deep tendon reflexes, distal leg weakness and wasting, clawing of feet and hammer toes as well as pes cavus foot deformity.
- Later there is weakness of hand muscles. It is slowly progressive.
- Diagnosis is by nerve conduction studies showing a demyelinating neuropathy and confirmed by DNA analysis showing duplication in *PMP22* gene.

Investigations of neuromuscular disorders

- EMG and nerve conduction studies.
- Repetitive nerve stimulation and single fibre EMG (myasthenia).
- Raised CK (muscular dystrophies) and lactate (mitochondrial myopathies).
- Tensilon test (myasthenia—rarely performed).
- Muscle biopsy.
- Muscle MRI scan.
- Brain MRI scan (congenital muscular dystrophy).
- DNA analysis (SMA, myotonic dystrophy, CMT, Xp21 muscular dystrophies).

Management

This is largely supportive. Three main areas of management are:

Managing orthopaedic complications

- Tendon release and lengthening for contractures (see 📖 p433).
- Use of orthotic appliances (see 📖 p220).
- Scoliosis (see 📖 p416) managed by using body braces and spinal jackets and eventually insertion of metal rods to stabilize the spine.

Managing respiratory complications

- Advocating immunisation including seasonal influenza vaccination (see 📖 p620).
- Low-dose prophylactic antibiotics during winter months.

- Aggressively managing respiratory infections with a low threshold for using antibiotics, chest physiotherapy (see 🕮 p176), and use of assisted cough devices and non-invasive ventilation.
- Regular lung function monitoring is important as well as seeking early symptoms of hypoventilation (headaches, nausea, need for turning or propping in bed).

Managing cardiac complications
- Prophylactic use of beta blockers and ACE inhibitors can prevent development of cardiomyopathy.
- Regular monitoring of cardiac function is very important as well as monitoring for cardiac rhythm disturbances.

Further resources
Duchenne Family Support Group: ☎ 0800 121 4518 🖱 http://www.dfsg.org.uk
Jennifer Trust for Spinal Muscular Atrophy: ☎ 0800 975 3100 🖱 http://www.jtsma.org.uk
Muscular Dystrophy Campaign: ☎ 0800 652 6352 🖱 http://www.muscular-dystrophy.org
Myasthenia Gravis Association: ☎ 0800 919 922 🖱 http://www.mga-charity.org
Myotonic Dystrophy Support Group: ☎ 0115 987 0080 🖱 http://www.myotonicdystrophysup-
   portgroup.org

Spina bifida (neural tube defects)

- Developmental spinal disorder in which contents of vertebral canal prolapse through a defect in the vertebrae.
- This can take various forms depending on which part of the neuraxis is involved such as:
  - Meningocoele (meninges only).
  - Myelomeningocoele (spinal cord and meninges).
  - Lipomyelomeningocoele (intra/extra dural fat, meninges, and spinal cord).
- This is often associated with other developmental anomalies such as lipomas, dermoid cysts, neurenteric cysts, diastematomyelia (cord split by bony or fibrocartilaginous spur).
- There are other anatomical anomalies like a low lying spinal cord or a tethered spinal cord, a syrinx or low placed cerebellar tonsils (Chiari malformation).
- Hydrocephalus is seen in 80% of children with myelomeningocoele.

Aetiology

Is varied and often complex.

Genetic factors

- Such as folate-dependent metabolic pathway gene defects, e.g. methyl tetrahydrofolate reductase deficiency.
- Syndromes such as 22q microdeletion.

Environmental factors

- Nutritional folic acid deficiency, AEDs, maternal diabetes, etc. all play a role.
- Incidence of neural tube defects is about 6 per 10,000 live births with a larger proportion being fetal losses.
- There is about a 5% recurrence risk of non-syndromic neural tube defects in siblings of affected cases which significantly reduces with pre-conceptional folate supplementation.
- Antenatal diagnosis is by anomaly scanning at about 20 weeks' gestation showing ventriculomegaly and vertebral arch defects, fetal MRI scans, and raised maternal serum alphafetoprotein levels.

Management

(Also see 📖 p426)
Is symptomatic and multisytemic.

- At birth the defect is assessed as to whether there is skin cover. This determines time of repair with open defects needing to be closed earlier.
  - Open defects: a mixed upper and lower motor neuron picture is seen on examination. Bladder and bowel involvement (see 📖 p162) needs urologic input and investigations. There is often associated scoliosis (see 📖 p416) and talipes (see 📖 p422).
  - Occult defects: are often heralded by skin pigmentation, dermal sinuses, or hair over the spine.

- An MRI scan determines the anatomical level of the lesion. The neurological level is often higher than the anatomical level and is a prognostic indicator of future disability.
- It is important to assess antigravity movement, spinal reflexes, and sacral sensations as well as sphincter tone.
- Associated Chiari malformations (see 📖 p263), syrinx, and hydrocephalus (see 📖 p264) need attention.
- Syndromes such as VACTERL (vertebral, anal, cardiac, tracheal, (o) esophageal, renal, limb anomalies) associations warrant investigations to look for other system involvement.
- Mild to moderate learning difficulties (see 📖 p117) often exist and need addressing.
- Talipes and scoliosis need orthopaedic intervention and monitoring or surgical correction (see 📖 p422 and p436).
- Neurogenic constipation (see 📖 p84) often exists and needs appropriate treatment. Bladder dysfunction (see 📖 p162) is usual and results in incomplete emptying against sphincter resistance leading to vesico-ureteric reflux and nephropathy.
- Other associated problems to monitor:
  - Development of hydrocephalus and ventriculo-peritoneal shunting (see 📖 p264).
  - Detethering of the spinal cord.
  - Addressing psychosocial issues (see 📖 p373).
  - Monitoring growth.
  - Development and nutrition (see 📖 p86 and p87).

Prognosis

- The neurological level of lesion is the main predictor of future needs.
- Ankle dorsiflexion predicts walking outdoors and independent transfers. Presence of knee extension predicts household ambulation and standing for transfers. Presence of trunk stability and hip flexion predicts non functional ambulation and wheelchair use (see 📖 p186).
- There is usually no overt LD.
- Hydrocephalus, shunt infections, renal failure and surgical interventions determine mortality and morbidity.

Further resources

ASBAH (Association for Spina Bifida and Hydrocephalus): ☎ 0845 450 7755 🖰 http://www.asbah. org

Colostomy Association: ☎ 0800 328 4257 🖰 http://www.colostomyassociation.org.uk

ERIC (Education & Resources for Improving Childhood Continence): ☎ 0845 370 8008 🖰 http://www.eric.org.uk

IA® (The ileostomy & internal pouch support group): ☎ 0800 0184 724 🖰 http://www.the-ia. org.uk

The Bladder and Bowel Foundation: ☎ 0845 345 0165 🖰 http://www.bladderandbowelfoundation.org

Chiari malformation

- A downward displacement of posterior fossa contents through the foramen magnum.
- There are different types of Chiari malformation based on degree of involvement of the posterior fossa structures.

Chiari I malformation

- Is where cerebellar tonsils descend below the foramen magnum.
- There may be a secondary syrinx in the spinal cord.
- A large displacement is often symptomatic with occipital headaches (worsened by cough, straining, or bending down), cerebellar signs, limb paraesthesiae, and reduced pain sensation due to the syrinx.
- These need a decompression of the foramen magnum.

Chiari II malformation

- Is when there is additional malformation of the pons and the pons and 4th ventricle are abnormally low.
- This is often associated with spina bifida.

Chiari III malformation

- Is where there is herniation of posterior fossa contents through a posterior meningocoele.

Hydrocephalus

- Increased volume of CSF spaces in the brain eventually causing raised intracranial pressure.
- This may be non-communicating or communicating.
- Incidence is 5–8 per 10000 births.

Obstructive hydrocephalus

Can be due to various causes such as:

- Aqueduct stenosis: genetic (X-linked L1CAM), acquired from intrauterine infections.
- Dandy–Walker malformation: cystic dilatation of 4th ventricle with vermis hypoplasia.
- Tumours and cysts, e.g. medulloblastomas, giant cell astrocytomas, colloid cyst of 3rd ventricle, ependymomas.
- Vascular malformations: arteriovenous malformations, aneurysm of vein of Galen.
- Intraventricular haemorrhage: premature babies with grade 3 and 4 intraventricular haemorrhage develop progressive ventricular dilatation.

Communicating hydrocephalus

- Post infectious, e.g. meningitis.
- Post haemorrhagic, e.g. intraventricular haemorrhage, post-traumatic, subdural and subarachnoid haemorrhage.
- Venous sinus thrombosis.
- Craniosynostosis and achondroplasia.
- Neural tube defects, e.g. myelomeningocoele, encephalocoele, and Chiari malformations.
- Other conditions associated with hydrocephalus are: DS (see 📖 p387), myotonic dystrophy, NF1 (see 📖 p250), Hurler syndrome, agenesis of corpus callosum, septo-optic dysplasia, etc.

Symptoms and signs of hydrocephalus

- Increasing head circumference crossing centile lines.
- Bulging anterior fontanelle.
- Headache, vomiting, increased drowsiness, sun setting eyes, prominent scalp veins.
- Papilloedema is a late and unreliable sign.
- Irritability and poor feeding.
- Visual disturbance.

Investigations

- Congenital hydrocephalus can be diagnosed antenatally by ultrasound scan or fetal MRI scan.
- Ultrasound scan if fontanelle is open.
- CT scan.
- MRI scan.

Treatment
- In neonates: diuretics, serial ventricular taps and lumbar puncture.
- Shunt: ventriculoperitoneal (mostly), ventriculoatrial , ventriculopleural and lumbo peritoneal shunts (rarely).
- Endoscopic 3rd ventriculostomy: for obstructive hydrocephalus mainly due to aqueduct stenosis.

Shunt complications

Infection
- 10% overall incidence of infection.
- Presents with fever, drowsiness, irritability, vomiting.
- Infection screen and shunt tap by neurosurgical team often required for diagnosis.
- Requires long courses up to 6 weeks of intrathecal and intravenous antibiotics.
- Externalization of shunt for the duration of antibiotic therapy followed by shunt replacement is often required.

Shunt block or disconnection
- 60–80% of shunts inserted in infancy require revision within 10 years.
- Symptoms are similar to infections but are less acute.
- They include lethargy, headache, visual disturbance, behaviour change, intermittent vomiting, and occasionally seizures

Over drainage
- Symptoms are lethargy, headache initially worse on sitting up and improved by lying down.
- CT or MRI will show slit ventricles and tonsillar descent.
- Intracranial pressure monitoring is required for diagnosis.
- Treatment is by inserting shunts with programmable high resistance valves.

Associated problems
- Learning difficulty (see 📖 p117).
- Fine motor impairment and tremor (see 📖 p136).
- Epilepsy (see 📖 p240).
- Visual impairment (see 📖 p275).
- Shunt migration, colonic perforation, peritonitis.
- Endocrine disturbances—precocious puberty.

Further resource
ASBAH (Association for Spina Bifida and Hydrocephalus): 📞 0845 450 7755 🖥 http://www.asbah.org

Benign intracranial hypertension

- This causes raised intracranial pressure in the absence of any space-occupying lesion.
- Symptoms and signs are headache, papilloedema, vomiting and VIth nerve palsy.
- Normal imaging is mandatory before a lumbar puncture is performed.
- A lumbar puncture reveals opening pressure of >30cm of water.
- There is an association with obesity and recent weight gain. Other associations for which a history should be sought is use of oral contraceptives, tetracyclines, retinoids, steroids, vitamin D and A.
- Treatment is by serial lumbar puncture to reduce closing pressure to <16cm.
- Diuretics such as acetazolamide or furosemide are often used.
- Lumbo-peritoneal and ventriculo-peritoneal shunting as well as optic nerve sheath fenestration may be needed.
- Visual fields and function need close monitoring (see 📖 p271).

Acquired brain injury

Aetiology
- Trauma, e.g. road traffic accidents, non-accidental head injury.
- Infections, e.g. meningitis and encephalitis.
- Neoplastic, e.g. leukaemia and brain tumours.
- Inflammatory and demyelinating, e.g. multiple sclerosis.
- Degenerative, e.g. metabolic and genetic conditions such as Parkinsonism, brain iron deposition, leucodystrophies.
- Vascular, e.g. strokes from thrombosis or haemorrhage.

Management
Depends upon underlying aetiology. Principles of acute management are:
- Neurosurgical intervention to relieve compression. This may involve drainage of collections of blood or pus or craniotomies.
- Fluid and electrolyte management
- Maintenance of normal oxygenation and BP are critical.
- Cerebral oedema needs treating with mannitol or steroids and intracranial pressure monitoring is important.
- Aggression (see 🕮 p334 and p369) and confusion is often seen in the phase of recovery from coma. Effects of sedative drugs and their withdrawal may play a part. Drugs such as risperidone and methylphenidate may be helpful.
- A multidisciplinary team of PTs, OTs, dieticians, and SLTs is needed to deal with associated problems of spasticity (see 🕮 p431), contractures, mobilization (see 🕮 p186 and p225), and feeding (see 🕮 p88).
- Aggressive treatment of seizures (see 🕮 p240) is very important and will affect long-term outcomes.
- Longer-term management includes graded rehabilitation into 'normal' life.
- Neuropsychology assessments (see 🕮 p215) are important to determine level of function especially before re-integration into school life and curriculum.
- Even in the face of minimal brain trauma, behavioural, emotional, and attentional problems (see 🕮 p126) can impair function significantly and need to be actively looked for.
- Post-traumatic epilepsy and headaches (see 🕮 p235) can appear months or years later. Psychosocial issues often surface and need psychology or psychiatric intervention (see 🕮 p373).

Acquired spinal cord injury

Aetiology
- Trauma.
- Inflammatory and demyelinating conditions, e.g. transverse myelitis, abscess.
- Vascular, e.g. anterior spinal artery infarction, spinal arteriovenous malformation.
- Compression, e.g. space-occupying lesion, syringomyelia, vertebral fractures.

Management

Acute
- Consists of neurosurgical intervention to remove cord compression.
- High-dose intravenous steroids (methylprednisolone, hydrocortisone) to reduce inflammation.
- Supportive measures such as ventilation, catheterization (see 🕮 p162).
- Management of constipation (see 🕮 p84) and treatment of spasticity (see 🕮 p431).
- Immobility poses risk of deep venous thrombosis and prophylactic subcutaneous heparin may be required.
- Prevention of contractures is important by adequate physiotherapy (see 🕮 p179) and use of orthotic appliances (see 🕮 p220).

Long term
- Includes managing spasticity by using medication such as baclofen and diazepam.
- Skin and nail care is important if there is sensory involvement (see 🕮 p96).
- Bladder and bowel management becomes important (see 🕮 p162).
- Psychosocial aspects (see 🕮 p373) need addressing as loss of ambulation in particular and loss of independence can have significant impact on affect and social interaction.

Further resources
Colostomy Association: ☎ 0800 328 4257 ℘ http://www.colostomyassociation.org.uk

ERIC (Education & Resources for Improving Childhood Continence): ☎ 0845 370 8008 ℘ http://www.eric.org.uk

IA® (The ileostomy & internal pouch support group): ☎ 0800 0184 724 ℘ http://www.the-ia.org.uk

The Bladder and Bowel Foundation: ☎ 0845 345 0165 ℘ http://www.bladderandbowelfoundation.org

Vision

Smooth seas do not make skilful sailors.

African proverb

Delayed visual maturation

- The visual pathways can take a few months to mature in some cases. Parents often describe the visual responses as 'inconsistent' or 'the child appears to look through me rather than at me'.
- As long as the eyes are structurally normal, there are no abnormal eye movements, and there are no other developmental concerns, such babies can be observed up to 6 months of age.
- Most cases improve spontaneously by 6 months. If there is no improvement, a brain scan and electrodiagnostic testing (electroretinogram (ERG) and visual-evoked potentials (VEPs)) are indicated.

Examination and assessment of visual acuity (red reflex, cover, and acuity tests)

- Visual acuity tests for children must be appropriate for the age and development of the child as shown in Table 7.1.
- The clinic-based tests would form part of the paediatric assessment (see 🕮 p9), and can alert paediatricians and GPs to eye conditions that need referral to an ophthalmologist.

Table 7.1 Visual acuity tests for children

Age	Clinic-based (informal) tests useful for paediatricians, GPs, as well as ophthalmologists	Formal tests of visual acuity
Neonate	Fixing and following, interest in human faces, response to bright lights.	Preferential looking tests where the child is presented with 2 cards—1 plain and 1 with stripes of varying widths (Teller cards). The expected response is shift of gaze towards the striped cards.
Young infants	Interest in human faces, social smile, stranger anxiety, steady fixation, reaching for bright objects.	Cardiff acuity cards is a preferential looking test similar to Teller cards, with familiar objects such as birds instead of stripes.
1–2 years	Interest in toys and smaller objects, stranger anxiety.	Kay picture cards have familiar objects like car, bird and the child names the object or matches it to the corresponding image on a card held by the parent by pointing.
2–3 years	Visual behaviour when navigating around room, ability to detect small objects.	Sheridan Gardner test involves single letters rather than rows of letters, and the child points to the corresponding letter on a hand-held card.
>3 years	Visual behaviour when navigating around room, ability to detect small objects.	Snellen or logMAR[a] visual acuity test involves row of letters of reducing size. For preschool children, the illiterate E or Landolt C test can be used.

[a] LogMAR: logarithm of minimum angle of resolution—a measure of visual acuity, i.e. ability to discriminate fine detail

Testing the visual field

- This can be a challenge in young children, and formal testing is only possible for the older cooperative child.
- Formal tests include the automated perimetry, e.g. Humphrey, or manual such as Goldman.
- For the younger child, tests are more observational, where the clinician places objects (typically bright toys) randomly in various positions in the visual field, and observes the child's response (normally a rapid head and eye movement in the direction of the toy).
- Valuable information can also be gathered from observing their ability to navigate around obstacles placed in the clinic, e.g. stepping over or avoiding a large toy placed on the floor.

Testing binocular vision

- Binocular vision is the ability of the higher visual centres in the brain to simultaneously process the visual signals from both eyes to produce a single image.
- It is important for both eyes to point in the same direction to produce a similar image on both retinas, and create a single 3-dimensional image with depth and distance perception (stereopsis).
- There are several age-appropriate tests to detect the presence and level of binocular vision such as the Lang test, TNO (Netherlands Organisation for Applied Scientific Research) and Titmus tests, Wirt fly test, and the synoptophore—often referred to by children as 'putting the lion in the cage test'.
- There are advantages to having good binocular vision, but lack of binocular vision does not usually limit ability at sport or schooling, and rarely, if ever, restricts choice of career.
- A squint (see 🕮 p281) can potentially interfere with the development of binocular vision, and it is desirable to detect and correct a squint early for these reasons.

External examination

- A visual inspection of the eyes and eyelids can reveal dysmorphic features (see 🕮 p384) like low set or slanted eyelids and palpebral fissures, wide-set eyes (telecanthus), and lid colobomas.
- Abnormal head posture because of nystagmus (see 🕮 p283) or squint, ptosis (droopy eyelids), squint or abnormalities of eye size, e.g. enlargement of the eye in glaucoma, or developmental abnormalities like microphthalmos will also be evident on external examination.

Direct ophthalmoscopy

- The direct ophthalmoscope is a very useful screening tool for the paediatrician as well as the paediatric ophthalmologist (Figs 7.1 and 7.2).
- It can be used in the clinic, community, or bedside and enables a quick assessment of the clarity of the ocular media by checking the red reflex (see 🕮 p273 and p277). It can be held some distance (1–2 feet/0.3–0.6m) away from the child for this test to minimize apprehension.
- Cataracts, corneal opacities and scars, as well as retinal conditions such as tumours (retinoblastoma) can be detected with this simple test. It is

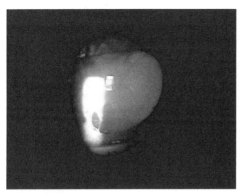

Fig. 7.1 Red reflex testing.

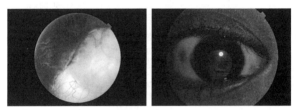

Fig. 7.2 a) Chorioretinal and b) iris coloboma.

important to remember that it might be more difficult to see a bright red reflex in heavily pigmented fundi (e.g. in Asian or Afro-Caribbean patients) as more light is absorbed and less reflected back and this is one of the common causes of referral to the ophthalmologist with an absent red reflex.

Testing for squint (strabismus) and eye movement disorders

- Although examining the eye with a penlight to assess the centration and symmetry of the light reflex (Hirschberg corneal reflex test) is an acceptable technique to look for ocular misalignment (squint (see 🕮 p281)), the definitive test is the cover test where each eye is covered in turn and the fellow eye observed to look for any corrective movement. This corrective movement will be outward in the case of a convergent squint, and inward for a divergent squint, or up or down in case of a vertical squint.
- It is also useful to check the range of eye movements, and is best done by asking the child to follow a penlight or a toy.

Refraction and the role of the optician/optometrist (general ophthalmic services)

- Refractive errors are common in childhood, and significant errors should be corrected with glasses (or contact lenses where appropriate) to provide clear vision, ensure optimum visual and general development (see ☐ p48), and prevent amblyopia (lazy eye).
- It is recognized that ex-premature children (see ☐ p289), children with developmental delay (see ☐ p117) including from birth hypoxia, and with multisystem disorders or genetic syndromes such as trisomy 21 (see ☐ p387) have a higher than usual incidence of refractive errors.
- For younger children, it is usual to assess their refractive status by objective means (retinoscopy performed by ophthalmologist or optometrist); while older children can have subjective testing where they can try different lenses while reading down the chart to see which one provides the clearest vision.
- In the UK, the community (high street) optometrists offer refraction and vision assessment for children (funded by the state) under the general ophthalmic services (GOS). This is a valuable screening service, and cases requiring the opinion of an ophthalmologist are referred on to the hospital eye service (HES).
- Prescriptions are issued on a HES (P) form which also serves as a voucher to reimburse the dispensing optician the cost of standard spectacles such that every child with an associated eye condition is able to access spectacles.
- Children with refractive errors whose eyes are otherwise healthy usually obtain their spectacles from opticians (self-funded unless entitled to benefits (see ☐ p292 and p514)).

Fundus examination

- Examining the fundus in a child takes considerable patience and skill.
- It is easier after pupillary dilatation with eye drops. Tropicamide, cyclopentolate, and atropine are all parasympatholytic agents (relax the pupillary sphincter), and phenylephrine is a sympathomimetic agent (stimulates the pupillary dilator muscle), with varying degrees and duration of action).
- Atropine is rarely used in practice, the commonest agent is cyclopentolate.
- Most ophthalmologists will use the indirect ophthalmoscope (head mounted device with a hand held lens), but it should be possible for some clinicians to examine the optic disc and central retina through the undilated pupil, particularly in light-eyed children with larger pupils.

Vision impairment

Visual impairment (or vision impairment) is vision loss to such a degree as to qualify as an additional support need through a significant limitation of visual capability resulting from either disease, trauma, or congenital or degenerative conditions that cannot be corrected by conventional means, such as refractive correction (see 📖 p286), medication, or surgery.

Incidence and causes of childhood visual impairment

- Visual impairment in childhood can be classified according to time of occurrence of the inciting event:
  - Prenatal: common causes are hereditary, chromosomal defects, intra-uterine infections, teratogens (drug abuse etc.).
  - Peri- and neonatal: commonest if prematurity and perinatal hypoxia.
  - Childhood: nutritional, tumours, infection, trauma (accidental and non-accidental) (see 📖 p447).
- The various causes can also be classified according to the anatomical site of involvement.
- The relative incidence of these causes varies between the developed and developing world.
- Disorders of the globe or anterior segment, corneal disorders, glaucoma, and cataract are relatively more prevalent in developing countries, while optic nerve and cerebral visual pathway disorders are more important causes in developed countries. Retinal disorders are common in all countries.
- Retinopathy of prematurity (ROP) is an important contributor in moderately developed countries where neonatal care has improved with greater infant survival, but without the screening services needed to treat ROP (see 📖 p289).
- The prevalence of childhood (0–15 years) blindness varies from 0.3 per 1000 children in European countries, to 0.8 in Asia, and 1.24 in Sub-Saharan Africa.
- There are approximately 60 blind children per million (child and adult) population in developed countries and 10 times this number in developing countries.

Degree of visual impairment

- There are 2 levels of visual impairment recognized in the UK—sight impaired and severely sight impaired. However, it is important to remember that these are only categories for the purposes of determining eligibility for extra help from SS (see 📖 p292).
- Broadly speaking, a sight impaired individual will be expected to experience difficulties undertaking tasks related to employment, and some activities such as driving.
- Such individuals will either have significant loss of visual acuity (central vision) or a significant loss of visual field (peripheral vision) but not both.
- Thus, cases with moderate to severe loss of visual acuity 6/18 to 6/60, but retaining a full field of vision *or* mild to moderate loss of visual acuity (≤6/18) but with extensive visual field loss are included.

- The severely sight-impaired individual might in addition to this, also experience difficulties with ADLs such as accessing public transport, crossing the road safely, cooking, etc (see 📖 p188). Such individuals have severe loss of visual acuity ≤6/60 with a full visual field, or moderate to severe loss of visual acuity with loss of visual field as well.

Table 7.2 Criteria for certification of sight impairment in the UK

	Visual acuity	**Visual field**
Sight impaired	6/60–6/18	Normal field of vision
Sight impaired	≤ 6/18	Loss of field of vision
Severely sight impaired	3/60–6/60	Normal field
Severely sight impaired	6/60–6/18	Loss of field of vision

Effect of vision impairment on motor function, social interactions, cognition

- The majority of children with visual impairment have additional disabilities, particularly with cortical visual impairment.
- Visual input is useful when learning and performing simple motor tasks such as walking and running, and important for performing complex tasks such as writing, eating, etc. Visual impairment in children will interfere with motor development, and this is an important consideration in dealing with GDD as well as children with multiple sensorimotor impairment (see 📖 p57 and p117).
- Children with CP (see 📖 p67) might have associated cortical visual impairment which might impair their mobility further.
- Maintaining eye contact, recognition of familiar faces, stranger anxiety, and social smile are all important in social interaction, and require a certain level of visual function. Early-onset visual impairment in children can interfere with these functions, and social interaction, with resultant delay in developmental milestones (see 📖 p48 and p57).
- Sleep (see 📖 p168) and behavioural disorders are common in severe visual impairment and can cause considerable stress to the family. These children are also prone to blind mannerisms such as eye poking, head nodding, finger flicking, and light gazing.
- Visual impairment from disorders of the cerebral cortex (cerebral or cortical visual impairment) can result not only in poor visual acuity and/or visual field loss, but also deficits of visual processing and cognition (see 📖 p213). The diagnosis of intellectual deficits in visually impaired children is difficult, and should only be made by trained child psychologists (see 📖 p215).
- Associated speech (see 📖 p202), hearing (see 📖 p296), and learning difficulties (see 📖 p117) are not uncommon, particularly when resulting from ante or perinatal events such as prematurity, intra-uterine infections and birth hypoxia.

Early intervention (see 📖 p59 and p60) by services such as the sensory support services and vision impairment team from local authorities can be of help in such cases. Such children receive excellent care from teams at children's development centres (see 📖 p22), with multiprofessional input (see 📖 p20 and p23) including community paediatricians, OTs, SLTs, audiologists, orthoptists, PTs, psychologists, and social workers.

Investigating a child with vision impairment

- A *thorough clinical examination*, with emphasis on objective assessment of ocular and visual function is essential. Age-appropriate visual acuity tests must be employed, and visual fields tested where possible.
- The *red reflex test* (see 📖 p272 and p273) is a very useful screening test for the non-ophthalmologist to detect any media opacities such as cataract or corneal problems, and can also alert the observer to life threatening conditions such as retinoblastoma.
- *Visual behaviour* and parental observations are very important, as are also any abnormal eye movements. Detailed retinal and optic nerve examination are important, and every child must undergo *cycloplegic refraction* after instilling eye drops to dilate the pupil.
- *Examination under anaesthesia* might be necessary in some cases, especially if the examination is difficult in the wake child, or the findings are very subtle.
- If the older child presents with acquired visual loss and there is no ocular explanation, one must bear in mind the possibility of functional (non-organic) visual loss. This is more common in boys than girls, often between 7–12 years age.
- Electrophysiological tests of vision including the *ERG* and *VEPs* can be very useful in diagnosing subtle retinal dystrophies and optic nerve disorders, and also disorders of the visual pathways.
- *Neuroimaging* should be performed where indicated, especially if the visual loss cannot be explained by the ocular examination and electrophysiology, or there is suspicion of intracranial or retro-ocular pathology.

The deaf–blind child

Dual sensory impairment is a major disability in a child, and can significantly impact learning, social, and communication skills.

Causes

- Congenital or infantile sight and hearing impairment can be due to congenital rubella, severe prematurity, CHARGE syndrome, and genetic disorders such as Norrie's syndrome, trisomy 13, Cockayne, Zellweger, and infantile Refsum syndromes, osteopetrosis.
- Early-onset sight impairment with subsequent hearing impairment is seen in Alstrom syndrome, Norrie syndrome, some types of Lebers congenital amaurosis, and X-linked ocular albinism.
- Late-onset (juvenile) loss of vision with subsequent hearing loss is seen in Refsum syndrome, Wolfram (DIDMOAD) syndrome, Alport syndrome and neurofibromatosis type 2 (NF2).
- Congenital hearing loss with subsequent sight impairment is seen in rubella, Norrie, Alstrom and Cockayne syndromes, some forms of Usher syndrome, osteopetrosis, and Stickler syndrome.

Management

- Early diagnosis of dual sensory impairment (hearing and sight) is important to ensure early intervention (see 🕮 p59 and p60) and enable achievement of their full potential. Support groups such as SENSE in the UK can be involved at an early stage.
- Clinicians seeing a visually impaired child must enquire about and test for hearing loss (see 🕮 p300), and, similarly, parents of children with early-onset hearing loss should watch for any signs of visual difficulties, particularly if more than one individual is affected in the family.
- All these children must have regular refraction (see 🕮 p286), and ERG testing might be indicated in some cases.
- Considerable input is needed into these children's educational needs (see 🕮 p524), with psychosocial support.

Further resource

SENSE: 🖑 http://www.sense.org.uk

Colour blindness

Recognition, impact on learning, career counselling, etc.

- The ability of humans to perceive light of differing wavelengths as colours is subserved by several types of cone photoreceptors in the retina.
- The 3 types of cones (red, blue, and green) contain different visual pigments that respond to a range of wavelengths (trichromatic theory of colour vision), and the differential output of the 3 families of receptors is processed by the retinal ganglion cells and visual cortex in an antagonistic way (red vs green, blue vs yellow, black vs white) to generate the sensation of colour.
- Colour blindness is the lack or loss of ability to perceive colour. It can be congenital or acquired.

Congenital colour blindness

- *Monochromatism* is a rare type of colour blindness, where none of the cone cells function properly or only one type works as it should. This results in no colour vision—all you see is black, white, and shades of grey.
- *Achromatopsia* is a retinal disorder where there are no cones, and, as a result, no colour perception, with poor vision and nystagmus.
- *Dichromatism* is when 1 of the cones is missing. Anomalous trichromatism is when all 3 cones are present but there is a fault in 1 of them making the individual less sensitive to certain colours. Depending on which cone is faulty, this will cause reduction in or absence of red green or blue sensitivity.
- Red cone and green cone defects are the commonest type of congenital colour blindness, and are known as red–green colour blindness.
- The genes that code for the pigment in the red and green sensitive cones are located on the X chromosome. Defects in this gene can result in *red–green colour blindness*.
- The pattern of inheritance is X-linked recessive. As females have 2 copies of the X chromosome, the healthy gene on the other X chromosome compensates for the defective gene on the faulty X chromosome, with resultant normal colour vision. Males, on the other hand, have only 1 copy of the X chromosome and if the gene is faulty, they suffer from red–green colour blindness.
- 8% of the male population are colour blind, and although they can perceive the difference between red and green colours, neither are perceived as red or green in the same way as normal individuals.

Acquired colour blindness

- Optic nerve disorders and some retinal disorders can result in loss of colour sensitivity. Sensitivity is usually lost across the colour spectrum, and manifests as desaturation of colours.
- Red is usually most affected with optic nerve disorders, and blue green in retinal disorders.

Colour vision tests
- The Ishihara colour test charts are very useful in assessing congenital colour blindness, and less useful in acquired defects.
- Other tests such as the Farnsworth Munsell 100 hue test or D15 panel are more useful in acquired defects.

Impact on learning and choice of career
- Congenital colour blindness affects the ability to distinguish between red and green, the colours used in traffic lights and signalling systems. Normal colour vision may be a prerequisite for certain professions such as pilots and coastguards.
- There is very little impact on schooling. There is no impact on ability to drive because the red-blind individual can differentiate between red and green, but does not perceive red and green as other normal individuals would. There is therefore no difficulty in recognizing traffic lights.

Squint

- The term *squint (or strabismus)* refers to misalignment of the eyes. The ocular system is designed for both eyes to point in the same direction in all positions of gaze. The eyes should therefore remain and move parallel to each other thus avoiding double vision, and allowing binocular (stereoscopic or 3-dimensional) vision.
- A squint may occur in the primary position, i.e. looking straight ahead, or only in certain directions of gaze. Depending on the direction of misalignment, squints may be horizontal, vertical, or both.
- *Pseudo squint*—some children might appear to have a squint despite accurate ocular alignment. Such cases will have a normal cover test (see 📖 p273), but might have an abnormal corneal light reflex test (Hirschberg test). This is referred to as a pseudo-squint, and could be due to abnormal separation of eyelids, or unusual facial configuration.
- An inward turn of the eye is a *convergent squint (esotropia),* while an outward turn is a *divergent squint (exotropia).*
- Vertical squints are described as right or left *hypertropia* depending on which eye rests higher.

Causes of squint

- *Refractive:* due to an underlying refractive error (see 📖 p286). The commonest situation is a convergent squint associated with a moderate to high hypermetropic refractive error (also referred to as accommodative convergent squint). Another commonly encountered scenario is when one of the eyes has a high refractive error (hypermetropic or myopic) and is amblyopic (lazy eye) with poorer vision, and the amblyopic eye drifts in (convergent) or out (divergent).
- *Non-refractive:* the cause of non refractive childhood squints is poorly understood, but is believed to be due to defective central control of eye movements. This is the commonest cause, and includes most divergent squints, and infantile esotropia.
- *Mixed:* where there is a refractive and non-refractive element to the squint
- *Neurogenic:* due to nerve palsy (IIIrd, IVth, or VIth) or skew deviation following intracranial pathology such as tumours or trauma. *Duane syndrome* and *Moebius syndrome* are other causes of squint where there is an underlying innervational defect.
- *Myogenic:* the cause here is under action (weakness) or restriction (tightness) of one or more muscles. Common causes are myasthenia (see 📖 p257), trauma including orbital fractures, and orbital masses.

Neonatal ocular misalignment

- It is not uncommon for babies' eyes to wander in or out for the first 2–3 months while the fixation system is still developing. This is referred to as neonatal ocular misalignment, and can be observed unless there are concerns about the child's vision.
- Persistence of ocular misalignment beyond 3 months warrants referral to the ophthalmologist.

Consequences of squint

- The child's visual system is immature and a squint can interfere with development of binocular vision as well as affect the visual acuity in the squinting eye.
- Adults who develop a squint will experience double vision (diplopia). Children rarely develop diplopia—instead the brain shuts out the image from the squinting eye. This might result in deterioration in visual acuity in the squinting eye, referred to as amblyopia or lazy eye. This loss of acuity is reversible if treated in time.
- Another mechanism adopted by the developing visual system is to suppress the image from the squinting eye and disrupt the binocular vision. This could result in loss of the ability to use both eyes together. If treated in time, this can be recovered, but is sometimes irreversible.
- The child might adopt an abnormal head posture, such as a face turn or head tilt to control the squint

Treatment of squint

- Correct refractive error with spectacles or contact lenses (see 📖 p286).
- Treat underlying medical conditions such as myasthenia (see 📖 p257).
- Treatment of amblyopia—with occlusion (patching) of the better seeing eye to force the weaker eye to be used, with improvement in visual acuity. Atropine drops (penalization) can also be used instead of patching in some cases to blur the vision in the better seeing eye.
- Surgery if spectacles do not correct the squint, to preserve/restore binocular vision, and to improve cosmesis.

Urgency of referral

- ▶ Any child presenting with a squint should be referred to either the community or hospital orthoptists (allied health professionals who deal with squints along with ophthalmologists) or optometrist, and should receive an eye examination, particularly red reflex testing as described on (see 📖 p273).
- ▶▶ Sudden onset squint with diplopia in the older child would merit an urgent referral (see 📖 p272, p273, and p277).

Nystagmus

- *Nystagmus* is rhythmic repetitive to-and-fro movement of the eyes.
- *Nystagmoid* (searching movements) on the other hand are random, non-repetitive movements.
- Nystagmoid movements indicate extremely poor visual function of central origin (posterior visual pathway).

Types of nystagmus

- Nystagmus may be congenital or acquired.
- *Congenital idiopathic motor nystagmus* appears shortly after birth, and is usually due to a disorder of the ocular stabilization (motor system); as a result of defective pause neurons in the brainstem centres controlling eye movement and gaze.
- *Congenital sensory nystagmus* is usually due to ocular causes such as severe congenital retinal dystrophy or severe optic nerve hypoplasia, and may be accompanied by some nystagmoid movements.
- Congenital nystagmus is also a feature of all forms of albinism.
- Nystagmoid movements usually indicate a visual disorder affecting the posterior visual pathway.
- Acquired nystagmus could be due to sensory or motor causes.
- *Acquired sensory nystagmus* can be due to central retinal dystrophies (cone or cone rod dystrophy) or early onset optic atrophy from conditions such as optic pathway gliomas.
- *Acquired motor nystagmus* can occur following head injury, brain tumours, demyelinating disorders, ICH, hydrocephalus (see 📖 p264), and some neurometabolic disorders (see 📖 p155).

Effect on vision

- In cases with sensory nystagmus, the poor vision is the primary problem and is responsible for unsteady fixation and nystagmus.
- In cases with congenital motor nystagmus, the visual system compensates for the constant eye movement by blurring the image to negate the constant movement of images on the retina, resulting in reduced visual acuity.
- The mature visual system is less capable of compensating, and older children with acquired motor nystagmus might experience oscillopsia (the sensation of constantly moving images) which can be a very distressing symptom.

Examination of the patient with nystagmus

- It is important to characterize the nystagmus as it may help with the diagnosis, prognosis, and in planning treatment.
- When testing visual acuity in nystagmus, it is important to test with both eyes open (binocular acuity) as the binocular acuity is significantly better than uniocular acuity and of more relevance to daily activities. This is due to the stabilizing effect of each eye on the fellow eye.

Types of nystagmus

Latent or manifest nystagmus

- Manifest nystagmus is present all the time while latent only presents when 1 eye is covered (binocularity is disrupted).

Uni- or multiplanar

- If the plane of movement of the eyes (horizontal or vertical) remains constant in all directions of gaze, it is described as *uniplanar* and if it varies with gaze it is termed *multiplanar*.
- Uniplanarity is suggestive of idiopathic congenital motor nystagmus.
- Multiplanar nystagmus is acquired and may need further investigation.

Pendular or jerk

- The nystagmus is described as pendular when the to-and-fro movement is of equal amplitude and speed in either direction.
- Jerk nystagmus on the other hand is asymmetric with respect to fixation and is faster in one direction than the other. It thus has a fast and slow component. The direction of jerk nystagmus is conventionally described as being in the direction of the fast component.

Direction

- The direction of the nystagmus must be noted and may be of diagnostic value.
- Horizontal: the commonest cause is congenital idiopathic motor nystagmus. It can also occur with internuclear ophthalmoplegia (INO).
- Vertical: may be pendular or jerk (down-beating—in cerebellar lesions or up-beating in midbrain lesions).
- Rotary: where the eye move in a circular pattern.
- Cyclorotatory: where the nystagmus is torsional, the eye rotating about its own axis.
- See-saw: where one eye elevates and intorts and the other depresses and extorts followed by the opposite corrective movement. This is typically seen in chiasmal lesions, e.g. craniopharyngioma.

Dissociated nystagmus

- If the speed and amplitude of nystagmus is different between the two eyes, it is described as dissociated. The classic example of dissociated nystagmus is the abducting nystagmus seen in INO.
- Rarely, nystagmus may be uniocular. Although this may be congenital, it is important to exclude a unilateral optic pathway glioma.

Null point and head posture

- Jerk nystagmus is often associated with a certain position of the eyes where the nystagmus is dampened (lowest intensity).
- The best visual acuity is achieved with the eyes in this position. This point is called the null point and is usually in or near the straight ahead position.
- If the null point is to either side of the midline, the subject may adopt an abnormal head posture. This is typically a face turn in horizontal jerk nystagmus away from the null point, thus rotating the eyes towards the null point where the nystagmus is dampened.

- The null point position is usually adopted only when performing fine visual tasks and may not be readily apparent.
- A null point is typically seen with congenital idiopathic motor nystagmus.

Fatiguability
- The nystagmus may be persistent or rapidly fatigable.
- Rapidly fatiguing nystagmus is of lesser clinical significance.

Large or small amplitude (fine or coarse)
- The amplitude (degree of excursion of the eyes in each nystagmus cycle) must be noted.
- The greater the amplitude, the poorer the visual acuity.

Fast or slow
- This refers to the speed of movement of the eyes. It is not of great clinical significance.

Dampening on convergence
- Certain forms of nystagmus dampen on convergence. This is typically seen in congenital idiopathic motor nystagmus.

Investigating a patient with nystagmus
- Not every child with nystagmus needs a head scan.
- All such cases should be referred to an ophthalmologist to look for a cause.
- ▶ Acquired nystagmus merits urgent referral and a head scan.

Treatment of nystagmus
- Certain forms of congenital nystagmus can be improved with eye muscle surgery to reduce abnormal head posture or improve vision by dampening nystagmus,
- Some drugs like baclofen can help with acquired nystagmus.
- Most types of nystagmus are not amenable to any form of treatment.

Refractive errors in childhood

- In the normal eye, the cornea and lens focus a clear image on the retina resulting in normal visual acuity. The normal eye is a perfect visual system where the power of the cornea and lens are matched to the length of the eye, i.e. distance to retina, so that the images is in focus when the eye is at rest.
- Any imperfections in this complex optical system will result in a defocused image and affect visual acuity (Table 7.3).

Table 7.3 Types of refractive errors

Name	What happens	What does the child see	How is it corrected	Associations
Myopia (short sightedness)	The image is focused in front of rather than on the retina. The cornea is too curved, or the eye is too long (more common).	Clear for near, blurry for distance.	Concave spectacle or contact lenses.	Ocular: retinal dystrophies. Systemic: collagenopathies e.g. Stickler syndrome, Marfan syndrome. Chromosomal disorders, e.g. DS.
Hypermetropia (long sightedness)	The image is focused behind the retina. The cornea is too flat or the eye too short.	Blurry all the time, both distance and near.	Convex spectacle or contact lenses.	Ocular: microphthalmos, nanophthalmos. Systemic: micro syndrome, Leber's congenital amaurosis (congenital retinal dystrophy often associated with developmental delay).
Astigmatism	The cornea is an abnormal shape, like a rugby ball rather than a football. The image is stretched.	Unclear all the time. Circles appear like oval.	Cylindrical spectacle lenses or toric contact lenses.	DS, craniofacial syndromes.

(Continued)

Table 7.3 (Continued)

Name	What happens	What does the child see	How is it corrected	Associations
Presbyopia	The lens cannot change shape to shift focus from distance to near.	Blurry for near only.	Reading glasses.	Does not occur in children.

- The incidence of clinically significant refractive errors (requiring the use of spectacle correction) in childhood is approximately 5% (The Baltimore Pediatric Eye Disease Study).

Refractive surgery in children

- As a general rule, refractive surgery can be considered when the refraction has been stable for a few years, usually past the adolescent years, i.e. after 18 years.
- It is unsuitable for children as the eye is still growing and the refractive error is changing.
- There are very few situations such as extremely high unilateral hypermetropia or myopia where spectacles cannot be given due to the extreme asymmetry and the child is contact lens intolerant. Such cases will rapidly develop amblyopia, and there are a few studies exploring the role of refractive surgery in such situations.

Child abuse

- Child abuse (see 📖 Chapter 12 Child Abuse) is a general term that encompasses several mechanisms of damage to children including neglect, emotional, physical and sexual abuse, and induced illness, i.e. Munchausen syndrome (see 📖 p451).
- NAI or abusive head injury are terms commonly used to describe physical abuse often involving shaking injury with or without impact. This form of abuse can affect the eyes and all children with suspected NAI should receive an eye examination including dilated fundoscopy by an experienced ophthalmologist (also see 📖 p447).
- The ophthalmologist will look for external evidence of trauma, and retinal haemorrhages.
- Such cases often end up in court and accurate documentation with retinal photography where available is very useful.
- The ophthalmic findings are crucial to the overall assessment and the ophthalmologist may be asked to provide an opinion on whether the eye findings are consistent with, and specific for NAI (see 📖 p444).
- Another less common situation where the ophthalmologist may be involved is neglect, where the child might not have received appropriate care from parents or professionals.

The child who is losing vision or failing at school

- Most childhood ocular disorders manifest in the first few years of life.
- A different approach is necessary for the child who complains of, or is noted to have progressive reduction in vision during childhood. These conditions often but not invariably present in slightly older children.
- There are broadly 4 groups of disorders with this presentation:
  - Refractive error (see 📖 p286): progressive myopia is the commonest cause.
  - Retinal dystrophies: can manifest in the 1st or 2nd decade.
  - Neurometabolic disorders (see 📖 p155): might present with visual loss as well as neuroregression.
  - Learning difficulties: such as dyslexia (see 📖 p147) or dyspraxia (see 📖 p136).
- Less common causes include glaucoma, cataract, corneal problems like keratoconus and hereditary optic atrophy.
- ▶ Such cases need referral to an ophthalmologist.

Visual effects of 'prematurity'

Depending on the degree, prematurity may be associated with eye and visual problems.

These include:

Retinopathy of prematurity

- Retinal development continues through gestation and vascularization is completed near term.
- Premature birth interferes with normal retinal vascularization with risk of abnormal retinal vascular proliferation that can cause retinal scarring and/or detachment (ROP).
- Babies born before 32 weeks' gestation or birth weight ≤1500g are at risk of ROP and fortnightly screening eye examinations are recommended (UK ROP guidelines May 2008, Royal College of Ophthalmologists and RCPCH).
- Most cases do not require treatment but ROP beyond a certain threshold will require prompt laser treatment of the avascular retina to reduce risk of visual loss.
- Laser treatment can result in loss of peripheral field of vision and this must be borne in mind when assessing the child's special needs (see 📖 p294).

Strabismus

- There is a higher than expected incidence of squints (see 📖 p281) in ex-premature babies and some centres will screen such children for the first few years although practice varies considerably.
- These children are often under the care of a community paediatrician and can be referred to the ophthalmologist if there is any suspicion of a squint.

Refractive errors

- There is a relatively high incidence of refractive errors (see 📖 p286) in ex-premature children.
- High myopia is more common than hypermetropia and astigmatism.
- There is some debate as to whether children who have received laser treatment for ROP are at greater risk of myopia.

Cortical visual impairment and developmental delay

- There is a greater incidence of cognitive impairment (see 📖 p117) in ex-premature children.
- As expected, visual difficulties are more common compared to term births and include visual field defects, visual processing deficits and binocular vision abnormalities.

Habilitation of a child with vision impairment

- Every child with visual impairment has the potential to become an independent and productive member of society.
- It is therefore imperative that adequate resources are made available to ensure they achieve their full potential.
- The goals may be different depending on the degree of multisensory impairment and any interventions must therefore be tailored to the individual.

Living skills

- Each local authority in the UK has specially trained staff usually called *rehabilitation workers* or *rehabilitation officers* who can support sight impaired children in a range of ADL, such as using public transport (mobility officers) cooking, and leisure activities.
- Rehabilitation workers may be part of a special team working with people with a sight or hearing loss or based with a local voluntary society for blind and partially sighted people.
- Not every local council employs rehabilitation workers, and the local authority can 'buy in' any service needed.
- Most local authorities offer a *registration card* which can help to prove entitlement to certain concessions. A registration card in England should follow the guidelines laid down by the Association of Directors of Adult Social Services.

Schools for the visually impaired

- Most local education authorities in the UK support schools for the visually impaired.
- Some schools are best suited for otherwise able children with visual impairment, while some deal with multisensory impairment and others with visual impairment and learning difficulties (including ASD).
- Many of these schools are situated next to schools for sighted children (see 📖 p524), and visually impaired children receive tutoring in both sections. Indeed, many sight impaired pupils can receive excellent education in mainstream schools with additional help where needed (integrated schooling).
- The teaching programme (see 📖 p533 and p534) should be tailored to the individual child's needs, and it is important that educational authorities allocate adequate resources for such institutions.
- The process of visual impairment registration includes data collection on the number of children registered by postcode to enable equitable regional allocation of resources.
- Children receive training in living skills (see 📖 p191 and p193) such as cooking, mobility (see 📖 p186), and educational techniques employed depend upon the level of vision.
- Large print educational materials, closed circuit TV (CCTV), touch typing, and Braille are some of the techniques employed in such schools.
- Children are also encouraged to develop tactile skills (see 📖 p194) and the use of white canes.

Low-vision aids

- Every child with visual impairment should be referred for low-vision assessment and provided with aids where appropriate (see ☐ p225). These aids include hand and stand magnifiers and CCTV among others.
- This service is provided by many hospital eye departments, some community optometrists, the RNIB (Royal National Institute of Blind People) and some charities.

Guide dogs

- The Guide Dogs charity (no government funding) is responsible for approximately 8000 guide dogs all over the UK to assist sight impaired individuals to improve their mobility and independence.
- There are currently 4500 dog owners with 780 new guide dogs provided each year.
- Any individual with sight loss, even if not registered sight impaired can own a guide dog for a nominal cost of 50 pence, with all equipment, training, vet bills, and dog food included.
- Children can have buddy dogs, in preparation for a guide dog as an adult.

White cane

- A white cane is used by many people who are blind or visually impaired both as a mobility tool and to make others aware of their visual disability.
- Children are usually introduced to the cane between 7–10 years age.

Higher education (university or vocational)

- Higher education (see ☐ p171) places greater demands on visually impaired individuals and is less organized than schooling for visually impaired children.
- Educational material is not easily available in large print or Braille and considerable resources need to be allocated to ensure accessibility for visually disabled individuals.

Certification and benefits

- Any individual, child or adult, in the UK with sufficient visual impairment is eligible to be registered sight impaired (partially sighted) or severely sight impaired (blind).
- This is a process initiated by the consultant ophthalmologist by completing a Certificate of Visual Impairment (CVI); this is called BP1 in Scotland.
- A copy of this form is sent to the patient, GP, local social services, Department of Health, and the Royal College of Ophthalmologists (for epidemiological studies).
- The ophthalmologist uses a combination of visual acuity and field of vision to judge eligibility to be registered and at which level. If the child has good visual acuity, there must be significant loss of visual field to qualify, and similarly if the visual field is full, the visual acuity must be very poor to be registered.

The criteria for severely sight impaired (blind) registration are:

- Best corrected (i.e. with glasses or contact lenses if needed) visual acuity of less than 3/60 with a full visual field *or*
- Best corrected visual acuity between 3/60 and 6/60 with a severe reduction of field of vision, such as tunnel vision *or*
- Best corrected visual acuity of ≥6/60 with a much reduced field of vision, especially the lower half.

The criteria for sight impaired (partially sighted) are:

- Best corrected visual acuity of 3/60 to 6/60 with a full field of vision.
- Best corrected visual acuity of up to 6/24 with a moderate reduction of field of vision or with a central part of vision that is cloudy or blurry.
- Best corrected visual acuity of up to 6/18 if a large part of the field of vision is missing, e.g. hemianopia.

The benefits of sight impairment registration

- The process of registration enables the affected individual (or parents if the individual is a child) to access extra support from social services and entitles them to certain concessions, but does not in any way place any restrictions on the individual.
- SS carry out an assessment of needs to identify what changes are needed to the individual's living situation to help adapt to the sight loss, and help with home life, mobility, work and education (also see 📖 p514). This varies from region to region.

Sight impaired/partially sighted individuals are entitled to the following:

- Free NHS sight test and glasses.
- Discounted rail travel.
- Local bus schemes.
- Exemption from BT Directory Enquiry charges.
- Information in accessible formats.
- Leisure concessions.

- Council tax disability reduction.
- Welfare benefits: people who are registered as severely sight impaired/blind or sight impaired/partially sighted are not automatically entitled to any welfare benefits, this is subject to age and other circumstances (see 📖 p514). These include:
  - Attendance Allowance.
  - Disability Living Allowance.
  - Carer's Allowance.
  - Employment and Support Allowance.
  - Tax Credits.
  - Pension Credit.
  - Housing Benefit.
  - Council Tax Benefit.
  - Exemption from 'non-dependants' deductions.

In addition, severely sight impaired individuals are entitled to the following concessions

- Blind person's personal income tax allowance.
- Reduction of 50% on the television licence fee.
- Car parking concessions: the Blue Badge Scheme.
- Free postage on items marked 'articles for the blind'.

Statementing (SEN) for a child with visual impairment

The process of statementing

- A statement of special educational needs (SEN) commonly referred to as a 'statement' sets out the child's needs and the help they should receive.
- The local authority usually makes a statement if they decide the child either doesn't seem to be making progress under School Action or School Action Plus or needs a lot of extra help (also see 📖 p524).
- The local authority should normally write and tell parents whether they are going to write a statement within 12 weeks of beginning the assessment.
- The statement is reviewed annually; with ongoing parental, school and clinician input to ensure that any extra support given continues to meet the child's needs.

The role of SSS/VI team

- The *vision impairment (VI)* or *sensory support services (SSS)* team comprise a network of teachers for the visually impaired and other professionals (see 📖 p531 and p533) who provide a link between the family and the local educational authority and schools, and provide extra help for the visually impaired child at home and school to achieve their full potential.
- This includes early intervention (see 📖 p59 and p60) for babies with eye conditions to ensure maximum visual activities and stimulation.

Further resources

LOOK: ☎ 0121 428 5038 🖳 http://www.look-uk.org
National Blind Children's Society: ☎ 0800 781 1444 🖳 http://www.nbcs.org.uk
Royal National Institute of Blind People (RNIB): ☎ 0303 123 9999 🖳 http://www.rnib.org.uk
The Partially Sighted Society: ☎ 0844 477 4966 🖳 http://www.partsight.org.uk
The Royal College of Ophthalmologists: 🖳 http://www.rcophth.ac.uk
Vision Aid: ☎ 01942 790 865
Victa Children Ltd. (Information & grants for equipment & aids: ☎ 01908 240 831 🖳 http://www.victa.org.uk
VI Scotland: 🖳 http://www.viscotland.org.uk

Chapter 8

Audiology

As was his language, so was his life.

Seneca, 5 BC–65 AD

Classification and definitions

- *Threshold of hearing*: lowest intensity of sounds an individual can hear.
- Sound pressure levels are measured in decibels (dB, log scale).
- *Audiogram* documents thresholds relative to normal threshold of hearing at 250Hz and 500Hz; 1, 2, 4, & 8kHz (in dB HL, where HL = hearing level).

Frequency Low: <500Hz; Mid: 500Hz–2kHz; High: 3–8kHz.

Severity of hearing impairment

Average hearing level: threshold in better ear at 0.5, 1, 2, 4kHz, averaged
- Hearing impairment (HI) = average hearing level ≥25dB HL.
- Mild: 20–40dB HL.
- Moderate: 41–70dB HL
- Severe: 71–95dB HL
- Profound: >95dB HL
- Deaf: no response >120–125dB at any frequency. Extremely rare.

Audiogram *shape* may be described, e.g.:
- *Low-frequency ascending*: >15dB HL difference from poorer low frequency thresholds towards better high frequencies, e.g. otitis media with effusion (OME).
- *High-frequency sloping*: 15–29dB HL difference (gently) or >30dB HL difference (steeply sloping) between mean of 0.5–1kHz, and mean of 4–8kHz, e.g. sensorineural hearing loss (SNHL).

Type of hearing impairment

(See Fig. 8.1)
- *Conductive*: outer/middle ear. Bone conduction (BC) thresholds normal, with average air–bone gap of ≥15dB.
- *Sensorineural*: inner ear/cochlear nerve. Average air–bone gap <15dB.
- *Mixed*: combined conductive and sensorineural components. BC thresholds >20dB HL, and ≥15dB average air-bone gap.
- *Central*: CNS rostral to cochlear nerve.

Other descriptions

- *Asymmetrical*: >10dB HL difference between ears in ≥2 frequencies (average of better ear should be >20dB HL, otherwise = unilateral).
- *Progression*: >15dB HL decline within 10 years in average hearing level.

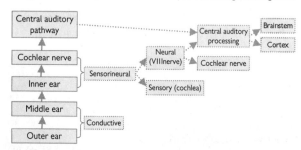

Fig. 8.1 Types of hearing impairment according to anatomical lesion.

Epidemiology of permanent childhood hearing impairment

This section does not include fluctuating impairment due to OME.

Prevalence

- Most common sensory impairment in the developed world.
- Incidence of HI detectable at or soon after birth is ~1–1.5 per 1000 live births in UK (with profound ~1 per 4000).
- ▶Prevalence at primary school age ~3.5 per 1000, increasing with age, plateauing at 9 years. Possible explanations:
  - Some forms acquired after birth.
  - Some milder congenital losses not detected until later.
  - Other inherited causes (AD) present as late onset or progressive.

Risk factors

Joint Committee on Infant Hearing (American Academy of Pediatrics, 2007) outlines 11 risk factors. 3 account for ~40–60% of cases:

- Family history of PCHI.
- NICU admission >5 days, or any of: ECMO, assisted ventilation, ototoxic medications, hyperbilirubinaemia requiring exchange transfusion.
- Craniofacial abnormalities, e.g. external ear, temporal bone anomalies.

Others include:

- Carers' concerns about hearing, speech/language, developmental delay.
- *In utero* infections and postnatal infections.
- Syndromes associated with HI or clinical findings suggestive of these.
- Neurodegenerative disorders.
- Head injury, particularly basal skull or temporal bone.
- Chemotherapy.

Aetiology

In 16–55% of cases aetiology is unknown (most probably genetic).

Environmental causes (acquired) (≤50%)

Prenatal

Congenital infections are commonest acquired cause worldwide.

- *Congenital cytomegalovirus* (CMV): commonest cause of acquired neonatal HI in developed countries. Risk of permanent childhood hearing impairment (PCHI) in symptomatic newborns is 22–65%, in asymptomatic it is 8–10%. May fluctuate, progress or be late onset. Early valgancyclovir may reduce HI.
- *Congenital rubella syndrome* (CRS): largely eradicated in developed world. Reduction in MMR uptake puts women born outside UK at risk of infection in pregnancy. In countries without vaccine, CRS still biggest cause of acquired congenital SNHL.
- *Congenital toxoplasmosis*: ~10–26% of these cases have PCHI.
- *Other congenital infections*: herpes, syphilis, varicella.
- *Maternal drugs*: alcohol, aminoglycosides, quinine, thalidomide.
- *Maternal disease*: diabetes, hypothyroidism.

Perinatal (see 📖 Risk factors p297)

Accounts for up to 27% of children with PCHI. Largest group relates to NICU admission—7-fold risk of PCHI. Unclear whether prematurity is an independent risk factor or due to:
- Low birth weight.
- Kernicterus.
- Severe birth asphyxia.
- Assisted ventilation ≥5 days.
- Infection: severe sepsis, neonatal meningitis.
- Ototoxic drugs.

Postnatal

- *Bacterial meningitis*: most frequent cause of acquired SNHL in childhood (6.5% of all cases). Incidence 7–31% depending on pathogen and other risk factors, e.g. CSF glucose <2.2mmol/L, age <1 month or >5 years. *Strep. pneumoniae* main organism. Often bilateral, severe or profound and rapid onset, but may be unilateral, progressive or fluctuating.
▶ Test early before cochlear ossification occurs to maximize chances of implantation. Early steroids decreases morbidity.
- *Viral infections*: measles, mumps, rubella, meningitis, HSV, VZV, HIV.
- *Otitis media*: uncommon cause of PCHI in developed world, but may mask underlying SNHL.
- *Ototoxic drugs*: aminoglycosides, radiotherapy, loop diuretics, and platinum-containing chemotherapy, e.g. carboplatin.

Genetic causes (>50%)

Huge heterogeneity; mutations in 300–500 genes can cause hearing loss.

Non-syndromic (~70% of genetic deafness)
- AR non-syndromic: ~40% of profound PCHI.
- Up to 50% of AR non-syndromic SNHL due to Connexin 26 gene mutations. Given populations have specific mutant variants.
- Aminoglycoside-induced deafness: screen for A1555G mitochondrial mutation, which increases susceptibility.

Syndromic (~30% of genetic deafness)
>400 syndromes have known association with SNHL.
- Autosomal recessive syndromes:
  - Pendred: bilateral widened vestibular aqueducts ± cochlear hypoplasia (Mondini malformation), plus goitre (older children) or abnormal perchlorate discharge test, commonest form of syndromic SNHL.
  - Usher: pigmentary retinopathy ± vestibular dysfunction, variable phenotype, Types 1, 2, and 3. Commonest cause of deaf-blindness.
  - Others: Alstrom, Jervell and Lange-Nielsen, Hurler, Cockayne.
- Autosomal dominant syndromes:
  - Waardenburg syndrome: types I–IV, with pigmentary abnormalities of hair, iris, skin ± dystopia canthorum.
  - Branchio-otorenal (BOR) syndrome: preauricular pits, and branchial, renal and external ear abnormalities.
- X-linked syndromes: Alport, Hunter, Norrie.
- Craniofacial syndromes associated with conductive hearing loss: Treacher Collins, Stickler, BOR, CHARGE association, Goldenhar.

Screening

Rationale for hearing screening
- Prelingual severe/profound HI incompatible with speech and oral language development; moderate HI may be detrimental.
- Any HI can impact on educational achievement, employment, and social development.
- Early detection and habilitation is cost-effective.

Rationale for newborn screening
(See 📖 p554 for screening)
- Late diagnosis delays speech and language acquisition.
- Sensory deprivation affects neural development.
- Speech and language outcomes better if aided <6 months.

Background

Health visitor distraction test
- Poor sensitivity (10–20% of congenital losses detected), poor specificity.
- Average age of identification >2 years (too late), and very costly.

Targeted newborn hearing screening
- Option only where funding or access limited; costlier per child tested.
- Tests a small 'at-risk' group, but in reality achieves <50% identification.
- 'At risk' group: NICU ≥48 hours, family history PCHI, syndromes.

England NHSP (Newborn Hearing Screening Programme)
- Pilots established 2001/2; universal by 2006. Uses objective tests:
  - TEOAEs (transient evoked otoacoustic emissions) on *all* babies: may be absent in first 24 hours of life (ear canal debris). Will miss auditory neuropathy spectrum disorders (ANSD).
  - AABR (automated auditory brainstem response) on babies who *fail*: absent/abnormal in auditory neuropathy and in delayed maturation.
- Not all PCHI is present at the time of screening; milder losses missed.
- ▶ Passed NHSP does *not* mean child cannot have HI.
- Early intervention has drawbacks, e.g.:
  - High parental anxiety.
  - 'Delayed maturation' may make audiological certainty difficult.
  - False sense of security if passed.
  - Identification does not mean intervention.

Subsequent screens
- To identify the increased prevalence from 1 (at birth) to 2 (for children aged 9–16 years) per 1000, reactive testing is recommended, if:
  - Parental/professional concern re: hearing or speech development.
  - Recurrent ear infections.
  - Upper airway obstruction.
  - Developmental/behavioural problems.
  - Bacterial meningitis.
  - Temporal bone fracture.
- Continued annual surveillance for children with DS, congenital cleft palate, or craniofacial anomalies.
- School entry screening: 'sweep' test at 0.5, 1, 2, & 4 kHz, with pass level 20–30dB HL.

Principles of testing

Approach to testing

- Battery of tests used to:
  - Assess site of lesion.
  - Follow progression.
  - Monitor effects of rehabilitation.
- Test choice dependent on history and differential diagnosis.
- Consider age and developmental level of child in choosing tests (see Table 8.1, and remember this applies to *developmental* age).
- Quiet, sound-proofed room with no reflective surfaces or lighting that casts shadows which may provide visual clues.

Table 8.1 Schema for applying tests to different aged children

Birth–6 months	6–24 months	24 months–5 years	>5 years
Otoscopy, tympanometry, and acoustic reflexes			
OAEs	OAEs	OAEs	—
—	VRA/DT	Play audiometry	PTA (>7 years?)
ABR/Frequency-specific ABR/ASSR	ABR/Frequency-specific ABR/ASSR	Speech audiometry Toy discrimination test	?+ other tests

Development of auditory behaviour

- 1 year: extreme distractibility.
- 2 years: inflexible attention to concrete aspects of the environment.
- 3 years: flexible, shifting attention control.
- 4 years: child chooses to control his attention.

Testing children with complex needs

- 40% of deaf children have an additional problem, often significant eye problems.
- Behavioural testing preferable—frequency specific information, no need for sedation or general anaesthetic.
- Be flexible:
  - Use of eye deviation instead of head turn (as long as repeatable).
  - Longer sound stimulus.
  - Expect slower/delayed response.
  - Involve carers.
- Modified distraction testing may be best option, utilizing how child typically responds to sound.

Behavioural testing (subjective)

- Cornerstone of testing—information about whole auditory pathway.
- Confirms thresholds obtained using electrophysiological techniques.
- Demonstrates observable response to sound.
- Identifies later onset or progressive loss missed by newborn screening.

Distraction test (DT): 6–18 months

- Child sitting upright on carer's knees, not leaning back against carer.
- Distractor at small table in front captures and releases attention.
- Tester presents frequency-specific stimuli 1m from child's ear at 45° angle behind, e.g. Manchester rattle, warble tones.
- Distractor determines response from head turn or facial expression.

Limitations

- Child may randomly check behind; requires distractor vigilance.
- Beware auditory (e.g. jewellery) or visual (e.g. reflection) clues.
- Sound field tested, therefore only tests hearing of better ear.
- Strict adherence to distances and sound levels necessary for validity.
- Less effective in older children who learn to expect sound from clues.
- Can only screen to 30–35dBA.

Visual reinforcement audiometry (VRA): 6 months–2½ years

- Head turn in response to sound is reinforced with visual reward, e.g. dancing teddies, revolving lights.
- Condition by introducing sound and visual reinforcer together.
- Can test individual ears using inset ear phones, and bone conduction.

Limitations

- After 2–3 years children less motivated by reinforcer; reduce habituation by giving breaks and short duration of reinforcer.
- Ensure correct distance, angled placement of speakers and calibration.

Play audiometry: ≥2½ years

- First condition child to produce play response to sound, e.g. put man in a boat, by modelling this when presenting a moderate level sound.
- Obtain minimum repeatable response level for different frequencies.
- Test individual ears using headphones, and bone conduction.

Limitations

- Younger children may be unable to wait until sound is heard.
- May need to change activity frequently to maintain attention.

Pure tone audiometry: >5–6 years (reliably from 7 years)

- BSA have published standard recommended procedures.
- Dependent on behaviour, attention, and listening skills.
- May need to mask; this requires attention and cooperation.

Speech discrimination tests: ~2½ years and older

- Valid and relevant indicator of functional hearing.
- Toy Discrimination Test (McCormick Toy Test): 7 pairs of similar sounding words, presented alongside various toys that child can identify, e.g. tree/key.
- Manchester junior word list and Manchester picture vocabulary test.

Electrophysiological testing (objective)

- When behavioural tests not possible (too young or challenging to test), to confirm behavioural thresholds or as a screen.
- Non-organic loss.
- Necessary for diagnosis of ANSD.
- Does not tell us whether child can hear.
- May need sedation or general anaesthetic.

Tympanometry

- Important component of test battery at all ages, testing middle ear function.
- Simple, quick, and requires little skill.
- Records compliance of middle ear and tympanic membrane mobility.
- Main system of classification described by Jerger (1970) (see Fig. 8.2).

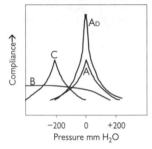

A   normal
A_D disarticulation of ossicular chain
B   middle ear effusion, drum perforation or impacted wax
C   negative middle ear pressure, e.g. after URTI or in OME.

Fig. 8.2 Jerger classification of tympanograms

Acoustic reflexes

- Tests function of auditory system from middle ear to brainstem.
- Stimulation of stapedius muscle contractions in response to loud sounds, ipsilaterally and contralaterally, produces characteristic patterns giving clues to site of lesion.

Otoacoustic emissions (OAEs)

- Weak sound signals of cochlear origin, due to outer hair cell motility.
- Recorded by microphone fitted into ear canal.
  - TOAEs in response to clicks or tone bursts.
  - DPOAEs (distortion-product OAEs) generated on simultaneous presentation of 2 pure tones of different frequencies.
- Highly sensitive, and specific to sensory hearing loss i.e. cochlear.

Auditory evoked responses

Auditory brainstem responses (ABR)

- Electrophysiological response elicited by transient acoustic stimuli (click or tone burst), detected by skin electrodes.

- Waves I–VII generated by areas of auditory pathway from distal auditory nerve (wave I) to cortex.
- Maturation of wave forms occurs with age.
- Necessary to diagnose ANSD.
- Automated ABR (AABR) used in newborn screening and removes need for human interpretation.
- Influenced by conductive hearing loss—all wave latencies increased.

Auditory steady state response (ASSR)

- Electrophysiological response elicited with amplitude and frequency modulated pure tones.
- Can be used to obtain frequency specific objective thresholds, particularly in young children and infants.
- Useful in combination with ABR; should not be used in isolation as non-specific.

Electrocochleography (ECochG)

- Records 3 components via transtympanic needle electrode:
  - Cochlear microphonic (CM) ⎱ originate from inner and outer hair cells
  - Summating potential (SP) ⎰
  - Compound auditory nerve action potential (AP)—distal afferents of cranial nerve VIII.
- Useful as adjunct to ABR in neonates for identification of wave I, which occurs synchronously to AP component of ECochG.
- Valuable contribution to identifying site of lesion in ANSD, i.e. cochlear vs retrocochlear.
- Limited widespread clinical use because requires general anaesthetic in young child.

Cortical electric response audiometry (CERA)

- Arise from rostral regions of auditory CNS, including thalamus, hippocampus, internal capsule, and cortex.
- Identification of central hearing loss in combination with ECochG and/ or ABR.
- Objective assessment of frequency-specific hearing thresholds in older children, particularly disabled.
- Limited application in young children as depends on awake but relaxed state.

Aetiological investigation of PCHI

Rationale
- To answer the question 'Why is my child deaf?'
- Identify associated problems, e.g. visual impairment in Usher syndrome.
- Identify treatable conditions, e.g. congenital CMV infection.
- Prevention of progression, e.g. A1555G mutation.
- Inform prognosis and understanding of natural history.
- Genetic counselling and family planning.
- Plan communication and educational needs, e.g. Usher syndrome.

History
(See 📖 p6)
- Presenting condition: parental concern, onset, progression.
- Associated features or concerns: speech, balance, locomotor delay, irritability, vomiting, tinnitus, infections, headache, visual behaviour.
- Ototoxic drugs, e.g. chemotherapy, loop diuretics, aminoglycosides.

Obstetric history
- *Pre-pregnancy health*: disease, e.g. epilepsy or diabetes, drugs (long-term, abuse), alcohol (how much, when), overseas, conception.
- *Prenatal*: general health, drugs, alcohol, hospital admissions, unexplained fevers, infection contact, blood tests (immunisation, rubella).
- *Perinatal*: gestation, delivery, condition at birth, birth weight, SCBU/NICU, length of stay.
- *Postnatal*: SCBU/NICU (including noise exposure), ventilation, jaundice, infection, haemorrhage, drugs, e.g. loop diuretics, aminoglycosides.

Developmental history
Smiling, communication, vocalization, sitting, walking (vestibular).

Past medical history
Infections, e.g. meningitis, drugs, noise, head injury, ear symptoms.

Family history
- Hearing loss—complete 3-generation family tree.
- Speech/language/learning delay.
- Health issues, e.g. renal disease, autoimmune disease, vision.
- Distinguishing features, e.g. hair (early greying ?Waardenburg syndrome), eyes, teeth, hands, ears, palate.
- Consanguinity (clarify exact relationships).

Examination
(See 📖 p9)
- 'Eyeballing': eye contact, smiling, posture, proportions, obvious dysmorphisms, play, movement, vocalizations, communication.
- Head: shape, hair (any changes?), fontanelles, circumference.
- Face: dysmorphisms, asymmetries, relative sizes.
- Nose: dents, nasal bridge.
- Mouth: size, lip shape, philtrum, palate and teeth.
- Eyes: colour, shape, iris (coloboma?), eyelashes, red reflex, conjugate eye movements, nystagmus, fundoscopy if possible.
- Ears: size, shape, setting (low?), pre-auricular pits, sinuses, and epidermoids, otoscopy looking at ear canal and tympanic membrane.

- Neck: size and shape, pits/sinuses/scars, cysts and swellings (branchial?).
- Trunk: spine, chest, heart position and sounds, organomegaly, skin.
- Limbs: tone, power and co-ordination, proportion, digits, nails, creases.
- Vestibular system: head position and eye movements, and:
  - Babies: Farmer's test, Moro reflex, parachute reflex.
  - Infants and children: rotation (VOR), truncal stability and righting, gait (walking, running, bending), assess on a slope or on foam.
- Observe family including general features, skin, eyes, ears, hands, gait.

Investigations

British Association of Audiovestibular Physicians (BAAP) and British Association of Paediatricians in Audiology (BAPA) have published guidelines (available on their website www.baap.org.uk) for investigation of:

- Infants identified through the newborn screening (2008).
- Severe to profound permanent hearing loss in children (2008).
- Bilateral mild to moderate permanent hearing loss in children (2009).
- Children with permanent unilateral hearing loss (2009).

Level 1 investigations (must do):

- Urine dipstick (haematuria, proteinuria, e.g. Alport syndrome)[a]
- Urine testing for CMV DNA PCR, or serology >1 year[ac]
- Hearing thresholds in 1st-degree relatives.[ac]
- MRI of inner ears and internal auditory meati (CT if clinical evidence to suggest abnormality of petrous temporal bone, or conductive loss).[b]
- Connexin 26/30 mutation testing (isolated sensorineural hearing loss).[b]
- Ophthalmic opinion, e.g. retinopathy, cataracts, chorioretinitis.[ac]

Level 2 investigations (consider, depending on history and examination):

- Referral to clinical geneticist, e.g. consanguinity, syndromes.
- Vestibular investigations, e.g. motor delay, fluctuation or progression.
- m.1555 A>G mitochondrial mutation, e.g. history of aminoglycosides.
- Pendrin, e.g. FHx of thyroid disease, or goitre.
- ECG, e.g. sudden death in family, Jervell and Lange-Nielsen syndrome (long QT)—caution interpretation in neonates; needs repeat after 4 months.
- Serology, e.g. maternal history: CMV, rubella, syphilis, e.g. history of tick bites or trip to endemic area such as New Forest: Lyme disease.
- Renal ultrasound, e.g. external ear anomalies, Mondini defect on MRI.
- Referral to developmental paediatrician, e.g. developmental delay.
- Haematology, though unlikely to provide a cause for hearing loss.
- Thyroid function, e.g. Pendred syndrome (dysfunction usually later life).
- Renal function, e.g. Alport syndrome, Alstrom syndrome.
- Immunology tests/autoimmune, e.g. FHx.
- Metabolic tests, e.g. in context of developmental delay.
- Clinical photography, e.g. any dysmorphic features.
- Chromosomes, e.g. dysmorphisms, consanguinity, developmental delay.
- Urine test including organic and amino acids.
- Guthrie neonatal blood spot, e.g. positive CMV serology of older child.

a. All these are also Level 1 for mild/moderate hearing loss.
b. Also strongly recommended as Level 1 for moderate losses.
c. Level 1 for unilateral hearing losses; also consider Level 2.

Middle ear disease

Causes of conductive hearing loss

By far the most frequently encountered cause of middle ear disease and conductive hearing loss in children is otitis media with effusion (OME). However, there are other causes:

- Craniofacial abnormalities, e.g. Crouzon, Treacher Collins, Goldenhar, Stickler, Down syndromes.
- Other craniofacial anomalies cause mixed CHL and SNHL, e.g. BOR.
- ME anomalies, often associated with EAC malformations, e.g. microtia.

Definitions

- *Acute otitis media* (AOM): rapid onset, fever, bulging erythematous TM; may be associated with middle ear effusion (MEE).
- *Otitis media with effusion* (OME): fluid in middle-ear cleft without signs of inflammation, may precede or follow a bout of AOM:
  - Otoscopy: fluid levels, bubbles, dull retracted TM.
  - Tympanogram: type B, or type C in early OME.
  - Early on, low frequency loss predominates; later audiogram flattens.

Epidemiology of OME

- Up to 80% of children have had OME by age 4 years (then declines).
- Point prevalence at 2 years is ~20%, and at 5 years is ~15%.
- *Risk factors*: passive smoking, bottle feeding, low socioeconomic group, attendance at nursery, FHx, allergy.

Sequelae of OME

- Mild to moderate hearing loss, often fluctuating, usually mild.
  - Early onset affects language development and speech clarity.
  - Later onset impacts on attention, listening, and concentration.
- Eventually behaviour may be disruptive.
- Prolonged early OME may cause later auditory processing difficulties.
- Balance difficulties (clumsiness and frequent falls) or vertigo.
- *Complications*: TM perforation, tympanosclerosis, ossicular involvement, TM retraction pockets, otorrhoea, cholesteatoma.

Management

At least half of cases resolve within 3 months and 95% within a year (unless there are underlying comorbidities).

- Depends on duration, degree of hearing impairment, and secondary effects, e.g. language development, behaviour, balance problems.
- If mild loss ≤30dB HL and no secondary problems, recommend watchful waiting for 3 months.
- Otherwise, refer ENT, but caveat: grommets give short-term benefit but no clear long-term benefit for language, behaviour, or cognition.
- Advice: appropriate seating position in class, ensuring eye contact.
- No evidence for oral or nasal steroids, antibiotics, antihistamines, or decongestants, and these may cause harm.
- Purpose-manufactured autoinflation nasal balloons may help.
- Consider hearing aids as alternative to surgical management.

Neural and central hearing loss

Encompassing hearing dysfunction arising in inner hair cells, VIIIth nerve or CNS connections, also described as 'retrocochlear hearing disorders'.

Auditory neuropathy spectrum disorders (ANSDs)

- Originally called 'auditory neuropathy'. See Table 8.2 for diagnosis.
- Group of heterogeneous disorders with similar auditory test results:
  - Disordered synchronization of sound with intact pre-neural hearing.
- Audiogram usually 'odd': patients may describe a 'smear' of sounds.
- Difficulties worse with speech than environmental sound.
- Can identify speech sounds, but cannot understand the words.
- Due to abnormalities in auditory nerve or lower part of brainstem.

Table 8.2 Diagnostic criteria for ANSD

Test	Result
ABRs	Absent or severely abnormal
Cochlear microphonics	Normal
Pure tone thresholds	Normal to severe impairment
OAEs/DPOAEs	Normal
Contralateral suppression of OAEs	Absent
Stapedius reflexes	Absent

Aetiology

Largest group will be NICU graduates due to perinatal risk factors. High-risk newborns should therefore have ABRs and/or CMs as well as OAEs.

- *Genetic* causes, e.g. non-syndromal (otoferlin gene, delayed maturation), or syndromal: NF2, HMSN, Refsum's, Arnold–Chiari, Usher.
- *Congenital* causes, e.g. asphyxia, RDS, LBW, CP, hyperbilirubinaemia; toxins such as thalidomide.
- *Acquired* causes, e.g. infection: HSV, CMV, basal meningitis; immune: Guillain–Barré, SLE; demyelination; neoplasia; metabolic; vascular.

Auditory processing disorder

- Impaired neural function with poor recognition, discrimination, separation, grouping, localization or ordering of non-speech sounds.
- Does not solely result from deficit in attention, language, or cognition.
- Estimated to affect ~5% of school-aged children.
- Diagnosis incorporates interaction between hearing and listening.
- Comorbidity common: learning, speech, language, attention and/or reading difficulties, e.g. dyslexia (see 🔲 p147), ADHD (see 🔲 p126), ASD (see 🔲 p107), FASD.
- Cause usually unknown, but includes neurological disorders, e.g. Moyamoya; maturational delay, e.g. auditory deprivation (OME6).
- Difficulties understanding sounds when listening to speech, reading, remembering instructions, staying focused while listening and difficulties hearing in noisy places despite normal hearing thresholds.
- Tests: spectral discrimination, temporal resolution, binaural interaction.
- Managed with hearing training programme plus educational advice.
- See websites 🕸 http://www.apduk.org and 🕸 http://www.ihr.mrc.ac.uk.

Balance and vestibular disorders

Structure and function of the vestibular system

Vestibular labyrinth comprises: 3 semicircular canals (detect rotation), utricle, and saccule (otolith organs, which detect static head motion with respect to gravity, head tilt, and linear acceleration). Primary functions:

- Orientation of the body with respect to gravity.
- Balanced locomotion and body position.
- Gaze stabilization during head movements.

Control of balance requires:

- Visual input.
- Proprioception.
- Graviceptor input from muscle, joints, tendons.
- Labyrinthine input.
- Central cortical and cerebellar functions.
- Musculoskeletal system.

Epidemiology of vestibular deficit

- True prevalence difficult to estimate; 'balance problem' is non-specific.
- Vertigo or dizziness is reported in 8–14.5% of school children in surveys, but fewer consult doctors.
- 30–40% of deaf children have vestibular hypofunction (higher in profoundly deaf).

Commonest causes of vestibular dysfunction (apart from hearing loss):

- Migraine: prevalence 2.7–10%, causes 25% of episodic vertigo (see 📖 p235).
- Benign paroxysmal vertigo of childhood (BPVC): brief vertiginous episodes 1½–5 years, causes up to 20% of vertigo.
- OME (see 📖 p306).
- Cranial trauma.
- Other causes include: ophthalmological problems, ototoxicity, vestibular neuritis, labyrinthitis, epilepsy (see 📖 p240), episodic ataxia, toxic, psychogenic, auto-immune disease, and rarely (importantly) posterior fossa tumours.

Impact of vestibular dysfunction

- Poor gaze stability affects reading.
- Motor delay impedes exploration, learning, social integration.
- Repeated vertigo episodes can cause anxiety and school absence.

Presenting history

- Imbalance plus delayed gross motor skills (sitting, walking), *or*
- Episodic dizziness/vertigo, suggested by:
  - Suddenly cries out, drops to floor, crawling or clinging to parents.
  - Pallor, sweating, vomiting, screaming.
  - Child lies very still, face down, eyes closed, wedged against cot side.
  - Descriptions like: world going round, sky falling.

Vestibular examination

Neurotological examination

- Eye movements: range of ocular motility, strabismus, cover test.
- Spontaneous nystagmus: 30° (not more) right and left, up and down.

▶ Vertical and direction-changing nystagmus → urgent neuroassessment.
- Smooth pursuit: symmetry, broken or not, e.g. neurological lesion.
- Saccades: over/undershoot, e.g. brainstem or cerebellar lesions.
- Optokinetic nystagmus (using rotating drum): asymmetry indicates central vestibular abnormality.
- Halmagyi head thrust: short sharp head acceleration through small arc, holding child's head, asking them to fixate in distance. Tests vestibulo-ocular reflex. Unreliable <5 years.
- Dynamic visual acuity: read Snellen chart with head still, then oscillating sideways: deterioration of ≥3 lines indicates bilateral vestibular failure.
- Hallpike manoeuvre for positional vertigo/nystagmus.

Assessment of postural control
- Observation of posture, stance, gait, and coordination during play.
- Hop, kick ball, walk downstairs. Unable to look around when running.
- Righting reflexes, stance, gait (Romberg's and Unterberger's tests in children >4 years).
- Standing on foam mattress, eyes closed.
- Heel-toe walking: peripheral vestibular disorder may veer to one side.

Examination of a neonate
- Muscular tone: vestibular areflexia results in floppiness with good kick.
- Moro (≤6 months): tests utricular function.
- Farmer's test (≤6 weeks): hold baby in outstretched arms facing tester, rotate them around. Eyes open and deviate in direction of rotation. Tests semicircular canal function.

Vestibular testing
Dependent on age, cooperation, and operator patience and sensitivity. Lack of normative data for children. Visual motor skills mature in teens.
- Caloric testing: 'gold standard' for peripheral vestibular lesions.
- Rotational testing (sitting on parent's lap).
- VEMPs (vestibular evoked myogenic potentials): assess otolith function.
- Posturography: functional balance assessment, not a vestibular test.

Management and compensation
- Management involves facilitation of compensation, i.e.:
  - Correct visual deficit.
  - Avoid vestibular suppressants (e.g. cinnarizine, cyclizine) except in very short term; they interfere with compensation.
  - Psychological health.
  - Physical exercise, ideally customised exercise programme delivered by physiotherapist + supervision, or Cawthorne-Cooksey exercises.
- Compensation for stable unilateral losses is highly efficient.
- *Other factors affecting compensation*: impaired proprioception and musculoskeletal function, autonomic symptoms, inadequate or inappropriate CNS activity, e.g. cerebellar damage, head injury, medical or psychological co-morbidity, fluctuating dysfunction, e.g. migraine, OME.
- Advice regarding potentially dangerous situations, e.g. swimming in the dark or underwater, running in the dark or on uneven ground.

Amplification

Aims of amplification

- *Rehabilitation*: facilitates communication, aims to ↓ or compensate for post-lingual HI; *Habilitation*: for HI present at birth, or prelingual.
- Aim to identify loss and commence habilitation by 6 months of age.
- Amplify speech so that it is audible, intelligible and comfortably loud.
- Babies amplified <6 months have better outcomes; no age too young.

Principles of hearing aid fitting

- Stability of the hearing aid (HA) is dependent on the quality of ear mould (good ear impression) and feedback management system.
- Materials for ear mould: silicone better for babies and young children as softer and less feedback, acrylic for older or milder losses.
- Power of HA dependent on level of HI, e.g. ≤60dB HL → medium power, 60–80dB HL → high powered, >80dB HL → super powered.
- SNHL/mixed: non-linear, selective amplification (frequency specific).
- CHL: may need only linear amplification with no digital processing.

Digital aids vs analogue

- ≥95% of HAs fitted in the UK are digital; children rarely have analogue.
- Microphone and receiver convert sound to electricity to sound.
- Digital HAs covert signal to numerical form before processing it.

Advantages of digital HAs

- Feedback cancellation/reduction.
- Noise reduction/attenuation.
- Increased signal to noise ratio (SNR) due to directional or dual microphone.
- Can have different amplification strategies within the same HA.

Commoner types of hearing aid

- Behind-the-ear (BTE): by far most popular for infants/young children as more reliable, less feedback, easier FM compatibility.
- In-the-ear (ITE): cosmetic appeal, better for milder loss (feedback).
- Bone conduction: CHL or mixed losses with multiple aetiologies, e.g. atresia, ossicular abnormalities, malformations.
- Bone-anchored hearing aid (BAHA): permanent alternative to BC aid.
- Middle ear implantable HAs: SNHL and mixed losses with microtia, intractable feedback or allergic reactions to moulds.

Process of hearing aids provision

Audiological assessment (aim to obtain ear specific thresholds, air and bone conduction) → selection of HAs and ear moulds → fitting → verification → evaluation to assess functional benefit to child (not easily predicted) → validation → HA orientation and counselling → HA follow-ups.

- Prescription targets generated from behavioural thresholds (≥6m).
- Generally good correlation between ABR and behavioural thresholds (except in ANSD), where behavioural testing not possible.

Selection of HAs is multifactorial, should not simply fit the audiogram and may require trial and error approach and constant re-evaluation.

Cochlear implants

What is a CI?

- Electronic device designed to replace the inner ear.
- Provides the profoundly deaf with access to hearing sensations.
- Electrode array implanted into cochlea stimulates auditory nerve fibres.
- Implant package secure in mastoid bone under the skin.
- Externally worn microphone and speech processor.
- For child who obtains little/no benefit from conventional amplification.

Specialist multidisciplinary team comprises: Consultant audiological physician (not all teams), consultant ENT, audiological scientist, specialist SLT, teachers of the deaf (ToD), clinical psychologist, and admin.

Children considered

- *Post-lingually deafened*, ≥3years, e.g. meningitis, head injury, cytotoxic drugs.
- *Pre-lingually deaf*, e.g. born deaf, postnatal illness in first 2 years of life.
- ▶▶ Meningitis causes labyrinthitis ossificans: refer *urgently* to enable CI.

Factors important in assessment predicting use and success

- *Age* (pre-lingual loss): ideally ≤2 years; >4 years gain little benefit.
- *Duration of deafness* (post-lingual and progressive losses): ideally <5 years; ≥8 years of great concern.
- *Anatomy and radiology*: very abnormal CT/MRI, e.g. complete ossification, or very abnormal middle ears, will be a challenge or unsuitable.
- *Medical issues*: do these affect a child's potential to use a CI?
- *Audiological results*:
  • Aided levels: should be >50–60dB(A); <40–45dB(A) is too good.
  • Unaided levels: >100dB HL get most benefit; <85dB HL too good.
- *Functional hearing*: consistency with audiological results important.
- *Use of hearing aids*: wearing HAs for 50% of waking hours (ideally all).
- *Communication skills*: consistent with type/time of HI or delayed?
- *Cognitive/non verbal skills*: is there severe general or specific delay?
- *Behaviour*: major behavioural problems impact ability to use CI.
- *Other vital factors*: family support and commitment, parental/child expectations, educational environment, availability of local SLT and ToD, child's learning style, ease of access and record of attendance.

Switch on and mapping

- 'MAP' is individual listening programme stored in speech processor.
- Set up gradually on an individual basis over a number of sessions.
- A great deal of intensive regular post-implant habilitation is needed.

Some other points to remember

- Critical period for speech acquisition between 18 months–3 years.
- Ethical dilemma and sensitive discussion for children born to Deaf signing parents in Deaf community reluctant to 'cure' their child.
- A child with a CI will always be a deaf child not a hearing child.
- Optimum age of implant for prelingually deaf child is probably ASAP.
  ❶ *But* potential for later unpredictable comorbidities, e.g. autism.
- Increasingly children with complex needs are receiving CIs; benefit may be limited but of functionally significant value.

Education and communication options

The listening environment

Speech perception is a developmental skill; all children need higher level of audibility and signal-to-noise (S/N) ratio to perceive speech than adults. Several factors impact on achievement of clear speech signal:

- Reverberation, e.g. plaster ceilings & walls, linoleum, high ceilings.
- Background noise (more importantly, S/N ratio), e.g. heating, traffic, fish tank, chatter. Worse for EAL children, and HI (incl. unilateral).
- Reverberation and poor S/N ratio have synergistic negative effect.
- Distance from speaker and whether the speaker is facing the listener.

Assistive devices

- Enhance speech signal for face to face communication, e.g.:
  - Hardwire system for classroom with group of HI children together.
  - Loop system more of use at home, cinema, or public spaces.
  - FM system: microphone worn by teacher, receiver worn by child.
- Can be used with CI and HAs, gives clear advantage in speech perception, listening behaviour and enhances S/N ratio.
- Soundfield systems act like public address, with loudspeakers.
- Emerging wireless technologies in use and under development.

Choices in education

Teachers of the Deaf (ToD)

- Crucial role in every aspect of HI child's development, management, education, including comorbidities and planning in school.
- Qualified teacher with mainstream experience, plus postgraduate masters/diploma in Audiology and Deaf Education.
- Manage transitions, HAs, CI and work with families, nurseries, schools.

School choices

- Local mainstream with intervention from advisory ToD ± SSEN: local, good speech models, may be poor access to ToD, acoustics, isolation.
- Mainstream school with, e.g. DRB (Deaf Resource Base), PHU (Partial Hearing Unit), HIU (Hearing Impairment Unit): ToD on site, hopefully good awareness, acoustics and support in class (including signed).
- School for the Deaf: small classes, often 'deaf plus' (i.e. other difficulties), SLT on site, good acoustics, deaf peer group, but may be far from home, isolated from hearing world, poor speech models.

Communication options

- Bilingual/British Sign Language (BSL): dynamic complex language in its own right; promotes +ve Deaf identity, but big commitment for family.
- Total communication, e.g. SSE (Sign Supported English), with integration of spoken and signed codes; flexible but difficult for child to focus.
- Oral-Aural and Auditory-Oral: uses residual hearing to maximum, appropriate spoken language experience, with or without lip reading.

Speech and language development

Requirements for normal language development

- Clear speech models by enthusiastic competent language users.
- Opportunities to hear, read, use, and practise; conversation, songs, TV.
- Clear explanations, definitions and support and encouragement.

Normal sequence of language development

(See 📖 p52)

- *Pre-canonical* stages (0–6 months) characterized by crying, cooing, and gooing, then vocal play, e.g. raspberries, squeals, growls, shouts.
- *Canonical* stages involve babbling (7–8 months), e.g. bababa, then reduplicated and variegated babbling (7–12 months), e.g. baba, babi.
- *Lexical* stages:
  - 12–18 months: single words, up to 50% intelligible.
  - 18–20 months: vocabulary spurt, rapid ↑ after 50 words acquired.
  - ~24 months: syntactic spurt, expansion of 2 word utterances.
  - 24–28 months: growth of grammatical morphemes, e.g. –ing, -s, the/a.
  - ~36 months: complex sentences with linking words.

Typically developing children often vary by ~6 months.

Factors affecting impact of HI on communication

- Type, degree, and stability of loss and aetiology.
- Ages at onset, diagnosis, and aiding.
- Consistency of aiding and acceptance of loss.
- Therapy/support, parent–child interaction and communication mode.

Effects of deafness on speech and language development

- Altered voice quality and reduced intelligibility.
- Reliance on gesture, visual cues, eye contact, body and facial expressions.
- Understanding of pragmatics (social use, context), semantics (meaning).

Conductive hearing loss

- Difficulties with attention and listening: fluctuating, tune out, tiredness.
- Speech delay, difficulties with phonological awareness and literacy.
- Language delay more likely to be longer term expressive, and may go on to develop APD features (see 📖 p307).

Mild HI may cause mild speech production and volume difficulties. Moderate HI may result in delayed language development, phonological processing, speech sound acquisition and subtle resonance, volume, pitch range and voice quality changes.

Severe and profound hearing loss

Speech perception, production and language skills significantly affected:

- Word endings missed, consonant/vowel discrimination.
- Phonological and phonetic errors, intelligibility variable; volume, quality, pitch, rhythm, intonation, rate may all be affected.

Role of speech and language therapist

(See 📖 p200)

- Identify communication skills; relate this to level of speech perception.
- Aid with differential diagnosis, monitor progress, plan and evaluate intervention, contribute to IEP or SSEN (see 📖 p524).

Psychosocial impact of hearing loss

Long-term implications
- Hearing impaired people are 3 times more likely to be out of work; those with hearing impairment and a speech problem are 8 times more likely.
- Psychological difficulties including low self-esteem, depression (see 📖 p350) and anxiety (see 📖 p354) are 2.5 times more common than in the hearing population.
- Initial diagnosis of a deaf child may be akin to bereavement or loss and trigger grieving process for parents and family.
- Psychological issues may underlie problems with compliance and attendance (see 📖 p375), poor hearing aid use, difficulties with testing.
- Evidence that difficulties limited to deaf children of hearing parents.

Education issues
- Most HI children are educated in mainstream schools where awareness about deafness may be patchy, with lack of similar peer group.
- Children may feel 'different', especially those with hearing aids.
- May be more bullying and teasing (see 📖 p342) in mainstream schools.
- Lack of access to Deaf community compared to Deaf schools or DRB.

Development of social skills
- Heavily dependent on a common language amongst peers, e.g. turn taking, understanding the rules of games.
- Difficulty keeping up with speed of conversations, understanding semantics and pragmatics, humour, laughing at wrong time, missing jokes.
- Delayed theory of mind skills in deaf children of hearing parents.
- All these may lead to social isolation.

Risk factors for psychological difficulties
- Lack of communication skills in child and between parents and child.
- Additional other disability, particularly ADHD (see 📖 p126).
- Poorer cognitive performance.
- Parental attitude: an insurmountable trauma or manageable challenge?
- Negative attitudes towards deafness in the family.
- Parental guilt, sadness or unrealistic expectations.
- Early diagnosis through NHSP (see 📖 p299) can affect bonding through grief at loss.
- Late diagnosis can also make adjustment very difficult.
- Baby's behaviour due to HL may affect attachment (see 📖 p346) and parenting style (see 📖 p371).
- Over protectiveness and difficulties boundary setting.

The Deaf community
- Medical model of deafness views it as an impairment thereby causing handicap and disability.

- In the Deaf community, it is a positive attribute; hearing loss in itself is not a disability as sign language enables equally free communication.
- Provides peer support, clear cultural identity and role models.

Successful parent child interaction, language development (be it sign or spoken), positive parenting, strong sense of identity and self-esteem, peer group and type of schooling, are all key features important in either protecting against or increasing risk of psychological difficulties.

Further resources

Deafblindness Sense: ☎ 0845 127 0060 🖅 http://www.sense.org.uk

Deaf Education through Listening & Talking (DELTA): ☎ 0845 108 1437 🖅 http://www.deafeducation.org.uk

Hereditary hearing loss homepage (for up-to-date overview of genetics of hereditary hearing impairment for professionals): http://hereditaryhearingloss.org/

Information for parents and professionals: 🖅 http://www.deafnessresearch.org.uk

National deaf children's society (NDCS) (for parents and professionals; all parents should be pointed in this direction): ☎ 0808 800 8880 🖅 http://www.ndcs.org.uk/

RNID: ☎ 0808 808 0123 🖅 http://www.rnid.org.uk

Mental health

The moon moves slowly, but it crosses the town.

African proverb

Introduction

Community paediatric teams and primary care professionals play a vital role in recognizing, evaluating, and managing a significant proportion of mental illness in children. Mental disorders are common in children and adolescents with a mean overall prevalence of 15.8%. Rates in general paediatric clinics have been reported to be as high as 28%. The majority of mental health problems are long-standing, often lasting >1 year, yet it is estimated that half of these children receive no professional help. Professionals need to be able to recognize mental illness, understand the nature and severity of the disorder, and know when to refer to specialist services.

The assessment of mental health in children can be challenging.
- Multiple environmental and psychosocial factors contribute to the child's presentation and parents, family, friends, and school may need to be involved in the assessment and treatment plan.
- The child's symptoms and response to stress must be interpreted in the context of the child's age and development level to avoid the risk of mislabelling normal behaviour as pathological.
- Children's symptoms can be transient, appear to lack the severity necessary for a diagnosis, and they frequently present with a range of symptoms which may either meet the diagnostic criteria for several conditions or not fit neatly into any categorical diagnostic system (ICD-10, DSM-IV). Comorbidity is common.

Despite these challenges the early recognition of problems and timely intervention can prevent and relieve a significant amount of suffering for both children and their families.

Working with child and adolescent mental health services

CAMHS structure

In the UK, service delivery is arranged in a tiered approach. Increasing complexity of mental illness is associated with a higher tier. Professionals are 'gatekeepers' for higher tiers. Higher tiers provide consultation to lower tiers.

- Tier 1: GP, health visitors, social services, school nurses, voluntary agencies.
- Tier 2: professional groups working as individuals: community paediatricians, clinical and educational psychologists, social workers, psychotherapists.
- Tier 3: 'Specialist CAMHS' (spCAMHS) multidisciplinary team, often includes: psychiatrist, psychologist, family therapist, mental health nurse, primary mental health worker, OT, child psychotherapist, social worker, dietician.
- Tier 4: highly specialized services: inpatient units, day services, intensive outreach and other specialist services: forensic, neuropsychiatry, LD.

UK mental health services use a 'Care Programme Approach' (CPA) to assess health and social needs, and formulate a care and risk management plan. A team member takes responsibility as 'care coordinator', providing the principle source of contact/liaison with the family and other agencies. Regular reviews occur (usually 3–6 months) and professionals involved in child's and families care may be invited to attend or copied into CPA review documentation.

Working with spCAMHS

- Meet the local psychiatric consultant/team at least once!
- Consider regular meetings: review cases that have physical and mental health needs, feedback on consultations for each other, agree referral pathways (particularly for emergency/urgent cases), review areas of good practice/need for improvement, and review overlap/division of labour, e.g. ASD/ADHD assessment and management.
- Regular communication prevents 'splitting' by parents.
- Consider joint paediatrician and psychiatrist clinics.
- Encourage paediatric and psychiatric trainees to sit in on clinics.
- Joint research and audit.

Referrals to spCAMHS

- Ideally there should be a local policy document regarding the nature and the severity of conditions seen by specialist CAMHS.
- Discuss the case with spCAMHS if uncertain whether to refer.
- Parents can feel that they have 'failed' if a psychiatric referral is required, so 'framing' the referral is important.
- Ensure the family understands the reasons for the referral and obtain assent.
- Consider the motivation of the family—poorly motivated parents may not engage with an assessment or treatment.

- Include what the child and parents want/expect from CAMHS in the referral information.
- Community spCAMHS time scale for assessments: 'emergency' within 24 hours, 'urgent' within 7 days, 'routine', within 4 weeks (often longer).

The psychiatric evaluation

Reviewing a child's mental health is a potentially time consuming but extremely beneficial intervention. When obtaining a psychiatric history the focus should be not only defining the current difficulties but assessing for other comorbidities for the child and family, conducting a mental state examination and formulating a treatment plan.

▶ History taking should be a cathartic and therapeutic intervention.

General approach

- Ask the family to introduce themselves.
- Use an initial period of 'unstructured' conversation as a 'warm up' focussing on engagement and observing the child, family and their interaction. Begin with neutral topics (hobbies, friends, school, pets).
- Family members may want you to 'side' with their opinion—adopt a neutral stance.
- Use active listening (brief summaries and paraphrasing to check understanding, use body language to convey attention, reduce interruptions).
- Spend individual time with the child.
- Outline the limits of confidentiality with older children and adolescents.
- Use single questions and language appropriate for the developmental level of the child.
- Age of child will influence approach with greater emphasis on drawing and play for children <6 years.
- Use drawings or pictures of emotional faces in books for children struggling to express themselves.
- Reference to a 3rd party ('I knew a boy who …') when children are struggling to express their worries.

Presenting complaint

What are the child's and family's understanding of the reasons for the referral? What would they like to get out of the session?

Problem:
- Antecedents, onset, duration and severity.
- Circumstances: pervasive/specific situations? Explore 'exceptions': what is different about those times when the problem is less prominent?
- Consequences: degree of emotional distress, social/academic functioning, family relationships, impact on development.
- Explore any global statements by obtaining specific examples of behaviour—when did that happen last? Tell me about that?
- What strategies have the child and family utilized to tackle the problem? What has been helpful?
- Review current support: friends, school counsellor, teacher, youth worker, extended family.

Review of other symptoms

Emotions

- Family may be unaware of the extent of the child's distress.
- Worries, fears, anxiety, depression, and somatization (abdominal pain, headaches).
- Suicidal ideation (have you ever felt so bad that you wanted to run away/end it all?).

Conduct

- Oppositional/defiant behaviour, lying, empathy, destructiveness, aggression (threats, verbal, physical, bullying).
- Do you ever get into fights at school?

Screen/review other problems

- Current level of functioning not covered in the presenting compliant.
- School: academic level and progress, motivation, special educational needs, bullying, relationship difficulties, school refusal/truancy, behavioural problems.
- Cognitive: memory, attention, concentration.
- Activity level, self-care, diet, exercise, sleep, play.

Past psychiatric history: previous diagnosis, duration and impact of interventions. Traumatic events, abuse and neglect.

Past medical history

Developmental history (see 📖 p6)

Family history: genogram, quality of relationships, family stresses and life events, family history of mental illness and current treatment.

Social history: housing, recent geographical moves, employment, social services input.

Alcohol, substance use and forensic history: assault, theft, fire setting, cruelty to animals, police involvement, youth offending service support.

Premorbid behaviour/personality

Future

- Hopes and aspirations in the short and long term.
- Hypothetical questions: if the problem went away what would you be doing? How would you know things had improved? What would other people see?
- 3 wishes/magic wand question.

▶ Always review the child's strengths: what strengths can the child and the family identify? How does the child react to their parent's comments?

Rating scales to explore generalized psychiatric symptoms or specific areas.

Observing the child

The Mental status examination (MSE) provides a systematic and structured approach for recording observations of the child.

Mental status examination

Appearance and behaviour

- Physical appearance, dysmorphic features, nutritional status, bruises, injuries, clothes (clean, unusual).
- Social responsiveness: shy, withdrawn, disinhibition, friendliness, reciprocity, rapport, can you 'connect' with the child?
- Interaction with carers: warmth, affection, ease of separation and reaction on reunion.
- Aggression, non-compliance, impulsivity.
- Nature of play: concrete, imaginary, main themes (e.g. loss, sexualized, violent, death), age appropriate.
- Non-verbal communication: eye contact, gestures, posture.
- Motor: hyper/hypo-activity, fidgeting, mannerisms, tics, stereotypies, gait, fine and gross motor difficulties.

Speech

Rate, rhythm, volume, prosody, immediate and delayed echolalia (repetition of phrases), neologisms (made up words). Appropriate for developmental level? Ability to 'chit-chat'/maintain reciprocal conversation.

Mood and affect

Subjective and objective mood, symptoms of depression (↓ energy, sleep, appetite, concentration, self-esteem and loss of interest in hobbies), range and appropriateness of affect.

Thoughts

- Content: view of self, world and future; preoccupations, fears, phobias, obsessions, compulsions and delusions (fixed, firmly held belief out of keeping with person's culture, content, e.g. persecutory, grandiose), fantasies, suicidal ideation and hopelessness.
- Form: poverty, flight of ideas (racing thoughts).

Perceptions

abnormalities in auditory, visual, and other sensory modalities. Types: altered perceptions—external object present, e.g. illusions and false perceptions—no external object present, e.g. hallucinations (occur in external space) and pseudo-hallucinations (inside head).

Cognition: concentration, orientation, short-term memory.

Insight: recognition of current difficulties and need for treatment, willingness to accept treatment.

Observing the family

- Parent–child interaction: overly close, distant, warm, punitive.
- Parental response to their child's distress. Emotional availability.
- Do the parents set effective limits/boundaries? How does the child respond?
- Problem solving skills during the session.
- Discrepancy between how the parents treat the child and siblings?
- Parental relationship: supportive, conflictual.
- Signs of mental illness in family members.
- Could the family interactions be maintaining the problem?

Summary

Key findings, including relevant 'negatives' that would make a diagnosis less likely. Risk: to self and others including self-injury, deliberate self-harm, aggression, vulnerability, child protection issues.

Psychological aspects of learning disability

1/3 of children with a mild LD and 50–70% of children with a moderate/severe LD (see 📖 p117) have psychiatric diagnoses. Any psychiatric disorder may occur but ADHD (see 📖 p126), ASD (see 📖 p107), stereotyped movement, e.g. rocking, DSH (head banging, biting) (see 📖 p352), and depression are especially common. Full diagnostic criteria may not be met and with increasing severity of LD more emphasis placed on observed behaviour. Children with LD (see 📖 p117) are more likely to experience poverty, social exclusion and adverse life events (maltreatment, physical health problems, bereavement).

Comorbid LD and psychiatric illness increases care-giver/placement strain considerably. Consider a coexisting psychiatric disorder before rationalizing behavioural symptoms as an integral part of the LD.

Factors predisposing to behavioural problems:
- Communication difficulties: speech and hearing impairments hinder understanding and communication of needs → social exclusion (see 📖 Chapter 8: Audiology).
- Non-verbal behaviours, e.g. hitting, self-harm used to attract attention (see 📖 p369).
- Limited coping strategies: receiving adult attention for shouting, aggression reinforces use of such behaviour when faced with a problem perceived as unsolvable.
- Undetected physical illness: e.g. infection, pain, constipation can lead to behaviours such as rocking or hitting painful body part.
- Boredom: self injury may serve to reduce boredom in severe LD.
- Epilepsy: both seizures and antiepileptic medication can worsen behaviour (see 📖 p240).
- Brain damage (mod/severe LD).
- Psychosocial factors (particularly mild LD): bullying (see 📖 p342), abuse, increasing self-awareness of limitations with age all increase risk of low self-esteem, anxiety and depression (see 📖 p350).
- Behavioural phenotypes: Prader–Willi (overeating (see 📖 p404)), Lesch–Nyhan (self injury), fragile X (social anxiety, gaze avoidance) see 📖 p403)).

Medication for behavioural problems

Use sparingly when other management strategies have failed. Very limited evidence base. Most used off licence. 'Start low, go slow', document target symptoms and review regularly. Increased sensitivity to adverse effects: extrapyramidal side effects, neuroleptic malignant syndrome, anticholinergic, worsening cognition with sedative medication or paradoxical disinhibition with benzodiazepines. Fluoxetine and low-dose risperidone can help via anxiolytic effect.

Sleep problems

(See 📖 p168)

Common, often present since infancy. Key factor in family breakdown. Both decreased need for sleep and difficulty falling asleep can occur. Improving sleep can improve behavioural problems. Sleep hygiene is mainstay of treatment. If inadequate, especially in autism, melatonin can be helpful.

Eating disorders
(See 📖 p356)
Pica (ingestion of inedible substances), regurgitation, under- and overeating common. Anorexia rare.

ADHD
(See 📖 p126)
Hyperactive subtype particularly common. Consider child's developmental level when deciding if hyperactivity and ↓ attention present. Symptoms should be present across several situations. Children with LD are more prone to medication side-effects particularly ↓ appetite.

ASD
(See 📖 p107)
Seen in 7.8–19.8% of LD. 66–80% ASD have LD. Behavioural problems are largely mediated through anxiety, often situational and worse at home.

Depression
(See 📖 p350)
Consider depression if new or increasing challenging behaviours particularly in adolescence or in absence of change in environmental factors. Less likely to express hopelessness, low mood. Appetite and sleep often affected (can ↑ or ↓) as are concentration (↓) and pleasure. Selective serotonin reuptake inhibitor (SSRIs) helpful. Adapted CBT may have a role depending on degree of LD.

Anxiety
(See 📖 p354)
In non-verbal children avoidance and agitation may suggest the diagnosis.

Psychosis
Not to be confused with 'self-talk' (common in LD). True psychosis rare. In LD visual and tactile hallucinations more common than complex delusions. Usually associated with ↓ functioning and altered personality. If suspected need EEG and brain imaging.

OCD
(See 📖 p332)
Repetitive actions, e.g. washing, tidying that reduce anxiety. Differentiate from stereotypies (repetitive, non-goal directed, e.g. rocking, hand-wringing).

Further resources
Foundation for people with learning disabilities 🖥 http://www.learningdisabilities.org.uk/
LD online, USA website on learning disabilities and ADHD 🖥 http://www.ldonline.org/

Autistic spectrum disorders: CAMHS aspects

(Also see 📖 p107–16, Pervasive Developmental Disorders)

Children with ASD have higher rates of mental illness and behavioural problems. ADHD (see 📖 p126), anxiety disorders (see 📖 p354), and depression (see 📖 p350) are common. If symptoms of mental illness are significant enough to warrant a comorbid diagnosis then management should follow the standard treatment protocols for the relevant disorder.

Children with ASD often present with clusters of symptoms that do not fit into diagnostic criteria and we will focus on their management in this section. Common difficulties include: aggression, agitation, anxiety, self-injury, repetitive behaviours, behavioural rigidity, sleep difficulties, 'ADHD-like' symptoms.

▶ There are no curative treatments for ASD and many of the interventions aimed at addressing the core symptoms of autism have insufficient evidence to recommend routine use.

Non-pharmacological interventions

Many of the 'generic' behavioural management techniques (behaviour therapy (see 📖 p210) and challenging behaviour (see 📖 p369) will be appropriate. However, the core symptoms of ASD and common coexisting learning disabilities must be taken into account when adapting these techniques.

- Systematically review possible precipitants for the behaviour, including: routine changes, transition from an activity of interest, anxiety, sensory overload, physical discomfort.
- Gather information: have there been changes that parents are unaware of (contact school, carers)?
- Exclude physical causes or exacerbating factors (pain, fatigue, sleep disorders, seizures, menstrual cycle).
- Reduce frustration by enhancing communication: use visual augmentation (pictures) (see 📖 p208).
- Encourage the use of: structured environments, predictable daily routines and consistent responses to behaviour at home and at school.
- Support from special educational services, including opportunities for social skills training at school (see 📖 p524 and p533).
- Parent support: training (see 📖 p371) and support groups for parents and siblings.

Pharmacological interventions

- Use to target specific behaviours that cause significant distress or impairments in functioning and education.
- ↑ risk of side effects and paradoxical effects so 'start low, go slow' and monitor closely.
- Symptoms often return upon discontinuation.
- Evidence supports the use of risperidone and aripiprazole for challenging and repetitive behaviours. Limited evidence to support the use of other medications, although they are frequently used.

Risperidone and aripiprazole
- Use: aggression, tantrums, irritability, repetitive behaviours. May help self-injury, stereotypies, behavioural rigidity, obsessional symptoms.
- Short-term treatment at low doses.
- High likelihood of side effects: weight gain, sedation.

Methylphenidate
- Use: hyperactivity, inattention, impulsivity.
- May ↑ risk agitation, irritability, emotional outbursts and stereotypic behaviour.

SSRIs (citalopram, escitalopram, and fluoxetine)
- Use: repetitive behaviours, anxiety, obsessions. May help depressive phenotype (social withdrawal, crying, reduced energy).
- Side effects: restlessness, insomnia.

Melatonin
- Use: sleep difficulties unresponsive to behavioural interventions.

Benzodiazepines
- Try to avoid as ↓ evidence to support use, potential paradoxical effect (disinhibition) and they are only suitable for short-term use.

Clonidine
- ↓ evidence to recommend routine use but may help hyperactivity, aggression, self-injury, sleep dysfunction.

Refer to CAMHS if there is a high likelihood of comorbid mental illness, or if family therapy or highly structured individual work for older/higher functioning individuals is required.

Asperger syndrome

(Also see 📖 pp107–16, Pervasive Developmental Disorders)

AS is an autistic spectrum disorder (pervasive developmental disorder). First described in 1944 by Hans Asperger the condition was 'lost' until it was rediscovered in the 1980s and incorporated into DSM-IV and ICD-10. AS is differentiated from autism by: lack of clinically significant delay in language development (single words ≤2 years, phrases ≤3 years), normal IQ.

4 main diagnostic classifications: ICD-10, DSM-IV, Gillberg, Szatmari.

✒ AS may be removed from DSM-V, being incorporated into a diagnosis of 'autism spectrum disorder', due to be published 2013.

Clinical features (adapted from ICD-10)

- Onset <3 years.
- No clinically significant general delay in spoken or receptive language or cognitive development.

Qualitative impairments in reciprocal social interaction:

- Impaired non-verbal behaviours (eye-to-eye gaze, facial expression, posture, gesture).
- Failure to develop peer relationships appropriate to developmental level that involve mutual sharing of interests, activities and emotions.
- Lack of social-emotional reciprocity (impaired or deviant response to other's emotions, lack of modulation of behaviour according to social context, weak integration of social, emotional, and communicative behaviours).
- Lack of spontaneous seeking to share enjoyment, interests, or achievements (↓ showing, bringing or pointing out objects to other people).

Restricted, repetitive and stereotyped patterns of behaviour, interests and activities:

- Encompassing preoccupation with one or more stereotyped and restricted patterns of interest (abnormal intensity or focus).
- Apparent compulsive adherence to specific, non-functional routines or rituals.
- Stereotyped and repetitive motor mannerisms (hand/finger flapping or twisting, complex whole-body movements).
- Preoccupations with parts of objects (odour, texture, noise, vibration).

- Prevalence: wide variation in estimates due to differing diagnosis criteria, M > F.
- Aetiology (see Autism 📖 p107).
- Family members—higher risk of ASD phenotype, 2–8% risk in siblings.

Assessment

- Average age at referral AS 47.5 months (autism 30 months).
- Referrals also common after commencing nursery/primary school when social interaction difficulties become more noticeable.
- No pathognomonic sign.
- Development history as for ASD (see Autism 📖 p107).

Enquire about:
- ↓ interest/desire for friendship and inability to initiate or maintain friendships → social isolation; better relationships with younger children and adults.
- Play with others: insist on taking the lead or overly passive.
- Behaviour at parties and when children visit the home—more interested in toys and food than peers?
- ↓ recognition of emotions and viewpoints of others.
- Sensitivities to noise, texture, odours, and taste.
- Motor clumsiness.
- Social rule breaking, e.g. need to always tell the truth.

Look for:
- Subtle speech and pragmatic language impairments—abnormal prosody/inflection voice, formal pedantic language, literal/concrete use of language with ↓ understanding of sarcasm, proverbs and implied intent.
- Content to discuss their topics of special interest.
- Tendency to talk 'at' you rather than 'with' you.
- Impaired 'chit-chat'.
▶ Eye contact, smiling and displays of affection/secure attachment to family members do not exclude a diagnosis of AS.
▶ Features in girls compared to boys: better social skills, areas of interest are less concrete/object orientated and more 'social', e.g. soap operas, celebrities, friends.

Investigations
- Screening and diagnostic tools (see Autism 📖 p107).
- Developmental ± psychometric evaluation for overall level of functioning and discrepancy between verbal and non-verbal performance.
- Physical examination: (see 📖 p9).

Differential diagnosis (Table 9.1)
Comorbidity (1/3 develop mental illness): depression, anxiety, ADHD, tic disorders, dyspraxia, aggression, oppositional behaviour, self-injury.

Table 9.1 Differential diagnosis

Disorder	Differentiating features
ADHD	Able to form, but not necessarily sustain, friendships. Appropriate. non-verbal communication.
Attachment disorder	History of adverse caregiving, improvement in social deficits in response to a more appropriate environment. Imaginative play preserved and lack unusual interests.
Elective mutism	Able to converse appropriately with family, normal non-verbal communication and imaginative play.

(Continued)

Table 9.1 (Continued)

OCD	Obsessions and compulsions are often accompanied by distress, social skills preserved, onset >4 years.
Social anxiety/phobia	Better social interaction with family and as a younger child, no restricted interests. ↓ anxiety with people they know.

Management

- Psychoeducation for child and family.
- Inform school—appropriate educational support and educational psychology assessment if appropriate.
- Support with accepting diagnosis—↑ awareness of difference from peers, bullying.
- Managing social situations—social stories groups at schools, help at home.
- Treat common comorbidity including tics and ADHD.
- Refer to occupational therapy for assessment if hypo/hypersensitivity or difficulties in motor development.
- Behavioural interventions (see 📖 p210).
- Refer to CAMHS if comorbid mental illness.

Prognosis

- Lifelong condition, some improvement with ↑ age.
- Much more likely to live independently, establish a family and to be employed compared to autism.
- Higher IQ improves prognosis.

Further resource

National autistic society: 🕭 http://www.autism.org.uk

Tic disorders

Description of tics

- Rapid, recurrent, non-rhythmic motor movement, or utterance (verbal tic).
- Involuntary, may be suppressed for short periods of time and may be preceded by premonitory sensation.
- Often occur in bouts, wax and wane in frequency and type of tic can vary.
- Precipitants include excitement, anxiety, fatigue and heat.

Classification

- *Simple:* single muscle group—eye blinking, head and shoulder jerks, facial grimacing, grunting, sniffing, throat clearing, coughing.
- *Complex:* multiple muscle groups—repetitive touching, squatting, echopraxia (copying actions), copropraxia (obscene gestures), self-injury, coprolalia (profane verbal tic, 10% TS), echolalia (copying heard phrases), palilalia (repeating own sounds).

ICD-10 classification

- Transient tic disorders, <12 months' duration, 6–20% children.
- Chronic motor or vocal tic disorder, >12 months' duration, 4% children.
- Tourette's syndrome/combined vocal and multiple motor tic disorder, >12 months' duration, 1% children.

Epidemiology

- Onset 4–8 years, 3:1 ♂:♀.
- Simple tics more common and develop earlier than complex tics. Motor tics more common and develop earlier than vocal tics.

Aetiology

- Tics occur in 10–15% 1st-degree relatives.
- Imbalance in dopamingergic system, basal ganglia implicated.
- Possible association with post streptococcal infection autoimmune response (PANDAS).

Assessment

Observe child during discussion of tics (discussion can often precipitate tics). Is there a video recording of the tics?

Explore:

- Onset, triggers, relieving factors, possible tic suppression and tic induced pain.
- Impact on emotional, social, academic and family functioning, especially interference with daily tasks, isolation, stigmatization, bullying and self-harm.
- Tic severity may not correlate with subjective distress.
- Comorbidity ADHD (79%), OCD (50%), depression (see 📖 p350), anxiety (see 📖 p354), learning difficulty (see 📖 p117), sleep disorders (see 📖 p168), conduct disorders, ASD (see 📖 p107).
- Physical examination. Myoclonus (see 📖 p238), dystonias (see 📖 p238), choreas, dysmorphic features, self-injury (see 📖 p352).

Differential diagnosis

OCD (see 📖 p332), ADHD (see 📖 p126), dystonia (see 📖 p238), stereotypies (earlier onset, fixed pattern, rhythmic, no premonitory urge), absence seizures (see 📖 p240).

Management

- Determined by impact on psychosocial functioning.
- Psychoeducation, support groups.
- Avoid caffeine (exacerbates tics).
- Try regular exercise, relaxation techniques, provide safe place in which to tic.
- Practising tics, e.g. before school: deliberate tic repetition for several minutes resulting in tic free period of >1 hour.
- Treat comorbidity.
- Medication: 35–50% tic reduction. Aim to reduce psychosocial impairment. Assess response over several months (tics wax and wane).
  - Clonidine (alpha 2 agonist). Reduces motor tics > vocal tics.
  - Risperidone (atypical antipsychotic). Greater evidence base but more side-effects than clonidine.
  - Alternatives: aripiprazole, haloperidol, atomoxetine (coexisting ADHD).

Prognosis

Average duration 4–6 years. 80% significant reduction in tics by age 18. Poor prognosis associated with comorbidity.

Further resource

Tourettes action, UK charity: 🖰 http://www.tourettes-action.org.uk/

Conduct disorder and oppositional defiant disorder

Definitions

- *CD:* aggressive, persistent, multiple antisocial behaviours that violate societal norms and rights of others, e.g. theft, property damage, physical aggression, cruelty to animals or persons, early/forced sexual activity, truancy, arson. Socialized or non-socialized according to whether the individual is part of a deviant peer group.
- *ODD:* repetitive, persistent pattern of negative, hostile, defiant and disobedient behaviour towards authority figures that is developmentally inappropriate and causes functional impairment. Easily provoked to anger, blame others, spiteful, vindictive.

Epidemiology

- CD: 4–9%, ♂:♀ 3:1, ↑ prevalence in ↓ socioeconomic groups.
- ODD: 1–16%, ♂ > ♀ in young children, ♂=♀ older children/adolescents. Onset usually by 8 years.

Aetiology

(Complex interaction of multiple risk factors especially inherited vulnerability, negative parenting and environmental factors)

- *Biological:* temperament (lack guilt, empathy), dyslexia, learning disability, low IQ, ADHD, CNS disorders, autonomic under-arousal, abnormal prefrontal cortex, prenatal toxin exposure, neurotransmitter abnormalities (serotonin, noradrenaline, dopamine), low cortisol, high testosterone, family history of CD/substance abuse/ADHD.
- *Psychosocial:* parenting style (harsh, inconsistent, ineffective, rejection of child), insecure/disorganized attachment, parental mental illness and substance misuse, family dysfunction, socioeconomic disadvantage, poor social information processing.

Differential diagnosis and comorbidity

ADHD, substance abuse, adjustment disorder, anxiety, depression, developmental disorder, learning disability, psychosis, chronic paediatric illness. ASD (2/3 children excluded from primary school have social and communication problems).

Assessment

- Multiple informants to assess behaviour in different settings (family, school, community, legal system—often low rate of agreement between informants).
- Empathic non-judgemental engagement of the young person to elicit their views and motivation for change.
- Description of current behaviour problems: nature, onset, duration, frequency, context, functional impact.
- Risk assessment if aggressive, sexual behaviour problems.
- Comprehensive history to identify aetiological factors (particularly family history, social history and parenting style and parents response to the behaviours).

- Identify comorbid conditions especially ADHD, substance misuse (very common and can improve symptoms and prognosis if treated).
- Physical examination with attention to neurological factors.
- Psychological assessment and/or review of school reports to assess IQ, language, reading and arithmetic skills.

Management

- Multimodal and multilevel interventions required (child, family, school, community). One-off, short-term, fear inducing treatments ineffective and can be harmful.
- Provide behavioural management advice (see 📖 p210 and p369).
- Parent management training: group based training. Most effective intervention for children < 12 years. *NICE recommends:*
  - Curriculum informed by social learning theory (↓ positive reinforcement of unwanted behaviour, e.g. giving child attention when misbehaving, ↑ positive reinforcement of desired behaviour, selective use of punishment, e.g. time-out, loss of privileges). Reinforcement and punishment should be consistent, contingent and immediate.
  - Individual treatment for families with especially complex needs.
  - Role play in session and homework (apply techniques to home situation between sessions).
- CAMHS input will depend upon local service arrangements and the presence of any comorbid mental illness.
- Child-focused individual interventions are only modestly effective, may not generalize and are less likely to be successful in adolescents. Include: CBT problem-solving skills, anger management, emotional recognition.
- Family therapy: little evidence.
- Pharmacological: only use if psychological interventions inadequate to control severe behaviour, or to treat comorbidity, e.g. stimulants for ADHD, antipsychotics (risperidone) for aggression.
- School based intervention: support for language, cognitive and social deficits. Specialist schools and residential treatments.
- Specialist foster placements for adolescents with chronic CD.

Prognosis

30–50% ODD develop CD. CD persists (40%) into adulthood manifesting as antisocial personality disorder, substance abuse, mood disorders, criminality, interpersonal difficulties, incomplete schooling, unemployment. Poor prognosis: early onset (<10 years), number and severity of behaviours, late treatment intervention, comorbidity (especially ADHD).

Encopresis and faecal soiling

Definition

The passage of normal stool in an inappropriate place in a child >4 years old and not due exclusively to a medical condition except through a mechanism involving constipation (DSM-IV).

Classification

- *Primary:* bowel control never established.
- *Secondary:* independent bowel control achieved for at least 6 months.
- *Retentive:* leads to constipation and overflow incontinence. Some consider this subtype more appropriately termed faecal soiling than encopresis.
- *Non-retentive:* deliberate soiling in inappropriate places. 'True' encopresis and the minority of cases.

Epidemiology

- 3:1 ♂:♀.
- 5% of 4-year-olds, 1-2% of 7-year-olds, and 1% of 11-year-olds.

Aetiology

- *Primary:* learning disability, dyspraxia, poor toilet training.
- *Retentive:* toilet fears/phobia in anxious children especially in public places, poor toilet training, multiple causes of constipation and painful defaecation.
- *Non-retentive:* regression secondary to psychosocial stressors, psychological distress that the child is unable to communicate directly, sexual abuse, conduct issues. There can be inappropriate deposition of faeces and smearing.

Assessment

▶ Very important to exclude an organic cause (anorectal malformations, Hirschsprung disease, neurological disorders, nutritional problem, thyroid disorders, inflammatory bowel disease, medication side effects) by history, physical examination and investigations.

Enquire about:

- Nature and pattern of soiling, antecedents, family reactions, and impact of attempted treatments.
- Environmental influence, e.g. bullying or anxiety about passing stool at school can lead to encopresis only occurring at home.
- Childs attitudes and access to toilets and reasons for avoidance, e.g. fear of monsters in the toilet.
- Developmental age of child.
- Stress or negative life events, e.g. parental separation, birth of sibling, starting school.
- Presence of emotional or psychiatric disorders, e.g. anxiety, phobia, ADHD, oppositional or conduct disorders.
- Presence of regressive behaviour including separation difficulties, clinging.

- Family dysfunction and parent-child conflict (can be cause and effect).
- Secondary low self-esteem, guilt and shame.

Management

- Treat constipation with fluids, dietary fibre, and stimulant and softening laxatives (see 📖 p84).
- Psychoeducation: explain it is a common condition.
- Address specific stressors and social difficulties: both causative and consequences, e.g. to reduce shame child should be able to leave class without asking to.
- Behavioural intervention: cooperation of both parent and child essential. Reduce punitive measures. If accident occurs reassure and help. Praise and reward charts for appropriate passage of stool. Regular post-prandial toileting for 10min without pressure to produce stool. Reading book or toy just for use on toilet.
- Family may require additional support from health visitors or social services to manage behavioural programme.
- Graded exposure and rewards for toilet phobia.
- Family therapy techniques: externalization of the problem as 'Sneaky Poo'. The child and family describe how 'Sneaky Poo' causes them both difficulties, helping to reduce scapegoating, and work together to 'out sneak Sneaky Poo'. Humour is used in this approach. Useful if there is an aggressive (smearing) component to encopresis. See website.

Prognosis

The majority or uncomplicated cases resolve by adolescence. Poorer prognosis associated with non-retentive subtype, significant family or social dysfunction.

Further resources

ERIC (Education and Resources for Improving Childhood Continence) UK children's charity dealing with bedwetting, daytime wetting, constipation and soiling and potty training. ✍ http://www.eric.org.uk/

Heins T, Ritchie K (1988) Beating sneaky poo: ideas for faecal soiling. 2nd Ed. Leaflet free to download ✍ http://www.dulwichcentre.com.au/beating-sneaky-poo-2.pdf

Enuresis

Definition

Repeated voiding of urine into the bed or clothes at least twice per week for at least 3 consecutive months in a child who is at least 5 years old, and not due exclusively to a general medical condition or medication (DSM-IV-TR).

Classification

- Primary enuresis (85%) (never acquired bladder control).
- Secondary enuresis (15%) (achieved bladder control for at least 6 months).
- Nocturnal, diurnal or both.

Epidemiology

- 4-year-olds: 12–25%, 8 year olds: 7–10%, 12-year-olds: 2–3%.
- <12 years old: ♂:♀ 1.5:1, >12 years old: ♂=♀.
- Nocturnal enuresis more common than daytime enuresis.

Aetiology/associations

- Genetic (70% have 1st-degree relative with functional enuresis), learning difficulties, behavioural and emotional difficulties, lower socioeconomic status, institutionalized care, abuse, psychosocial stressors, psychiatric disorder, e.g. ADHD.
- Secondary enuresis is most commonly associated with psychosocial factors.

Assessment

Essential to exclude organic cause of urinary symptoms (UTI, diabetes, constipation, structural abnormality, neurological problem, medication) by history, physical examination, urinalysis etc.

Enquire about:

- Toileting patterns and fluid intake.
- Onset, frequency, timing of wetting, impact of environment change. Keep diary record.
- Sleep and sleeping arrangements.
- Previous interventions, including duration, consistency of approach, and degree of success.
- Impact on the child and family, motivation for change.
- Aetiological factors as previously.

Management

- Psychoeducation and support groups.
- Practical measures: hygiene, mattress protectors, disposable products and changes of clothes.

NICE guidance 2010

Nocturnal enuresis

- Behavioural management: avoid punishment and criticism; reward charts and praise for appropriate fluid intake and toileting during

daytime, utilizing toilet prior to sleep, taking medication or utilizing an enuresis alarm.
- Enuresis alarm: 'bell and pad' sounds an alarm when damp. Slow response but reduced rate of relapse compared to medication. Assess response after 4 weeks. Terminate use after 2 weeks without wetting.
- Medication:
  - Desmopressin (synthetic antidiuretic hormone) : 1st-line medication in children >7 years. Low risk of side effects. Nasal spray, tablet, and melt. Rapid onset of action. Review after 4 weeks. Medication holiday after 3 months to review response.
- 2nd-line medication:
  - Oxybutynin (anticholinergic): short-acting. Elixir or tablet. Can be combined with desmopressin.
  - Imipramine (tricyclic antidepressant with anticholinergic effects): Low dose 3 hours before bedtime. Toxic in overdose so avoid in DSH and depression. Review after 3 months.

Diurnal enuresis
- Psychoeducation, behavioural programme with regular toilet times, bladder re-training.
- Oxybutinin.

Prognosis

Improves with age. Prevalence in 16-year-olds 1–3%. Small proportion will continue into adulthood.

Further resource

ERIC (Education and Resources for Improving Childhood Continence) UK children's charity dealing with bedwetting, daytime wetting, constipation and soiling and potty training. ℬ http://www.eric.org.uk/

Preschool behavioural problems

Behavioural problems while common in preschool children are difficult to classify (due to rapid rate of development between age 0–5) and the vast majority do not meet diagnostic criteria for the conduct, hyperactivity, and emotional disorders seen in older children.

Common problems

- Fears, worries, disruptive behaviour (aggression, tantrums), overactivity, inattention, soiling, sleep problems, eating problems, comfort habits (rocking, head banging, masturbation).
- Moderate/severe behavioural problems seen in 7%, mild in 15%.
- Comfort habits, sleep, appetite and toileting problems usually transient however others may persist. Problems identified age 3 persisted to age 8 in 73% boys and 48% girls.
- A history of preschool fears and worries, overactivity and disruptive behaviour often present in older children with emotional disorders, ADHD, ODD/CD respectively.

Management

Where problems are part of a psychiatric disorder management proceeds as described in relevant chapters. If problems are likely to be transient intervention may be unnecessary. A behavioural modification approach (Management of behavioural problems 📖 p210) is the mainstay of treatment.

Disruptive behaviour

Includes attentional and oppositional problems, ADHD, ODD. Most common problem behaviour in early childhood. ♂>♀ in >3-year-olds. Co-occurrence of ADHD and oppositional problems associated with persistence of problems into adolescence. Aetiological factors: individual factors, e.g. child temperament, ineffective parenting strategies (low quality parent-child interactions, inconsistent/harsh/unresponsive parenting), low quality, high volume day-care, other factors as for conduct disorder (📖 p334).

Sleep disorders

(Also see 📖 p168, sleep disorders and management)
Occur in ~1/3 of 0–3-year-olds. Large spread of normal sleep variations depending on parental attitudes and tolerance.

Insufficient sleep

- Circadian rhythm sleep disorders: causes include chaotic bedtime routine, ADHD, LD. Treatment includes re-establishing appropriate bedtime routine, melatonin.
- Upper airway obstruction: causes include tonsillar hypertrophy, obesity, structural abnormality. Associated with daytime somnolence, ↓ attention.

Parasomnias

- *Night terrors*: child wakes a few hours after sleep onset, afraid, inconsolable, partially or unresponsive to attempts to communicate. Child does not recall the disruption next morning.

- (Nightmares occur later in night, child is consolable, responsive to parent and may recall details on waking). Management: wake child 15min before terror usually occurs. Usually effective within a few nights.
- *Somnambulism* (sleep walking).

Eating/feeding problems

(See 📖 p356)

- *Food refusal:* means of child asserting independence. Multifactorial aetiology, child temperament, parenting skills, family stress, feeding experiences, parental anxiety over poor intake leading to bribes or increased attention and child learning to manipulate parents. Management: eat as a family to remove focus on the child, remove conflict, offer balanced meal and remove without comment if not eaten, praise for eating, reduce intake between meals.
- *Pica:* consumption of non-food items. Seen in autism (see 📖 p107), LD (see 📖 p117), and poor parental supervision (see 📖 p371).

Bullying

Definition

Intentional use of power and aggression that is repeated against another to cause distress or exert control. The power imbalance between bully and victim can be perceived or actual, physical, psychological or social. Bullying can be direct or indirect, physical or verbal.

- *Direct:* hitting, kicking, property destruction, sexual harassment, taunting, name calling.
- *Indirect:* exclusion from a group, manipulation of friendships, spreading rumours, cyberbullying (internet, text messaging).

Epidemiology

Bullying typically occurs at school. Prevalence is highest in boys in primary and early secondary school but decreases in both sexes with age. Boys engage more in physical and verbal bullying and indirect bullying is more prevalent in girls.

Characteristics of children who bully: aggressive, hot temperament, positive attitude to violence, lack empathy, home environment characterized by domestic violence, lack of parental affection and involvement. Antisocial personality disorder or ADHD may contribute to behaviour.

Characteristics of victims of bullying: quiet, anxious, unassertive, low self-esteem, physically weak or disabled, obese, poor social skills, socially isolated (few and poor quality friendships), over-protective/enmeshed family.

Note: there is no one clinical type of bully or victim and some children alternate between the two ('bully-victims' or reactive bullies).

Physical and psychosocial health problems associated with bullying

- Symptoms seen in both bullies and victims:
  - Physical symptoms (headache, stomach ache).
  - Psychosomatic symptoms (difficulty sleeping, bed-wetting).
  - Depression, anxiety, suicidal thoughts.
- Children who bully may misuse alcohol or substances and drop out of school. Victims may demonstrate school refusal or absenteeism and a drop in academic performance. 'Bully-victims' may experience the highest level of pathology.
- Can persist into adulthood.

Screening and assessment

Given the high prevalence, substantial health and psychosocial consequences of bullying and the reluctance of victims to seek help it is important that professionals are attentive to identifying children involved. Appropriate intervention can minimize short- and long-term consequences.

Consider bullying in any child possessing the characteristics of bully or victim just described or who present with the described physical and psychosocial problems. Follow-up with questioning about peer relationships and school functioning:

- Have you ever been bullied? How are you bullied? What about? Where? How often?

- What do you do when others pick on you? Have you ever told a teacher?
- How do you feel when you are bullied?

Frequent and prolonged bullying associated with greater health risks. Screen for psychiatric comorbidity: depression, anxiety, CD.

Children who admit to being bullied must be believed and reassured they were right to report it. Explain the potentially serious consequences to parents and encourage them to take action with school.

Management
- Multidisciplinary: parents, school, and mental health specialists. Essential that all disciplines understand the potentially serious health consequences and need for early intervention.
- Inform school and commence anti-bullying interventions.
- Essence of management is addressing relationship difficulties, e.g. social and cognitive skills training, anger management, assertiveness training and treating psychiatric comorbidity.

Further resources
Anti-bullying network, not-for-profit company: ℘ http://www.antibullying.net/
Parentline Plus, advice to parents regarding bullying: ℘ http://www.familyandparenting.org/ or helpline ☎ 0808 800 2222.

School refusal

Definition and clinical features
- Severe difficulty in attending school associated with emotional distress.
- Presentation varies with age. Children: somatic symptoms (GI, muscular, autonomic), tantrums, self-harm. Adolescents: anxiety and mood disorders (see 📖 p354).
- Onset can be acute or gradual. Refusal can be complete or partial.
- Explicit desire to not attend school, no attempt to conceal non-attendance.
- Willing to complete homework.

▶ Note contrast with truancy: lack school related anxiety, conceal non-attendance from parents, intermittent absence, avoid going home, disinterested in schoolwork (see 📖 p522).

Epidemiology
- Incidence 1–2%. ♂=♀.
- No association with intelligence or socioeconomic level.

Aetiology
- *Predisposing*: separation anxiety, social phobia.
- *Precipitating*: starting new school or following breaks from school (holidays or illness), life events (parental illness or separation, moving home), school fears (bullying, tests, group work, teacher).
- *Maintaining*: fear of explaining absence to peers, 2° gain (access to parent, TV, computer at home).

Assessment
- Frequency and timing of symptoms—present outside school hours?
- School related fears and other aetiological factors.
- Family history of dysfunction (conflict, enmeshment, ineffectual discipline), school absence in siblings, family's response to school refusal.
- Parental anxiety and illness.
- School academic and attendance reports, educational psychologist reports.
- Exclude physical cause of somatic symptoms.
- Tool: school refusal assessment scale-revised

Comorbidity: anxiety disorders, mood disorders, ADHD, learning difficulties, social interaction difficulties.

Differential diagnosis: truancy, child caring for ill parent.

Management
- Take a medical history and conduct a physical examination. If appropriate reassure parents that there is no physical illness.
- Emphasize the benefit of early reintegration to school. A coordinated, consistent approach involving the child, both parents and school is essential. Identify a teacher to assist with liaison.

Behavioural approaches
- Reduce incentives to remain at home (computer, TV, no homework) and reward attempts to attend school. Escort child into school to be met by an identified teacher.
- Rapid return (flooding): appropriate for short absence, can be highly stressful for children and parents.
- Graded return (systematic desensitization): appropriate for chronic school refusal.

Anxiety management
- Use in conjunction with a behavioural approach. Exploring the child's fears and recommending relaxation techniques.
- 'Self-help' literature for parents.
- Social skills training can be provided by Tier 1/2 CAMHS.
- Refer to specialist CAMHS if mental illness, severe anxiety or protracted school refusal.

Education
- Schools can refer to educational welfare/school attendance officers if parental condoned absence is suspected.
- Home tuition or off-site pupil referral units: consider in prolonged school refusal with comorbid mental illness. Risks encouraging school non-attendance.

Prognosis
- Short term difficulties: peer and family relationships, academic performance.
- 70% return to school. 1/3 experience emotional or social difficulties as adults.
- Poor prognosis: adolescent onset, duration >2 years, lower IQ, comorbid depression.

Attachment disorders

Definitions

Secure attachment: primary caregiver provides safe base for exploration. Child readily comforted if distressed. Child seeks and maintains contact with mother after period of separation.

Attachment disorder: significant abnormalities in social relationships, evident before age 5, associated with emotional disturbance, reactive to changes in patterns of rearing. 2 clinical syndromes: Reactive (inhibited) type and disinhibited type.

Clinical features

Reactive type
- Fearfulness and hypervigilance non-responsive to comforting.
- Look miserable, lack emotional responsiveness.
- Limited initiation of/response to social interaction.
- Ambivalent or contradictory social responses especially on parting or reunion.
- Growth failure.
- Associated with severe parental abuse/neglect (caution in making the diagnosis in the absence of abuse/neglect).

Disinhibited type
- Clingy infants, attention seeking and indiscriminately friendly children.
- Inappropriate approaches to unfamiliar adults, willingness to 'go-off' with stranger without checking back with primary caregiver, may seek physical interaction with stranger.
- Difficulty in forming close, confiding relationships with peers.
- Unconcerned by changes in caregivers
- Associated with institutional rearing from birth, extremely frequent changes in caregivers, absence of primary caregiver.

Both types: overactivity, reduced concentration, learning difficulties, aggression to self and others, low self-esteem.

Epidemiology

Prevalence low in general population but disinhibited attachment is significantly increased if institutional care from birth.

Risk factors

- *Caregiver:* young, isolated, inexperienced, depressed, substance addiction, family dysfunction, poverty.
- *Child:* difficult temperament (e.g. anxious), sensory impairment, intellectual disability.

Assessment

- Quality (appropriate, indiscriminate, inappropriate), level, frequency and pervasiveness of social interactions.
- Quality of care by current caregivers.

- Combination of caregiver interview and observed interactions including a degree of distress to activate child's need for caregiver (e.g. novel/scary toy).
  - Does he relate preferentially to parents rather than strangers?
  - Does he refer back to parents in play?
  - Does he move away and play independently?
  - Evidence of stranger anxiety?
  - Disinhibited behaviour, e.g. attempting to sit on clinicians lap.
- Important to distinguish from ASD (lack capacity for social relationships, difficulties does not remit in normal rearing environment, coexisting language disorder).

Differential diagnosis
ASD, PTSD, ADHD, anxiety disorders, selective mutism.

Interventions
- Social services input is often required due to the association with inadequate parental care.
- Provide a safe and emotionally secure care setting for the child, with consistent, positive emotional responses and appropriate behavioural management from caregivers. Young children can improve in enhanced caregiving environment.
- Enhance caregiver's understanding of child's behaviour, emotional sensitivity, and responses to child.
- Severely affected children may require residential placement.
- CAMHS referral to assess and treat comorbidity (anxiety, PTSD, ADHD).

Prognosis
- Enhanced caregiving improves reactive type, however, interpersonal difficulties often persist.
- Disinhibited type persists in a significant proportion despite enhanced caregiver environment.
- Increased risk of mental illness in adolescence, adulthood.
- Enhances to caregiving before age 2 improves prognosis.

Consequences of child abuse

Consequences of child abuse and neglect are multiple, varied and often persist into adulthood despite cessation of the abuse. It can be difficult to clearly distinguish between cause, effect and confounding factors. Abuse and its consequences share common risk factors. Which consequences are a direct result of abuse and which may have resulted from the disordered family environment?

Outcomes of different types of abuse (see 🕮 p440): physical, emotional, sexual, neglect are very similar (possibly due to overlap between different types of abuse:

Physical
- Non-organic failure to thrive, psychosocial short stature.
- Impaired brain development
  - Impaired physical, mental, emotional development.
  - Chronic stress → hyperarousal → vulnerability to sleep disturbance, psychiatric disorder.
- STDs

Cognitive
- ↓ verbal and non-verbal ability, ↓ academic achievement:
  - Consequence of neglect >abuse.
  - Combination of prenatal, postnatal (e.g. ↓ nutrition) factors and ↓ stimulation (↓ exposure to language and fewer opportunities for cognitive development).

Interpersonal difficulties
- Insecure and disorganized attachment often persist into adulthood.
- ↓ empathy.
- ↓ trust in others.
- ↓ peer relationships, ↓ ability to initiate and maintain relationships.
- ↑ negative and conflictual behaviour even with close friends.
- ↑ aggression (2° to hyperarousal, paranoia and ↓ empathy).

Behavioural problems
- Delinquency, teen pregnancy, juvenile and adult criminality and violence.
- Risk of juvenile arrest increased 59%, adult arrest 28%.
- Hoarding food. Overeating.
- Self-soothing when stressed: rocking, head banging, self injury, masturbation.

Emotional dysregulation
- Withdrawal, emotional blunting, emotional lability.
- Anger.
- Low self-worth.

Psychiatric disorder
- Depression, anxiety, eating disorders (♀>♂), PTSD, dissociative disorder, borderline personality disorder, alcohol and substance misuse, ADHD, conduct disorder (♂>♀).

- DSH ($\female$>$\male$), suicidal behaviour.
- 80% have at least one psychiatric diagnosis by 21 years.

Intergenerational transmission of abuse
- 30% of abused children become abusive parents.

Additional consequences of sexual abuse
- Guilt, feeling responsible for abuse or family break-up.
- PTSD.
- Helplessness and hopelessness.
- Inappropriate sexualized behaviour (sexualized play, seductive behaviour to strangers, public masturbation) → prostitution.
- Anxiety regarding sexual orientation ($\male$>$\female$) difficulty with adult sexual relationships.

Factors increasing impact of abuse
- Prolonged, frequent, coercive, violence, penetrative.
- Close relationship with abuser, denial of abuse by abuser.
- Response of non-abusive carer (believe/reject).

Factors diminishing the consequences of abuse
- *Individual factors:* 'resilience' (self-esteem, optimism, intelligence, creativity, independence).
- *Community factors:* access to caring adult, neighbourhood and family stability, positive social relationships, access to healthcare.

Management
- Range of consequences therefore need range of services and interventions. CAMHS and social services input.
- Treat child in context of family.
- Improving parental/carer competence, empathy and emotional availability.
- Abuse specific counselling for child/CBT (express feelings, clarify erroneous beliefs, reduce stigma, stress-management, emotional regulation skills).
- Manage and treat emotional, behavioural and psychiatric disorders.
- Neuropsychology testing to identify strengths and weaknesses and assist with improving school performance.

Further resource
MOSAC (UK charity supporting non-abusing parents and carers of sexually abused children): ℘ http://www.mosac.org.uk/

Depression

ICD-10 diagnostic criteria:

- Symptoms present for > 2 weeks
- Core symptoms: low mood, loss of pleasure and interest (anhedonia),
  ↓ energy.
- Additional symptoms: disturbed sleep, ↓ concentration, ↓ appetite,
  ↓ self-esteem, guilt, negative views of the future, self-harm or suicidal
  thoughts or acts.
- Severity determined by number of symptoms and impact on daily
  functioning (school, home, social):
  - *Mild:* 2 typical and 2 additional symptoms. Functioning with difficulty
    in some areas.
  - *Moderate:* 2 typical and 3–4 additional symptoms. Considerable
    difficulty in several areas of functioning.
  - *Severe:* 3 typical and 6 additional symptoms. Psychotic symptoms
    may occur. Significant functional difficulty in all domains. Unlikely to
    be attending school.

Presentation in younger children: describe low mood or guilt less frequently than adolescents. Presentation may be 'atypical' with irritability,
anger, somatic complaints (abdominal pain), eating difficulties and school
difficulties. Death and suicide themes may be present in play.

Epidemiology

- Children: prevalence <3% ♀:♂ 1:1. Adolescents: prevalence 2–8%, ♀:♂
  2:1.
- Risk factors: genetic (heritability 40%), low female birth weight, early
  onset female puberty, late onset male puberty, physical illness, illicit
  substance use, family dysfunction, traumatic life events.

Assessment

Interview child with parents and then alone. Enquire about:

- Impact of mood on academic and social functioning.
- Self harm, suicide plans, and attempts (Suicide and DSH 🕮 p352).
- Mood swings and hypomania (increased energy, reduced sleep,
  impulsiveness, rapid speech).
- Recent life events and relationship difficulties.
- FHx of mental illness.
- Family capacity to cope.
- Illicit substance and alcohol use.

Instruments: Mood and Feelings Questionnaire, Birleson depression self-
rating scale, Child Depression Inventory, Beck Depression Inventory.

Physical examination: chronic physical illnesses can cause or exacerbate
depression. Consider anaemia, hypothyroidism, diabetes, medication side
effects. Look for evidence of self harm. Consider the impact of weight and
acne on self-esteem.

Comorbidity: conduct disorders, anxiety disorders, illicit substance use,
ADHD, attachment disorders.

Differential diagnosis: anxiety disorders, acute stress reaction, bipolar affective disorder, organic conditions.

Management

- The management and the urgency of a referral to specialist services will be dependent upon the degree of risk and the severity depression. Discuss with CAMHS if unsure.
- Psychoeducation and advice on keeping child safe (removing sharps, medication and ensure family has emergency contact details for GP).
- 'Keep busy' (activity scheduling: TV, drawing, favourite music, walks, exercise), 'look after yourself' (regular healthy eating and sleep hygiene) and talk to someone (family, school counsellor/nurse, youth worker).
- A multimodal approach is required with support for child and family.
- Mild episode:
  - Self-help or counselling.
  - Consider tier 2 CAMHS referral.
- Moderate or severe episode:
  - Refer to tier 3/spCAMHS.
  - Psychological therapies (CBT, interpersonal psychotherapy, family therapy) are 1st-line treatment for first 12 weeks.
  - If insufficient improvement then fluoxetine is 2nd-line treatment in combination with therapy.
  - Sertraline or citalopram if fluoxetine ineffective or poorly tolerated.

Prognosis

- ~10% of adolescent depression follows a protracted course.
- Relapse rate of 40–60% necessitates follow-up for 12 months after symptom remission or 2 years if one or more previous depressive episodes.
- Recurrence in adulthood seen in 40–70% of depressed adolescents.

Further resources

Childline: ☎ 0800 1111 🕭 http://www.childline.org.uk

Get Connected, UK confidential helpline signposting to sources of help: ☎ 0808 808 4994 or 🕭 http://www.getconnected.org.uk

Young Minds, UK charity to improve mental health of children and young people. Downloadable publications on depression. 🕭 http://www.youngminds.org.uk/

Suicide and deliberate self-harm

Definitions

- Suicide: intentional taking of own life.
- Suicide attempt: non-fatal act undertaken with the intent of taking own life.
- DSH: deliberate act intending to cause harm to self but with a non-fatal outcome (cutting, over-dose).

Epidemiology

- DSH: ♀>♂ 4:1. Common (7–15%), true prevalence unknown as only minority (10–20%) present to services.
- Suicide: 3rd leading cause of death in 15–24 year olds (12% of all deaths). ♂>♀. Males use more lethal methods (hanging, guns), females (self poisoning).
- Suicidal phenomena rarer in <12 years, ♂>♀, hanging, suffocation, walking into traffic, throwing self down stairs most common (i.e. easily available, less complex but more lethal acts possibly due to less awareness of the finality of death).

Assessment

- Interview young person alone for part of the session.
- DSH:
  - Purpose: relieve negative affect, communicating distress/need for help, self-punishment.
  - Assess injury, medical risk.
  - Risk of further DSH/suicide.
- Suicidal thoughts
  - Common (experienced by 15–50% adolescents); become abnormal with when associated with intent/plan.
  - Assess intensity, frequency, duration of thoughts and any protective factor preventing acting on thoughts.
- Collateral information from parents/3rd party essential.
- ❶ Review current medication. SSRIs and atomoxetine can increase agitation and suicidality, particularly during the initial 1–2 weeks of commencing treatment.
- Physical examination: (see Depression 📖 p350).
- Investigations: Scale for suicide ideation (SSI), Beck scale for suicide ideation (BSI).

Risk factors for suicidal behaviour

- Past suicide attempts (strongest predictive factor for future suicide attempt).
- Seriousness of past attempts or plans.
- Psychiatric disorder: bipolar, depression, psychosis, anxiety, CD, ODD, substance misuse and chronic physical illness (90% completed suicides had psychiatric disorder especially depression).
- Personality: impulsivity, aggression, perfectionism, hopelessness.
- Family: parental mood disorder, suicide attempts, substance misuse, family violence, poor supervision and communication, trauma/abuse.

- Precipitating and maintaining stressors: relationship break-up, peer difficulties, school failure, bullying (especially <12 years), feeling marginalized.
- Exposure to DSH, e.g. in friends, media, video-sharing websites.
- Lack of coping skills or support.

Assessment of seriousness of DSH/suicide attempt

- Purpose of attempt: suicide, escape, get attention, manipulate environment?
- Expectations of outcome act: thought act likely/possibly/unlikely to result in death?
- Objective lethality of act (does not always correspond with child's expectations of act).
- Degree of premeditation: impulsive, contemplated?
- Final acts, e.g. saying good bye, suicide note?
- Behaviour at time of act: did they take precautions to avoid discovery? Attempt to get help afterwards?
- Ongoing suicidal ideation, regret act unsuccessful?

PATHOS overdose assessment tool (↑ features ≈ ↑ risk):

- **P**roblems > 1 month?
- **A**lone when overdosed?
- Pla**n**ed overdose for > **Three** hours?
- **HO**peless about future?
- **S**ad most of time prior to overdose?

Management

- Any untreated recent overdoses will require admission for physical assessment and treatment.
- Treat physical effects of self-harm, e.g. infection.
- Restrict access to means of DSH. Ensure adequate parental supervision and access to crisis lines if appropriate.
- Advise using distraction (music, exercise, phone friend, drawing) and talking to manage urges to self-harm.
- Referral for psychiatric assessment. Urgent assessment if serious intent, ongoing suicidal ideation, hopelessness, or significant symptoms of mental illness contributing to DSH.
- CAMHS management of recurrent DSH: treat underlying mental illness, try to avoid admission to inpatient CAMHS, CBT, DBT, improve self-esteem, and develop alternative ways to regulate emotions.

Further resource

National self-harm network, UK charity, has downloadable advice leaflets for young people: ℜ http://www.nshn.co.uk

Anxiety disorders

Anxiety disorders differ from normal fear and worry (common in children) in that they cause significant distress and impact on child's functioning. Normative fears change with developmental age from concrete external things (e.g. loud noises, strangers, the dark) to internalized abstract issues (e.g. social and academic performance, health). Anxiety disorders are the most common mental disorders of childhood (prevalence 6–20%).

Separation anxiety disorder

Developmentally inappropriate and excessive anxiety regarding actual or anticipated separation from attachment figures or home that results in impaired functioning. Associated with sleep disturbance, nightmares, somatization, school refusal, and oppositional/defiant behaviours on separation. Occurs in 3.5% children. ♀>♂. Associated with panic disorder and agoraphobia in adulthood.

Specific phobias

Marked fear that is out of proportion to the objective threat of a specific object or situation and leads to avoidance. Common phobias: animals, dark, thunderstorms, heights. Onset usually in childhood. Incidence 5%. ♀>♂. Good prognosis if treated.

Generalized anxiety disorder

Excessive and unrealistic concerns about competence, past and future. Anxiety is 'free-floating' and not limited to specific circumstances. Symptoms include restlessness, irritability, poor sleep and concentration, and over-activity. Symptoms must be present most days for several weeks. Sufferers are often perfectionistic and high reassurance seekers.

Onset in middle childhood/adolescence. Prevalence 2%. High rates of comorbidity (90%) with other anxiety disorders and depression. Poorer prognosis, often persists into adulthood.

Panic disorder

Repeated unprovoked episodes or severe anxiety with rapid onset and not restricted to any particular situation. Intense fear of impending doom, dying, losing control. Physical symptoms of anxiety are interpreted in catastrophic fashion. Onset in adolescence. ♀>♂. Prevalence 3–6%.

Panic attacks are a feature of agoraphobia: fear of a panic attack occurring in a place from which escape would be difficult. Leads to anticipatory anxiety and avoidance.

Social phobia

Anxiety in social situations (e.g. parties, eating or speaking in public). Fear scrutiny, ridicule, embarrassment and humiliation. Can lead to avoidance of social situations despite desire for social contact. Onset in early adolescence. Prevalence 5–15%. ♀>♂. Comorbidity 30–60% (anxiety disorders, mood disorders, substance misuse).

Risk factors

Genetic, temperament (timid, shy, emotionally restrained, reticent), parental anxiety disorder, overprotective and critical parenting styles, insecure attachment, negative life events, cognitive style (overestimate risk, underestimate coping skills).

Differential diagnosis

Adjustment disorder, acute stress reaction, PTSD, depression, ADHD, psychosis, PDD, hypothyroidism, hypoparathyroidism, migraine, asthma, caffeine, iatrogenic, endocrine and CNS disorders.

Assessment

- Differentiate unrealistic anxiety from fear of real threats, e.g. bullying.
- Use multiple informants.
- Situations in which anxiety experienced, severity of symptoms, impact on functioning, child and family coping skills.

Management

- Try psychoeducation and self-help first.
- Refer to CAMHS.
- CBT: 1st-line treatment, relaxation techniques, graded exposure to real or imagined anxiety provoking situations, cognitive restructuring, social skills training, relapse prevention.
- Medication (use only if partial response to psychotherapy) SSRIs.
- Involve parents (especially younger children): encourage consistency, avoid excessive reassurance, manage parents' anxieties.

Longitudinal course of anxiety disorders

Comorbidity with other anxiety disorders (60%), mood disorders and substance misuse. Severe symptoms with significant impact on functioning are associated with anxiety, mood and substance disorders in adulthood.

Obsessive compulsive disorder (OCD)

Obsessions: persistent thoughts, images, impulses (e.g. contamination, sexual thoughts, harm occurring to others) that are intrusive, distressing, time-consuming and senseless. Recognized as one's own thoughts.

Compulsions: mental or physical behaviours/rituals undertaken in an attempt to reduce the anxiety associated with obsessions (e.g. hand washing, checking, counting).
Symptoms present on most days for 2 weeks and impair functioning.

Prevalence: 0.5%. Onset in adolescence (pre-pubertal onset more common in boys, family history OCD).

Aetiology: genetic vulnerability, external stressors (meningitis, head injury, PANDAS, stressful life events). Differential diagnosis: normal developmental rituals, tic disorder, Sydenham's chorea, ASD.

Management: refer to CAMHS. CBT: exposure to intrusive thoughts coupled with response prevention, anxiety management. SSRI.

Eating disorders

(See 🕮 p341).

Although dieting and concerns regarding weight are frequent amongst adolescents the majority do not develop eating disorders.

Anorexia nervosa (AN) diagnostic guidelines

- Underweight: < 85% expected for age and height (either lost or never achieved) or BMI ≤ 17.5 (RCPsych proposed <2% centile in children).
- Self-induced weight loss: excessive exercise, vomiting, misuse of laxatives, appetite suppressants, diuretics.
- Body image distortion: fear of fatness.
- Endocrine changes: amenorrhoea, delayed or arrested puberty, loss of potency and sexual interest in males.

Bulimia nervosa (BN) diagnostic guidelines

- Persistent preoccupation and craving for food.
- Recurrent out-of-control binges (≥2/week for ≥3 months).
- Compensatory behaviour: vomiting, laxatives, appetite suppressants, diuretics.
- Fear of 'fatness'.
- Normal weight and menses.

▶ 50% children with ED do not meet full diagnostic criteria AN or BN (use terms 'Eating Disorders Not Otherwise Specified' (EDNOS) or 'atypical' AN or BN).

▶ 'Atypical' presentation more common <13 years: ↓ binge and purging, more premorbid anxiety, ♀~♂.

- AN: ♀:♂ 10:1, onset mid teens, prevalence 0.3%.
- BN: ♀:♂ 30:1, onset mid-late teens, prevalence 0.9%.
- Risk factors: family and twin studies support genetic component to aetiology (possible perfectionistic, harm avoidance and rigidity traits), dieting, athletes, performers (ballet, modelling).

Assessment

- Presentation: weight loss/growth failure of unknown cause, delayed puberty, symptoms of low weight (dizziness, syncope, fatigue, easy bruising, cold intolerance, SOB, palpitations, headache, GI symptoms, menstrual irregularities), complications of low weight, weight loss associated with chronic disease.
- Spend part of the session alone with child.
- The child will have been struggling with the disorder for several months or more, afraid of the consequences of informing others, and be reluctant to relinquish control. Guilt, low mood, poor self-esteem are common.

▶ 'ED' are secretive, skilled at hiding signs from family and professionals, and may reassure you that eating is under control. Avoid agreeing and minimizing symptoms.

- Talk through an average day of eating and drinking, calorie-counting, food avoidance.
- Family: dysfunctional family interactions; history of ED, obesity, OCD.

Physical examination for medical complications

Pale complexion, facial wasting, flat or anxious affect, muscle wasting, ↓ BP with postural hypotension, bradycardia, cardiac arrhythmias, murmur (mitral valve prolapse), failure to develop 2° sexual characteristics, dry skin, brittle hair, lanugo hair, cold extremities, swollen parotids, pitted dental enamel, Russell's sign (calluses on knuckles from self-induced vomiting).

Additional medical complications

↓ (K, Mg, PO₄, Na, Glu, Ca, TFT), ↑ (urea, cholesterol, LFT), anaemia, prolonged QT interval, oesophagitis, gastric reflux (see 📖 p83), constipation (see 📖 p84), cognitive deficits, growth retardation. Long term: infertility, ↓ bone density (see 📖 p99), osteoporosis.

Investigations

Screening questionnaires
- *SCOFF Questionnaire:*[1]
  - Do you make yourself **S**ick because you feel uncomfortably full?
  - Do you worry you have lost **C**ontrol over how much you eat?
  - Have you recently lost more than **O**ne stone in a 3 month period?
  - Do you believe yourself to be **F**at when others say you are too thin?
  - Would you say that **F**ood dominates your life?
- 1 point for every "yes"; >2 indicates a likely case of anorexia nervosa or bulimia, (sensitivity: 100%; specificity: 87.5 % in adults)[1]
- *Self-report questionnaires:* EAT (>13 years), ChEAT (8–13 years), EDI-2.

Bloods
- FBC, U+E, LFT, Ca, Mg, glucose, TFT, Fe, Folate, B12.
- ECG if CVS signs/symptoms.
- CAMHS to determine need for pelvic ultrasound ± bone densitometry.

Comorbidity: depression, social phobia, OCD, DSH, substance misuse (anabolic steroids in boys).

Differential diagnosis: see comorbidity; inflammatory bowel disease, malabsorption syndrome, hyperthyroidism, Addison disease, diabetes, malignancy, chronic infection.

Management

General
- Water or mouth wash post vomiting (brushing erodes tooth enamel).
- Psychoeducation, check bloods and refer to specialist CAMHS—sooner rather than later if organic causes are unlikely.
- Parents in denial/unaware of the eating behaviours may be reluctant to consider a psychiatric cause/referral to CAMHS. Try to avoid putting off the referral with unnecessary investigations.

---

1. Reprinted with permission from Morgan JF, Reid F, Lacey JH. The SCOFF questionnaire: assessment of a new screening tool for eating disorders. *British Medical Journal* 1999; **319**:1467.

Anorexia
- Family therapy 'Maudsley' approach:
  - Phase 1: parents initially take charge of meals, avoid debates regarding food at mealtimes, supportive approach.
  - Phase 2: ↑ weight associated with ↑ child responsibility for own eating.
  - Phase 3: weight restored, child development issues addressed.
- Individual sessions and dietician input.
- Eat (3 meals + 3 snacks)/day, aim for 0.5kg/week weight gain.
- Psychotrophic medication only for comorbid mental illness—low mood and anxiety usually improves as weight ↑.
- Intensive outpatient or inpatient treatment (only if failure of outpatient treatment, rapid and ongoing weight loss, medical compromise).

Bulimia
- More an individual approach due ↑ age.
- CBT, fluoxetine, family therapy.

Prognosis
- AN: 50% recover fully, 30% partial recovery, 20% chronic course, ~2% die suicide or starvation, good prognostic factors: early intervention, early onset, healthy relationships friends and family.
- BN: 50% recover, 25% partial recovery, 25% chronic course.

Further resource
BEAT, UK charity: ℠ http://www.b-eat.co.uk/Home

Somatizing disorders

Definition and classification

Persistent physical symptoms without a demonstrable physical cause resulting in distress and functional impairment. An identifiable stressor may or may not exist. Symptoms are not consciously produced.

Somatoform disorders

- Recurrent abdominal pain disorder (RAP): diffuse abdominal pain usually lasting few hours then remitting with normal abdominal examination. Can be accompanied by limb/joint pain.
- Persistent somatoform pain disorder.
- Dissociative/conversion disorders: loss of sensory or motor function or altered states of awareness associated with psychological distress.
- Chronic fatigue syndrome (📖 p361).
- Somatization disorder: persistent, multiple and variable physical symptoms, repeated requests for investigations. Refusal to accept medical advice that no organic cause.
- Hypochondriacal disorder: persistent preoccupation with having a serious illness.

Clinical features

- GI, neurological, and musculoskeletal symptoms most common.
- Young children: abdominal pain, headache.
- Older children and females: headache, loss of limb function and neurological symptoms.
- Polysymptomatic presentation increases with age.
- Presentation may mimic symptoms in family members.

Epidemiology

20–25% of childhood presentations with headache, abdominal or muscle pain attributed to somatizing. RAP (prevalence 10–15%), pain disorders, fatigue and dissociative disorders are most common. Somatization disorder and hypochondriacal disorder are rare in children and adolescents.

Aetiology

Predisposing: female, low IQ, depression/anxiety, personality (anxious, obsessional, perfectionist), low socioeconomic class, parental ill-health (somatization, chronic disease or disability, depression/anxiety) family dynamics (enmeshed, over-protective, poor conflict-resolution), abuse.

Precipitating: stressful life events, physical illness, anxiety, depression, academic, family, or social problems.

Maintaining: excess attention on symptoms (medical investigations, parental over-concern), difficulty in recovering without 'losing face', secondary gain (benefits of sick role), secondary physical changes, e.g. muscle wasting.

Differential diagnosis: adjustment disorder, factitious disorder (intentional fabrication of symptoms), unidentified physical disorder.

Comorbidity: (30–50%), depression, anxiety disorder, school refusal.

Management
- Therapeutic alliance is crucial.
- Establish family's attitude to and understanding of the symptoms.
- Stop investigations.
- Explain and reassure that no evidence of organic disorder while acknowledging the symptoms are real not 'put-on'.
- Present model of stress causing physical symptoms, e.g. tension headache. Explore stressors in child/family.
- Avoid conflict and confrontation. Aim for consensus with family on presentation and management while acknowledging diagnostic uncertainty.
- If child/parent convinced about physical aetiology avoid disagreement and focus on need for 'rehabilitative' treatment, e.g. graded return to previous level of functioning.
- Be positive regarding prognosis and outcome.
- Allow child to recover without 'losing face' rather than 'catching them out'.
- Consider referral to or joint working with CAMHS.
- CBT, problem solving skills training, positive reinforcement of health improvements, and removal of positive reinforcement of illness behaviour.
- Family work/therapy to improve communication and explore uncommunicated stressors.
- Possible role for antidepressants, analgesics.

Prognosis
Most improve but a significant proportion can persist to adulthood. Openness to psychological factors and engagement with treatment are good prognostic indicators.

Chronic fatigue syndrome/myalgic encephalitis

Definition
Generalized fatigue persisting after routine investigations fail to identify an organic underlying cause. Symptoms can fluctuate in severity and change over time.

Definition CFS/ME adapted from NICE guideline 2007
Fatigue has all of the following features:
- New or had a specific onset (i.e. it is not life-long).
- Persistent and/or recurrent.
- Unexplained by other conditions.
- Has resulted in a substantial reduction in activity level characterized by post-exertional malaise and/or fatigue (typically delayed, for example by at least 24 hours, with slow recovery over several days).
- Persists for at least 3 months.

And 1 or more of the following symptoms:
- Sleep difficulties (see 📖 p168).
- Muscle and/or joint pain that is multisite and without evidence of inflammation.
- Headaches (see 📖 p235).
- Painful lymph nodes without pathological enlargement.
- Sore throat.
- Cognitive dysfunction (e.g. impaired concentration, short-term memory, word-finding, organizing thoughts and information processing (see 📖 p213)).
- Physical or mental exertion exacerbates symptoms.
- General malaise or 'flu-like' symptoms.
- Dizziness and/or nausea.
- Palpitations in the absence of identified cardiac pathology.

Epidemiology
- Prevalence 0.05% <18 years. Slightly higher in girls, no difference between socioeconomic groups.
- Onset 11–14 years, gradual or sudden, often preceded by acute illness (influenza, gastroenteritis, glandular fever).
- Risk factors: mental illness (anxiety, depression), childhood trauma, sexual abuse (see 📖 p453).

Assessment
- Impact on child's functioning, current activity levels (>50% bed bound at some stage) and possible maintaining factors.
- Psychiatric symptoms, depression (50%) (see 📖 p350), anxiety (see 📖 p354), suicidal ideation, DSH (see 📖 p352), hopelessness.
- Ascertain child's problem solving skills.
- Impact on family (disruption, emotional, financial), family response to illness (over-involved, conflictual), FHx of chronic physical or mental illness.

- Physical examination: lymphatic, liver, spleen, and tonsillar enlargement. Palpation over nasal sinus, lying and standing BP and HR. Neurological examination.
- Investigations: no test is diagnostic, FBC and film, U&E, creatinine, Ca, LFT, glucose, TFT, ESR or plasma viscosity, CRP, CK, gluten sensitivity, ferritin. Viral serology if Hx infection (EBV-IgM, IgG, EBNA). Urinalysis.

Differential diagnosis

Infection (EBV, influenza, TB, HIV), neuroendocrine (diabetes, Addison's, hyper/hypothyroidism), haematological (anaemia, lymphoma, malignancy), psychiatric (depression, anxiety), neurological. Obstructive sleep syndromes (see 📖 p90), iatrogenic, fabricated or induced illness (see 📖 p451).

Management

- Establish collaborative relationship, avoid debates regarding cause, adopt pragmatic approach.
- Education and information provision including local and national support groups.
- Regular paediatric reviews (monitor progress, development of new physical/psychological symptoms, review diagnosis, support needs). Avoid frequent changes of medical practitioner with resultant anxiety and unnecessary investigations.
- Multidisciplinary management: paediatrician, liaison psychology service, OT, school and CAMHS (see 📖 p23).
- Functional management
  - Sleep: regular bed and wake times, reduce daytime napping.
  - Rest periods of 30min maximum with no sleeping, physical or mental exertion.
  - Healthy diet.
  - Relaxation techniques.
- Education: consider home tuition and gradual return to school.
- Referral to specialist service in severe cases
  - CBT: 12–16 sessions (alter pessimistic beliefs and maintenance cycles, reduce distress and symptoms (see 📖 p373)).
  - Graded exercise therapy (GET) and activity management (obtain baseline of activity, gradually increase, add in exercise, maintain activity levels at less than full capacity to avoid 'boom and bust'.
  - Family therapy.
- Medication: treat comorbid mental illness, melatonin for sleep difficulties.
- Relapse management: relapse part of normal recovery, generate plan before relapse occurs.

Prognosis

Average duration ~ 37–49 months with 12 months off school. 60–80% full or partial recovery.

Chronic illness and mental health

Psychiatric disturbance (anxiety/emotional disorder >behavioural) occurs in 20–50% of children with a chronic medical condition (see ⬚ Chapter 4: Neurodevelopmental Disorders). Risk of psychiatric disorder is increased in physical illness (↑x2), physical illness with disability (↑x3), CNS illness (↑x5). The link between physical and mental illness can be causal or coincidental (mediated via family/psychosocial factors).

Psychiatric disturbance includes: depression, anxiety, ↓ self-esteem, altered self-concept, anger, hyperactivity, conduct disorder and other disruptive behaviour, psychosis. Slight ↑ risk of DSH, suicidal ideation/attempts.

Factors that hinder adaptation to the illness are risk factors for psychiatric problems. Impact of risk factors is influenced by developmental stage of child and can change with time:
- Age at illness onset: early recurrent hospitalizations disrupting attachment, disruption to family/social/academic life in childhood, impede peer group attachments/intimate relationships in adolescence.
- Diagnosis: delayed, misdiagnosis, emotional issues ignored, uncertain prognosis.
- Illness: chronicity, degree of disability, functional loss, CNS involvement.
- Stigma (especially school age/adolescence): physical disfigurement, intrusive treatment regime /adverse effects.
- Personality: avoidant coping (poor adjustment, ↓ self-esteem, anxiety), denial (treatment non-adherence), over-acceptance of illness (↑ anxiety, illness takes over life).
- Parental response: inconsistent, overly attentive/controlling (adolescents need to take increasing responsibility for illness/treatment), parental depression/anxiety, family dysfunction, poor communication/emotional expressiveness.

Asthma
- Psychosocial stress (acute and chronic), emotional arousal (anger, depression) can precipitate symptoms and worsen prognosis.
- Asthmatics and their parents are more anxious than controls.
- Treatments (e.g. steroids) can precipitate emotional and behavioural disorders.

Diabetes
- Increased rates of psychiatric disturbance in type 1.
- Stress and depression associated with poor glycaemic control.
- Treatment non-compliance/recurrent hospitalizations with ketoacidosis associated with family conflict, parent-child conflict, depression.
- Adolescents in particular can struggle with balancing intrusive monitoring and treatment regime with desire for autonomy.

Epilepsy
(See ⬚ p240)
30% psychiatric comorbidity.
- Multiple causes: direct result of brain pathology/seizure, medication side effect, psychosocial (stigma, academic and social limitations).

- Risk of comorbidity increased by: neurological cause for epilepsy, high seizure frequency, cognitive impairments, family difficulties, young, male, low socioeconomic status.

Assessment
- Screen for existence of and risk factors for psychiatric morbidity.
- Cognitive assessment (impairments influence coping and problem-solving). Educational disability can result from school absence, reduced expectations of child.
- Social, academic function, quality of life. Family and child need opportunity to discuss social and psychological concerns in addition to physical ones.
- Non-illness related stresses facing the family (child's chronic illness associated with marital conflict, behavioural disturbance in siblings, financial difficulties).

Management
- Repeated education about illness/treatment including developmentally appropriate written information (aids treatment compliance).
- Most effective if both parents and child present with child fully included in discussions.
- Focus on and build on strengths (of both child and parents) to start with rather than negatives.
- Communication with other agencies.
- Contact with self-help organizations, other families with similarly affected children.
- Treat psychiatric comorbidity.
- Referral to CAMHS for severe, persistent behavioural/emotional problems.
- Individual therapy: counselling, narrative therapy, CBT, role play.
- Family work: enhance communication, facilitate acceptance/adaptation to diagnosis, allow ventilation of feelings.

Post-traumatic stress disorder

Definition
Psychological distress secondary to a traumatic event, e.g. RTAs, abuse (see 📖 p440), natural or man-made disasters, exposure to death, serious physical illness (particularly requiring hospitalization or invasive interventions).

Symptoms usually arise within 6 months of the trauma:
- Repetitive and intrusive recollections, thoughts, dreams, daytime images ('flashbacks').
- Emotional detachment or 'numbness'.
- Avoidance of activities or stimuli associated with trauma.
- Hyper-arousal (difficulty sleeping, concentrating, anger, hyper-vigilance).

Epidemiology
Children and adolescents: lifetime prevalence 3–10%, probably under-reported in children.

Risk factors
- Trauma: life-threatening, 'man made', proximity to trauma, duration of trauma.
- Individual: ♀>♂, pre-existing mental illness, history of neglect/abuse, low socioeconomic class, lack of social support, distressed/unsupportive adults.

Assessment
- Presentation varies with age and developmental stage. Younger children more frequently present with physical symptoms and repetitive play incorporating aspects of the trauma.
- Consider PTSD in children with new onset behavioural disorder, anxiety, agitation, aggression, or self harm (all possible signs of hyperarousal).
- Flashbacks or recalling traumatic memories may be accompanied by dissociative episodes which can be confused with absence seizures.
- Encourage the child to draw or play in the assessment.
- Enquire about:
  - Sleep disturbance, recurrent nightmares.
  - Coping strategies including self-harm and illicit substance use.
  - Were other family members traumatized?
  - Is child now in a safe environment?
- Physical examination to assess possible abuse or injuries if appropriate.
- Instruments: Children's Revised Impact of Event Scale (CRIES), Post-Traumatic Cognitions Inventory – child version (cPTCI) (🕸 http://www.childrenandwar.org/measures).

Comorbidity
Depression (see 📖 p350), behavioural disorder (see 📖 p210), sleep disorder (see 📖 p168), ADHD (see 📖 p126), self-harm (see 📖 p352).

Differential diagnosis

Acute stress reaction (negative life event, symptoms of distress resolve rapidly within 3 days), adjustment disorder (negative life event, e.g. bereavement, symptoms resolve within 6 months), anxiety (see 📖 p354), depression (see 📖 p350), ADHD (see 📖 p126), attachment disorder (see 📖 p346), conduct disorder (see 📖 p334), sleep disorder (see 📖 p168).

Management

Early detection and treatment within CAMHS is best.

- No clear benefit from single session debriefing immediately post trauma.
- Trauma-focused CBT. Consider group CBT if mass trauma.
- Family therapy. Children and parents may avoid discussing the trauma for fear of distressing each other. Depression, anxiety or PTSD in family members exposed to the trauma should be considered and treated. Parents may struggle with guilt, particularly if the child has been abused.
- Medication should not be routinely used. Consider SSRIs in severe PTSD or if comorbid depression or anxiety.

Prognosis

Most resolve completely within a year but some cases become chronic. Prognosis negatively influenced by severity of episode, lack of supportive parents, premorbid adversity and comorbidity.

Alcohol and substance misuse

Definition

Experimental and recreational use of illicit substances and alcohol is common in adolescence.

Harmful use: pattern of use causes mental/physical harm to user, is criticized by others and causes adverse social consequences.

Dependence syndrome: compulsion to take substance, withdrawal, tolerance, neglect of alternative interests, persisting use despite harmful consequences, reinstatement after abstinence. (Note: withdrawal symptoms less common in adolescents than adults).

Epidemiology

- Most common substances used by adolescents: tobacco, alcohol, cannabis, amphetamines.
- Prevalence: alcohol abuse 0.6–4.3% of adolescents, substance abuse 3.3% 15-year-olds, 9.8% 17–19-year-olds.
- Inhaled solvents used more frequently by younger teens (6–7% 11–12-year-olds).
- Polysubstance use is common. 75% of adolescents obtain substances from friends or relatives.

Aetiology/risk factors

Genetic vulnerability, dopaminergic system, impulsivity, low socioeconomic status, peer pressure, poor social skills, mental illness (conduct disorder (see 📖 p334), ADHD (see 📖 p126)), ineffective parenting (see 📖 p371), parental substance misuse, childhood sexual abuse (see 📖 p453), traumatic life events.

Clinical features

Common presentations include changes in: academic and social functioning, cognition (reduced concentration, psychotic symptoms, flashbacks), mood and behaviour (agitation, irritability, somnolence, withdrawal, impulsivity, hypervigilance, antisocial behaviour).

Assessment

- Interview the young person alone for part of session and explain limits of confidentiality.
- Pattern of alcohol/substance use: current amount, frequency of use, binges, range of substances, used socially or alone, features of harmful use or dependence.
- Risk: self-harm (see 📖 p352), suicide, unprotected sex, aggression (see 📖 p334), criminal behaviour, funding of habit (theft, prostitution).
- From family: premorbid functioning, parental alcohol/substance use, access to alcohol/substances at home. Have the parents raised their concerns with the adolescent?
- Physical examination: self-care, weight deficit, accidental injuries, DSH, infection, skin reactions, signs of nicotine and alcohol use, rash around mouth and nose (inhaling solvents from a bag), gynaecomastia (anabolic steroid use).

- Bloods in IV drug use: Hep B, C, HIV.
- Urine toxicology not routinely required.

Comorbidity
60–75%. Conduct disorder, ODD (see 📖 p334), ADHD (see 📖 p126), depression, anxiety disorders, PTSD (see 📖 p365), eating disorders (see 📖 p356).

Management
- Non-judgemental approach.
- Treat comorbid physical illness.
- Discuss/provide information about substances and associated risks.
- Encourage engagement with local drugs advisory service or specialist treatment services dependent upon severity of substance use. Treatment usually involves:
  - Address risk including safe sex.
  - Individual and group work incorporating cognitive and behavioural approaches (see 📖 p373).
  - Motivational interviewing: non-confrontational approach designed to lead adolescent to desire change (includes pros and cons of substance misuse, alternative means of achieving 'pros').
  - Relapse prevention: cue avoidance, social pressures, alternative coping strategies.
  - Harm reduction approach if abstinence impossible, advise use of safer drugs, clean needles, first aid.
- CAMHS referral for mental illness (see 📖 p319).

Prognosis
Most addictive behaviour terminated by adulthood.

Further resources
Drugscope, independent UK charity: ℘ http://www.drugscope.org.uk
FRANK, independent UK government funded website offering information and support: ℘ http://www.talktofrank.com/ (accessed 1/5/11)

Challenging behaviour

Challenging behaviour is an umbrella term used to describe a variety of different behaviours including: aggression, tantrums, destruction, sexualized behaviour, self-injury, stereotyped behaviours, running away. There is often a repetitive nature to the behaviours and they can interfere with functioning and development.

The term is more frequently applied to younger children, children with learning difficulties and autism.

In order to accurately interpret behaviour the developmental age of the child should be taken into account, e.g. tantrums in a 2-year-old are 'normal' but inappropriate for 10-year-olds. All children will at some point 'challenge' their carers or teachers, so obtaining a detailed history of difficulties is key to distinguishing 'normal' behaviour and the management of 'challenging' behaviour.

Assessment

Who perceives the behaviour as challenging, what is their understanding/ explanation of the origin and purpose of the behaviour, and why do they find it challenging/distressing?

Review potential causes of challenging behaviour: pain, distress, anxiety, gaining attention, inability to cope with change, sensory stimulation, self-soothing (sexualized behaviour), sensitivities to light/sound, boredom, communication with others (go away, come here, need help).

Utilize a functional analysis approach (see Management of behavioural problems 📖 p210).
- Look for patterns of precipitants and perpetuating factors. Consider keeping a behaviour diary.
- Is the behaviour pervasive or only present in certain environments or company?
- What is the child trying to communicate?
- How have carers, family members, and school responded to the behaviour?
- Range of interventions tried, duration, and consistency.

What is the child's explanation for the behaviour? They will have been asked this before by other adults and may be understandably wary of discussing the issue, particularly if they feel embarrassed or believe that you may tell them off or judge them. Children may often 'not know', be unable or unwilling to communicate why they behave in a certain manner, so need to approach the issue indirectly.

If possible see child alone for part of the session. Using drawings or models can help. A non-judgemental approach throughout the session can facilitate discussion.

Management
- Exclude physical cause for behaviour, comorbid mental illness, learning disability (see 📖 p117), and neurodevelopmental disorder (see 📖 p62).

- Assess risk to self and others.
- Intervention dependent upon most likely cause.
- Use behavioural interventions (Management of behavioural problems 📖 p210) and ensure that behavioural interventions involve a coordinated response from school and family.
- Consider the impact of:
  - Changes to physical and social environment.
  - Methods of enhancing communication—visual forms of communication pictures, objects, 'emotional' faces.

Anger management: parent management training and individual behavioural training (Conduct disorder and oppositional defiant disorder 📖 p334).

Sexualized behaviour: feedback regarding where and when the behaviour is appropriate, review causes including possible sexual abuse (see 📖 p453).

Self-injury: often used to communicate, behavioural treatments, enhance communication skills (functional communication training), (Suicide and deliberate self-harm (📖 p352), ASD CAMHS aspects (📖 p327)).

Education: SEN support including behavioural support services ± educational psychologist input (see 📖 p533).

Medication: only consider after behavioural analysis and interventions, identify which symptoms will be targeted, conduct a thorough risk benefit analysis before commencing, determine how the response will be measured and monitored (child's report, carer/school reports, questionnaires).

Refer to CAMHS if listed interventions inadequate.

Further resources

Challenging behaviour foundation: charity for children and adults with severe learning disabilities. Information sheets for managing behaviour at: ℬ http://www.thecbf.org.uk/
(See Further resources in 'Parenting' 📖 p371).

Parenting

Parenting is an immensely rewarding but at times challenging 'job'. A balanced authoritative parenting style that is flexible and meets the child's developmental needs will be most successful. Excessive authoritarian, permissive, or disengaged approaches are more likely to be associated with difficulties.

Supporting parents

- Use attentive listening when reviewing the parents concerns—it is itself therapeutic, increases the likelihood of parental change/following your advice, and models 'how to listen' to their children.
- Try to avoid judging and blaming the parent—it will not help the child or parent.
- The parents are part of the solution.
- Empathise—all parents get frustrated and parenting can be more challenging and stressful if a child is 'unwell'.
- Address parental guilt—may feel as if they have 'failed' or are responsible for child's illness, particularly if mental illness. Make time to explore parental concerns.
- Are the parents being too hard on themselves? Aim to be a 'good enough' parent rather than a perfect parent.
- Review the parental relationship—impact of illness, degree of cooperation, conflict, triangulation with child.
- Review parental closeness with child and advise as appropriate—too close leading to inhibition (enmeshment) or too distant.

General advice/approach

- Externalise—the behaviour is the difficulty rather than the child.
- Encourage a consistent approach from both parents that is also consistent over time.
- Encourage parents to 'tune in' to the child—what would it be like to be in their child's shoes? What is the child attempting to communicate? What are they feeling?
- Enjoy your child—spend time doing things together.
- Let the child know they are special—listen to them, express your affection, recognise and praise appropriate behaviour.
- Provide security and stability—routines and order will help reduce child anxiety.
- 'Time out' for parents—anger and frustration will alter a parent's response to a situation. Try to stay calm.

Advice for managing specific behaviours—see individual topics or management of behavioural problems topic (see 📖 p210).

Other sources of parental support:
- Self-help.
- Parenting programmes.
- Local and national support groups (see 📖 p372).
- Family, friends.
- Health visitors (see 📖 p540), GP, social services (see 📖 p546), school (see 📖 p542).
- CAMHS—family therapy (see 📖 p374).

Parental mental illness

- Is the 'unwell' child actually bringing their parents/family for treatment?
- Recognition is key, so always ask. Enquire about postnatal depression, affective disorders, past and current input from GP/mental health services, and any other FHx of mental illness.
- Consider genetic risk in child.
- Could there be a common aetiology, e.g. parental stress reaction caring for a seriously ill child, shared exposure to traumatic event.
- Review capacity of parent to cope with current situation and child. Parents often try to shield their children from their illness.
- Chronic difficulties such a parental personality disorders are often more damaging for children than acute episodes of illness.
- Individual assessment and treatment for parent—GP/mental health services.
- Family therapy—adult mental health team or CAMHS (see 📖 p374).
- Review the impact of the parental illness on the child.
- Review risk to children. Ensure your concerns are explained to the parent and communicated to other professionals (Child protection see 📖 p441 and p455).

Further resources

Incredible years website: ℜ http://www.incredibleyears.com/ParentResources/
Family and parenting institute: ℜ http://www.familyandparenting.org/
Young Minds Parents Helpline (offers information and professional advice): ☎ 0808 802 5544 or ℜ http://www.youngminds.org.uk/
Young Carers Net (UK website for <18-year-olds who look after someone in their family who has an illness, disability, drug/alcohol addiction or mental illness): ℜ http://www.youngcarers.net

Psychotherapeutic interventions

Psychosocial interventions are the 1st-line treatment for the majority of child mental illness. The choice of intervention is determined by the needs of the child and family, evidence base and local availability.

Behaviour therapy

(See Management of behavioural problems 📖 p210.)

Cognitive behaviour therapy (CBT)

- Structured therapy that focuses on the links between thoughts (cognitions), emotions, and behaviour in different situations.
- Changing cognitions will change emotions and behaviour.
- The therapist is a 'coach' working collaboratively with the child to develop a formulation of the problem and maintenance cycles.
- 'Socratic' questioning (encouraging the child to reach their own conclusions to reveal new perspectives) is utilised to identify and alter unhelpful cognitions associated with psychopathology.
- Common cognitive distortions include: black and white thinking, jumping to conclusions, mind-reading, magnification, personalizing, over-generalization.
- 'Homework' is used between sessions and includes 'thought diaries' and behaviour experiments.
- The behavioural component of CBT may be sufficient in itself, e.g. activity scheduling for depression.
- Usually individual therapy but group CBT possible. Parents can join sessions for younger children.
- Time limited, ~ 6–24 sessions.
- Recommended by NICE for depression, anxiety disorders, and bulimia nervosa.

Counselling

- A supportive, cathartic, client-led therapy that focuses on the discussion of distressing issues.
- Problem solving and advice can be incorporated.
- Children and adolescents can value the contact with an 'independent and non-judgemental' adult.
- Used in schools and local youth support organizations.
- Evidence base is limited.
- Commonly used to manage mild depression and anxiety, significant life events, relationships, school difficulties, and substance misuse.

Creative therapies

- These include art, play, music, and drama.
- Most suitable for younger children and those with learning and communication difficulties.

Dialectic behaviour therapy (DBT)

- Used to manage self-harm and emotional dysregulation.
- Incorporates elements of CBT, mindfulness, and problem solving.
- Both individual and group work.
- Not widely available.

Family therapy
- Family treated as a whole rather than just the child.
- ↓ feelings of guilt and 'scapegoating' in children.
- Sometimes only part of family seen.
- Therapist maintains neutrality.
- Use 'reflective team' and a one-way mirror.
- ↓ frequency sessions compared to other therapies, ~ 6–12 sessions over several months.
- Widely utilized, best evidence: eating disorders, depression.

Interpersonal psychotherapy (IPT)
- Focuses on relationship difficulties including conflicts and adapting to life events.
- >11 years, ~12 sessions.
- Used in depression, grief reactions and bulimia nervosa.

Parenting programmes
Provide group support and teach positive parenting skills (see 📖 p372, further resources).

Psychodynamic psychotherapy
- Brief or intensive (1–3 sessions/week over 1 year).
- Aim to gain insight into unconscious processes that maintain psychopathology.
- Parents can be seen separately in parallel with the child.

Treatment non-adherence

Treatment adherence is rarely complete. In children and adolescents with chronic conditions it is estimated at 58%, with adolescents adhering less than children (WHO). Non-adherence can result in mortality or chronic morbidity depending on the underlying medical condition.

Factors that may increase non-adherence

Illness and treatment related factors
- Chronic illness, relapsing-remitting course.
- Demanding, complicated, intrusive, long-term treatments.
- Suboptimal treatment response or delayed onset of action.
- Experiencing or fear of adverse events or painful treatments.
- Stigma/embarrassment associated with illness or taking medication.
- Illness or treatment impacting on social life.
- Fear of future, e.g. effect on relationships, sexual attractiveness.

Individual factors
- Reduced capacity in children to evaluate treatment benefit and consequences of non-adherence.
- Lack of acceptance of diagnosis and prognosis.
- Anger at illness directed towards parents and clinicians and their imposed treatment.
- Parent-child conflict and child's desire to exert autonomy by disregarding parental advice.
- Feeling overwhelmed by responsibility of managing own health. Non-adherence is a means of exerting control of a situation in which they feel disempowered.
- Psychiatric disorder: depression (hopelessness), poor insight, oppositional defiant disorder, ADHD (forgetting medication).
- Primary and secondary gain: avoid school, maintaining parental attention.

Parental factors
- Psychiatric disorder.
- Family conflict.
- Inadequate parental supervision.

Management

Open discussion of positive and negative aspects of treatment
- Psychoeducation utilising age-appropriate information both at time of diagnosis and transition to adolescence (a time of increasing responsibility for own condition). Check understanding.
- Avoid term 'non-compliance' (suggests deliberate antagonism and implies blame).
- Do the consequences of non-adherence justify an intervention?
- Empower child and family by involvement in treatment decisions, and acknowledge validity of their views on positive and negative treatment effects. Siblings can play important part in motivating the patient.
- Discuss strategies to manage side effects.
- Consider increasing the frequency of contact to enhance therapeutic alliance.

Suggestions to facilitate discussion based on motivational interviewing techniques:
- Write a list with the young person of pros and cons of treatment and no treatment. Do they assign greater importance to some factors over others? Review treatment related fears.
- Who from your family most wants you to receive the treatment? Who next? What do you think the reasons are?
- How would life be different in 1 year or 5 years' time without and then with the treatment?
- What advice would you give to a friend in a similar situation?
- Elicit aspirations. What would you need to do to achieve your goals? How would treatment influence this?

Practical measures
- Daily pill dispenser (dossette box), charts.
- Simplify treatment regime (e.g. sustained release preparations). Switch to more acceptable alternative treatment.

Other
- Identify and treat mental illness.
- Liaise with psychology service or CAMHS if individual or family work appropriate.
- Young people may respond better to non-professionals, e.g. support groups, contact with other young people with similar condition.

Resources

Mind: ☎ 020 8519 2122 ✍ http://www.mind.org.uk
The Mental Health Foundation: ☎ 020 7803 1100 ✍ http://www.mhf.org.uk

Anxiety

Anxiety UK: ☎ 0844 477 5774 ✍ http://www.anxietyuk.org
OCD Action (UK charity for OCD): ☎ 0845 390 6232 ✍ http://www.ocdaction.org.uk/

Autistic spectrum disorders

National Autistic Society: ✍ http://www.autism.org.uk

Bullying

Anti-bullying network (not-for-profit company): ✍ http://www.antibullying.net/
Parentline Plus (advice to parents regarding bullying): ✍ http://www.familyandparenting.org/ or helpline ☎ 0808 800 2222.

Child abuse

MOSAC (UK charity supporting non-abusing parents and carers of sexually abused children): ✍ http://www.mosac.org.uk/

Deliberate self-harm

National self harm network (UK charity, has downloadable advice leaflets for young people): ✍ http://www.nshn.co.uk

Depression

Childline (UK helpline provides a confidential telephone counselling service for children with any problem): ☎ 0800 1111 ✍ www.childline.org.uk
Get Connected (UK confidential helpline signposting to sources of help): F0808 808 4994 ✍ www.getconnected.org.uk
Young Minds (UK charity to improve mental health of children and young people): ☎ 020 7336 8445 Downloadable publications on depression: ✍ http://www.youngminds.org.uk/

Eating disorders

BEAT (UK charity): ✍ http://www.b-eat.co.uk/Home

Enuresis and encopresis

ERIC (Education and Resources for Improving Childhood Continence) UK children's charity dealing with bedwetting, daytime wetting, constipation and soiling and potty training: Y http://www.eric.org.uk/
Heins T, Ritchie K (1988) Beating sneaky poo: ideas for faecal soiling. 2nd Ed. Leaflet free to download: ✍ http://www.dulwichcentre.com.au/beating-sneaky-poo-2.pdf

Learning disabilities

Challenging behaviour foundation: charity for children and adults with severe learning disabilities. Information sheets for managing behaviour at: ✍ http://www.thecbf.org.uk/
Foundation for people with learning disabilities: ✍ http://www.learningdisabilities.org.uk/
LD online, USA website on learning disabilities and ADHD: ✍ http://www.ldonline.org/

Parenting, conduct disorder and oppositional defiant disorder

Incredible years website: ✍ http://www.incredibleyears.com/ParentResources/
Family and parenting institute: ✍ http://www.familyandparenting.org/
Young Carers Net (UK website for <18yr-olds who look after someone in their family who has an illness, disability, drug/alcohol addiction or mental illness): ✍ http://www.youngcarers.net
Parentline Plus ☎ 0808 800 2222 ✍ http://www.parentlineplus.org.uk

Substance misuse

Drugscope (independent UK charity): M http://www.drugscope.org.uk

FRANK (independent UK government funded website offering information and support): http://www.talktofrank.com

Tic disorders

Tourettes action (UK charity): ✆ 0845 458 1252 http://www.tourettes-action.org.uk/

Genetics

There is only one pretty child in the world, and every mother has it.
Chinese proverb

Introduction to clinical genetics

Clinical genetics is a speciality that integrates all aspects of medicine. It deals with both common and rare childhood and adult disorders. It is involved in the use of basic sciences to understand the origin and progression of a disease, which helps the development of screening guidelines and therapeutic options, when appropriate.

Role of a clinical geneticist

A clinical geneticist is a medical doctor trained in paediatrics and adult medicine.

The main role of a clinical geneticist is:
• To make a diagnosis (syndromic or non-syndromic).
• Discuss the natural progression and prognosis of the condition.
• Recommend screening and treatment measures.
• Counsel the family regarding reproductive risks.
• Discuss preconceptual advice, prenatal testing, and other appropriate reproductive options (such as artificial insemination by donor, egg donation, preimplantation genetic diagnosis), where appropriate.

Which patients to refer?

Many patients seen in a community paediatrics clinic have shared care with a clinical geneticist.

The common reasons for referral are:
• Developmental delay: may be global or be limited to specific skill areas (see 📖 pp44–5).
• Facial dysmorphism.
• Congenital structural abnormalities: including cardiac, palatal, limb, brain, kidney, skeletal, skin, bowel abnormalities.
• Growth abnormalities: proportionate or disproportionate growth restriction or overgrowth.
• Neurological abnormalities: hypotonia or hypertonia (see 📖 p233), microcephaly or macrocephaly (see 📖 p231), seizures (see 📖 p240), movement disorders (see 📖 p238, Abnormal movements), SNHL (see 📖 p307), blindness (see 📖 p275), cranial nerve abnormalities.
• Behavioural problems: including sleep disturbances (see 📖 p168), ADHD (see 📖 p126), ASD (see 📖 p107).
• FHx of an inherited disorder (see 📖 p153).

Chromosomes and genes

Within each of our cells, in the nucleus, there is double-stranded DNA which represents our genes. There are ~30,000 pairs of genes in each of our cells, which are packaged into chromosomes. Chromosomes also come in pairs (one maternal and the other paternal) and there are 23 pairs of chromosomes in each of our cells (except the gamets). The pairs are numbered 1–22 according to their size and banding pattern and these are known as autosomes. The remaining pair of chromosomes are the sex chromosomes. 46XX is the usual karyotype in females and 46XY in males.

Modes of inheritance

Autosomal dominant (AD)

- AD disorders are caused by abnormalities (mutations or deletions) in genes encoded on the autosomes.
- A mutation in 1 copy of the gene is sufficient to cause the phenotype.
- There is a 50% chance in each pregnancy that the offspring may inherit the mutation, as we pass on only 1 copy of each of our genes through the egg or the sperm.
- Examples include: NF1 (see 📖 p399), Noonan syndrome, tuberous sclerosis (see 📖 p401), achondroplasia, etc.

Autosomal recessive (AR)

- AR disorders are caused by mutations in genes on the autosomes.
- Mutations in both copies (maternal and paternal copy) of the same gene are needed in order to cause the disorder.
- AR disorders are caused when both parents carry a mutation in 1 copy of the same gene (they are called carriers).
- When both parents are carriers there is a 1 in 4 chance (25%) in each pregnancy that the baby may be affected.
- The sibling of an affected individual is at a 2 in 3 risk of being a carrier.
- More common in consanguineous families as a shared common ancestor may pass on the same mutation to both parents.
- Some AR disorders may be common even in the absence of consanguinity if the carrier frequency in the general population is high, e.g. cystic fibrosis (CF) with a carrier frequency of 1 in 20 or spinal muscular atrophy (SMA) with a carrier frequency of 1 in 50.
- Examples include: many metabolic disorders (mucopolysaccharidosis, organic acidurias, glycogen storage disorders, etc. (see 📖 p153)), CF, SMA (see 📖 p258).

X-linked recessive (XLR)

- XLR disorders are caused by abnormalities of genes on the X chromosome.
- As females have 2 copies of the X chromosome, abnormalities in 1 copy of the gene cause mild or no symptoms; hence they are called carriers.
- In males as there is only 1 copy of the X chromosome, abnormalities of the XLR gene are manifested and males are affected.
- Although a female carrier does not usually have any symptoms herself, she can have affected sons (there is a 50% risk in each pregnancy that any son she has will be affected) and carrier daughters (there is a 50% risk in each pregnancy that any daughter she has will be a carrier).
- Males with XLR disorder cannot pass the disorder to their sons as they will pass on the Y copy of their sex chromosome to them; all their daughters will be obligate carriers as they will have to pass on the X chromosome which carries the abnormality.
- Examples include: Fragile X syndrome (see 📖 p403), Duchenne muscular dystrophy (see 📖 p258), ATRX (alpha-thalassemia/mental retardation syndrome)(see 📖 p406) etc.

X-linked dominant (XLD)

- XLD disorders are also caused by abnormalities of genes on the X chromosome.

- Typically males are very severely affected resulting in spontaneous loss of pregnancy or neonatal death.
- Females are affected but will survive.
- When an affected female goes on to have children there is a 33% risk of having an affected female baby as affected males are less likely to survive.
- Examples include: Rett syndrome, Incontinentia pigmenti, etc.

Imprinting disorders

- Genomic imprinting is the normal mechanism by which certain genes are selectively expressed from the maternal or paternal copy of the chromosome.
- When this mechanism is disrupted (by uniparental disomy (UPD), where both copies of a chromosome are inherited from the same parent or by a defect in the imprinting centre), an imprinting disorder may be caused.
- Examples include: Angelman syndrome (see 📖 p404) caused by paternal UPD15, Prader–Willi syndrome (see 📖 p404) caused by maternal UPD15, Russell–Silver syndrome caused by imprinting alterations on chromosome 7 or 11, Beckwith–Weidemann syndrome caused by loss of methylation of *KvDMR* or *UPD11*, etc.

Mitochondrial

- Mitochondrial DNA is a double-stranded circular DNA which encodes 13 proteins all of which are subunits of respiratory chain complexes.
- Tissues with a high energy demand, e.g. skeletal muscle, cardiac muscle, CNS, pancreatic islet cells, liver and kidney, are most likely to be affected.
- Mitochondrial disorders are usually inherited from the mother as the fraction of paternal mitochondria in the fertilized egg is very small (0.1%) and is eliminated in early embryogenesis.
- When the mutation is present in only a few mitochondria in a cell, it is termed 'heteroplasmy' and when the mutation is present in all the mitochondria in a cell, it is termed 'homoplasmy'.
- Mitochondrial mutations show a threshold effect i.e. there is a threshold beyond which heteroplasmy causes disease.
- The threshold varies between different mitochondrial disorders, e.g. Leigh syndrome, NARP (neuropathy, ataxia, retinitis pigmentosa) (see 📖 p247), MELAS (myopathy, encephalopathy, lactic acidosis and stroke).
- Some mitochondrial disorders are caused by nuclear genes which regulate the function of the mitochondria, e.g. some autosomal recessive forms of cerebellar ataxia (see 📖 p247).

Multifactorial

- This type of inheritance is seen in isolated disorders such as:
  - Cleft lip ± palate (see 📖 p407).
  - Learning difficulties (see 📖 p117).
  - Behavioural problems (see 📖 p340 and p369) etc.
- They occur as a result of an interaction between environmental and genetic factors.

Genetic testing

- Different genetic tests are used depending on whether the chromosomes or the genes are being tested.
- Genetic testing should be carried out with appropriate counselling and consent of the patient/parent as the results may have implications for not only the proband but also for other family members. Care should be taken to maintain confidentiality.
- Genetic testing is offered to children for diagnostic purposes or if genetic testing will provide guidance for screening measures in children at risk of a familial disorder, e.g. bowel screening in children at risk of developing familial adenomatosis polyposis.
- Predictive testing of adult onset conditions is *not recommended* in children, e.g. myotonic dystrophy, hereditary motor-sensory neuropathy etc.

Chromosome tests

Karyotype
Is the basic chromosome test looking at the number and arrangement of chromosomes.

Fluorescent in situ hybridization (FISH)
- Is the test that uses specific fluorescent probes which align to a part of a particular chromosome.
- It is used when a specific chromosome deletion or duplication is suspected, e.g. 22q11 deletion in DiGeorge syndrome (see 📖 p396).

Comparative genomic hybridization or array CGH
- Is a relatively new test by which submicroscopic chromosomal aberrations (deletions or duplications) can be identified. However, these abnormalities are not always considered to be pathogenic, as very small aberrations may represent a normal variant.
- Parental testing is often required to clarify the pathogenicity of the finding.

Molecular tests
These tests are done when a single gene disorder is suspected. Either mutations (nucleotide substitution, deletion, or insertion) or abnormal copy numbers (deletions or duplications) in a single gene can account for a disorder.

Sequencing of a gene
- This is the test by which mutations in specific genes are looked for, e.g. tuberous sclerosis (see 📖 p251), NF1 (see 📖 p250), Rett syndrome (see 📖 p405).
- In order to request this test the gene for the suspected condition should be known and testing should be available either in a NHS laboratory or in a research laboratory.
- Caution should be exercised in the interpretation of results when the mutation is reported as a variant and the pathogenicity of the mutation is not clear.

Polymerase chain reaction (PCR)
- Is the technique by which a specific sequence of DNA from the patient is amplified using primers, DNA polymerases and DNA precursors

and compared against that of a standard DNA by running them both on a gel.

- A discrepancy in the size of the PCR product indicates a mutation or deletion of the gene, e.g. in fragile X syndrome (see 📖 p403), myotonic dystrophy (see 📖 p258).

Multiplex ligation-dependent probe amplification (MLPA)

- This is a multiplex PCR method by which gene deletions or duplications are detected. Many single gene disorders may be caused by a complete or partial deletion of the gene in a proportion of patients.
- Hence, when no mutation is identified in a clinically suspected disorder, MLPA should be considered to detect abnormal copy numbers, e.g. in a patient clinically suspected to have CHARGE syndrome but with no mutations detected in the *CHD7* gene.

Whole exome sequencing

- This is a new technique by which the coding sequences (exomes) of all known human genes are sequenced with an aim of finding the causative mutation/s in a gene.
- This test is currently available only in a research setting but is likely to become more widely available in the future.
- This test is useful when a genetic disorder is suspected but no genes have been identified so far to cause it.
- The limitation of this test is that it misses mutations in introns which may account for a patient's phenotype.

Whole genome sequencing

- This is also a new technique by which the entire genome (exons and introns of all genes) of a patient is sequenced with an aim of finding the causative mutation/s.
- The interpretation of the results of this test is complex and hence it is available only for research currently.

Approach to evaluation of a child with dysmorphism, congenital malformation and/or developmental delay

Facial dysmorphism can be a good clue to the clinical diagnosis in several syndromes. In some syndromes, e.g. DS, the facial features are typical and all affected individuals resemble one another (see 📖 p387). In other syndromes, the dysmorphic features may be more subtle or non-specific. Associated structural abnormalities and neurodevelopmental problems will provide further clues to the diagnosis in these cases.

Definitions of terms used

- *Syndrome:* is a set of developmental abnormalities occurring together in a consistently recognizable pattern, e.g. DS, Noonan syndrome, etc.
- *Sequence:* is a pattern of developmental abnormalities occurring as a consequence of a primary defect, e.g. Pierre Robin sequence, a triad of a wide U-shaped cleft palate, small chin, and relatively large tongue (glossoptosis), occurs as a consequence of a small chin, which prevents the normal sized tongue from descending and obstructs the closure of the palatal processes.

- *Association:* is a non-random collection of developmental anomalies that occur together more frequently than expected by chance, e.g. VACTERL (vertebral anomalies, anal atresia, cardiac anomalies, tracheo-oesophageal fistula, (o)esophageal atresia, renal anomalies, and limb defects).
- *Malformation:* is a structural abnormality that occurs due to an abnormal developmental process i.e. a primary error in morphogenesis (e.g. cleft lip).
- *Deformation:* is a distortion of normally programmed structures by a physical force, e.g. talipes caused by oligohydramnios.
- *Disruption:* is the abnormality caused by destruction of normally programmed structures, e.g. limb defects caused by amniotic bands.
- *Dysplasia:* refers to the abnormal cellular organization within a tissue which results in structural changes, e.g. renal cystic dysplasia.

History taking in dysmorphic syndromes
- *Family history:* 3-generation family history with a special focus on congenital abnormalities and neurodevelopmental problems; history of miscarriages, terminations, stillbirths, and neonatal deaths.
- *Pregnancy and delivery:* maternal health, bleeding, medications, alcohol/drug intake, investigations, fetal movements, liquor volume, gestation, and mode of delivery
- *Neonatal history:* Apgar score; birth weight, length; feeding difficulties, admission to special care baby unit, medical problems, congenital anomalies
- *Growth:* height, weight and head circumference.
- *Childhood medical problems:* hearing, vision, seizures, regression of milestones, involuntary movements, constipation/diarrhoea.
- *Developmental history and schooling history:* developmental delay and additional educational needs.
- *Behavioural issues:* social interaction and communications skills, obsessive or ritualistic behaviour, hyperactivity, poor attention span, sleep disturbances, self-harming, and involuntary laughter.

Examination
- *Face:* asymmetry e.g. Goldenhar syndrome, CHARGE syndrome, etc.
- *Hair:* texture e.g. curly, coarse hair in Noonan syndrome, colour e.g. blonde hair in Angelman syndrome, alopecia e.g. ectodermal dysplasia, premature greying e.g. Waardenburg syndrome.
- *Skull:* shape e.g. craniosynostosis in Apert syndrome, Crouzon syndrome, size e.g. microcephaly in Angelman syndrome, macrocephaly in Noonan syndrome.
- *Ears:* shape e.g. cup-shaped ears in CHARGE syndrome, size e.g. microtia in Treacher Collins syndrome, position e.g. low-set ears in DS, posteriorly rotated ears in Noonan syndrome, preauricular pits and tags e.g. branchio-oto-renal syndrome.
- *Eyebrows:* deficiency e.g. absent in ectodermal dysplaisa, interrupted in Kabuki syndrome, synophrys e.g. Cornelia de Lange syndrome, Waardenburg syndrome.
- *Eyes:* deep-set eyes e.g. Angelman syndrome, prominent eyes e.g. Crouzon syndrome, everted eyelids e.g. lateral eversion in Kabuki

syndrome, structural abnormalities e.g. microphthalmia, anophthalmia. Periorbital puffiness e.g. Williams syndrome, epicanthic folds e.g. DS, upslanting palpebral fissures e.g. DS, downslanting palpebral fissures e.g. Noonan syndrome.

- *Nasal bridge:* flat e.g. DS, Stickler syndrome, prominent e.g. autosomal recessive microcephaly.
- *Nose:* short e.g. fetal alcohol syndrome, Williams syndrome, hypoplastic alae nasi or pinched e.g. 22q11 deletion syndrome, anteverted nares e.g. Cornelia de Lange syndrome, prominent nasal tip e.g. tricho-rhino-phalangeal syndrome, protruding nasal columella e.g. Rubinstein–Taybi syndrome.
- *Philtrum:* length e.g. short in Mowat–Wilson syndrome, long in fetal alcohol syndrome, smoothness e.g. smooth in fetal alcohol syndrome.
- *Cheeks:* malar flattening e.g. DS, Treacher Collins syndrome, prominent cheeks e.g. Williams syndrome
- *Lips:* thickness e.g. thin upper lip in fetal alcohol syndrome, shape e.g. cupid's bow shape in Smith–Magenis syndrome.
- *Chin:* size e.g. micrognathia in Pierre Robin sequence, prominence e.g. Angelman syndrome, Sotos syndrome.
- *Neck:* webbing e.g. Noonan syndrome, Turner syndrome, sinus/fistulae e.g. branchio-oto-renal syndrome, low posterior hairline e.g. Noonan syndrome, Turner syndrome.
- *Thorax:* size e.g. small in Jeune syndrome, shape e.g. bell-shaped in Jeune syndrome, skeletal abnormalities e.g. pectus excavatum in Marfan syndrome.
- *Abdomen:* protuberant abdomen e.g. Beckwith–Weidemann syndrome, umbilical hernia e.g. Beckwith–Weidemann syndrome.
- *Back:* spine abnormalities e.g. scoliosis, lordosis.
- *Upper and lower limbs:* asymmetry e.g. Beckwith–Weidemann syndrome, disproportion e.g. skeletal dysplasias, brachydactyly e.g. short 4th and 5th fingers in pseudohypoparathyroidism, arachnodactyly e.g. Marfan syndrome, camptodactyly e.g. distal arthrogryposis, clinodactyly e.g. Russell–Silver syndrome, abnormal thumbs e.g. Rubinstein–Taybi syndrome, polydactyly e.g. Bardet–Biedl syndrome, wide sandal gap e.g. DS, nail hypoplasia e.g. fetal alcohol syndrome, unusual palmar or plantar creases e.g. single palmar crease in Down syndrome, deep plantar creases in mosaic trisomy 8.
- *Skin:* hypopigmentation e.g. ash leaf macules in TS, hyperpigmentation e.g. café au lait patches in NF1, hirsuitism e.g. Coffin–Siris syndrome, eczema e.g. Dubowitz syndrome, photosensitivity e.g. chromosomal breakage disorders.

▶ It is the facial gestalt and the pattern of associated abnormalities that guides the clinician to the diagnosis rather than a single dysmorphic feature.

The list of features is by no means exhaustive. For further reading see 📖 p586 and p596.

Common chromosomal syndromes: aneuploidy

Refers to abnormalities in the number of chromosomes, e.g. DS (trisomy 21), Edwards syndrome (trisomy 18), Patau syndrome (trisomy 13), Pallister–Killian syndrome (tetrasomy 12p).

Down syndrome or trisomy 21

Incidence

- Approximately 1 in 1000 live births. Approximately 60,000 people with DS are living in UK.

Aetiology

- DS may be caused by:
  - Full trisomy 21 i.e. maternal meiotic non-disjunction in 94% of patients.
  - Mosaicism in 2.4%.
  - Translocations in 3.3%. About 75% of the unbalanced translocations are de novo, and about 25% result from familial translocation.
- Advanced maternal age remains the only well-documented risk factor for maternal non-disjunction. The chance of having a child with DS increases with increasing maternal age:
  - At 35 years: 1 in 385.
  - At 40 years: 1 in 106.
  - At 45 years: 1 in 30.

Diagnosis

Prenatal screening

- A combination of the following 3 is used for screening in the general population to calculate the chance of having DS child:
  - Maternal age.
  - Ultrasound findings (thickened nuchal fold, shortened long bones, hypoplastic nasal bone, echogenic bowel, etc.).
  - Maternal serum markers (low AFP, raised human chorionic gonadotropin, low unconjugated oestriol uE3).
- If the screening result suggests an increased risk then following (invasive) tests are offered for more definitive answers:
  - Amniocentesis (performed at 14–16 weeks, >99% accurate).
  - Chorionic villus sampling (at 10–13 weeks, >95% accurate).

Postnatal studies

- FISH studies: for rapid diagnosis on the postnatal ward.
- Karyotyping: is essential to provide risk of recurrence and for genetic counselling.

Effects of extra chromosome 21

- Increased fetal loss, spontaneous abortions (reduced prenatal viability).
- Increased postnatal morbidity.
- Reduced physical growth (short stature, follow 2nd centile on normal growth charts).
- Delayed cognitive development.
- Intellectual disability.

- Dysmorphic physical features (see 📖 p390).
- Increased chance of congenital malformations.
- Increased risk of auto-immunity.
- Reduced humoral and cell-mediated immunity.
- Abnormal physiologic functioning.
- Premature senescence (cataracts, Alzheimer disease, etc.).

Clinical features
Well over 100 features have been described in DS.
- Cardiac:
  - Atrioventricular septal defect.
  - Ventricular septal defect.
  - Atrial septal defect.
  - Patent ductus arteriosus.
  - Tetralogy of Fallot.
  - Other complex congenital heart diseases.
  - Pulmonary hypertension.
- Respiratory:
  - Tracheo-oesophageal fistula.
  - Repeated aspiration (see 📖 p91).
  - Frequent chest infections (>10 times increase in pneumonia (see 📖 p94)).
  - Airway obstruction secondary to glossoptosis, large tonsils/adenoids (leading to arterial hypoxaemia, alveolar hypoventilation, pulmonary hypertension) (see 📖 p90).
- Gastrointestinal:
  - Duodenal atresia/stenosis.
  - Oesophageal atresia.
  - Anal atresia/stenosis.
  - GOR (see 📖 p83).
  - Hirschsprung's disease.
  - Meckel's diverticulum.
  - Increased risk of coeliac disease (reported prevalence 5–15% in DS population).
  - Chronic constipation (see 📖 p84).
- Orthopaedic/musculoskeletal:
  - Atlanto-axial instability.
  - Short long bones.
  - Hypoplasia of the middle phalanx (clinodactyly).
  - Short and broad fingers and toes.
  - Increased space between 1st and 2nd toe (sandal gap).
  - Hyperextensible (increased range of movements in most joints).
  - Joint instability (hips, patella).
- Neuropsychiatric:
  - Intellectual disability (IQ range in DS 20–85; normal range 80–110) (see 📖 p117).
  - Delayed cognitive development.
  - Seizures (5–10% of DS, infantile spasms are common during infancy) (see 📖 p240).
  - Depression (see 📖 p350).
  - Dementia (early onset, Alzheimer's type).

- Behavioural problems (obsessive tendencies, oppositionality, etc. (see 📖 p334)).
- Increased prevalence of autism and ASD (see 📖 p107).
- Increased incidence of congenital SNHL (see 📖 p307), ADHD (see 📖 p126), etc.
- ENT:
  - Hypoplasia of maxillary sinuses.
  - Frequent URTI (both viral and bacterial).
  - Middle ear effusions (OME) (see 📖 p94).
  - Conductive HL (secondary to the above).
  - Large adenoids, tonsils with hypotonia of neck musculature.
  - OSAs (sleep difficulties) (see 📖 p90).
- Eye:
  - Increased incidence of congenital cataract.
  - Keratoconus.
  - Nystagmus (see 📖 p283).
  - Squint (see 📖 p281).
  - Blocked nasolacrimal duct.
  - Increased incidence of conjunctivitis, blepharitis.
  - Increased prevalence of acquired lens opacities (see 📖 p275).
  - Increased prevalence of refractive errors (hypermetropia is more common) (see 📖 p286).
- Haematology:
  - Transient abnormal myelopoiesis (TAM) (leukaemic picture in the neonatal period, secondary to GATA1 mutation).
  - Increased risk of acute lymphoblastic leukemia.
  - Increased risk of acute myeloblastic leukaemia.
  - Decreased risk of solid tumours.
- Endocrine:
  - Congenital hypothyroidism.
  - Hashimoto's thyroiditis (causing hypothyroidism, rarely hyperthyroidism).
  - Diabetes mellitus (insulin dependent, autoimmune).
- Dermatology:
  - Dry skin/eczema (see 📖 p97).
  - Alopecia.
  - Vitiligo.
  - Folliculitis.
  - Recurrent skin infections (see 📖 p95).
  - Transverse palmar crease.
- Dental:
  - Delayed dental eruption.
  - Increased incidence of dental caries (see 📖 p165).
  - Malformed teeth.
  - Malocclusion.
  - Hypocalcified teeth.
- Immunology:
  - Impaired humoral immunity.
  - Impaired cell mediated immunity.
  - Increased auto-immune conditions (Hashimoto's thyroiditis, diabetes, coeliac, vitiligo).

- Reproductive:
  - Decreased fertility in both sexes.
  - Hypospadias.
  - Micropenis.
  - Undescended testicles.
- Abnormal physiologic functioning:
  - Hypersensitivity to pilocarpine.
  - Hyper-reactivity to methotrexate.
  - Predisposition to hyperuricaemia.
  - Increased insulin resistance.
- Dysmorphology:
  - Round face.
  - Flat facial profile (hypoplasia of the cheek bones).
  - Upslanting palpebral fissures.
  - Bilateral epicanthic folds.
  - Flat nasal bridge.
  - Small, low set ears.
  - Small mouth.
  - Relatively large tongue, protruding.

Investigations
- TFT (at birth, annually thereafter, 1/3 will develop hypothyroidism in their lifetime).
- Echocardiography (performed in all patients with DS soon after birth).
- Hearing test: soon after birth and then annually. SNHL (see 🕮 p307) and OME (see 🕮 p306) common.
- Vision test: screen for cataracts, then 1–2 yearly for lifetime (see 🕮 p275).
- Neck X-ray (for atlanto-axial instability): perform if there is suspicion of cervical cord compression.
- Coeliac screen: if growth falters.
- Immunoglobulin subclasses: to identify deficiency of IgG subclasses-if significant bacterial infections.
- Haematology: FBC. Bone marrow test if features of BM dysfunction

Medical care
- Annual health checks and follow-up: complete physical examination (for listed clinical features).
- Growth monitoring: weight faltering common in early years. Rule out hypothyroidism, coeliac etc. Involve dietician. Obesity is a preventable secondary handicap in later years. Encourage physical activity. Explore leisure facilities. Review caloric intake.
- Developmental assessments: annually in the early years, then before secondary school, before transition to college etc. Multidisciplinary assessments involving SLT (see 🕮 p202), OT (see 🕮 p188), PT (see 🕮 p176), etc. as required, more often in early years.
- Sleep: enquire snoring, restless sleep etc. OSA is common (see 🕮 p90). Refer to respiratory colleagues for sleep study. ENT colleagues for airway obstruction.
- Surgical interventions/operations: for heart anomalies, adeno-tonsillectomy, other congenital anomalies, etc. Anaesthetists pay

attention to atlantoaxial instability. Antibiotic prophylaxis for certain heart lesions (e.g. MVP), dental procedures.
- Vaccination: recommend all routine vaccinations (see 📖 p620) plus annual flu vaccinations in early years, pneumococcal vaccines.
- Liaison and referral to following specialists is common:
  - Neurologist (epilepsy (see 📖 p240), cervical cord compression, etc.).
  - Orthopaedic surgeon (hip dislocation, scoliosis (see 📖 p416), feet anomalies (see 📖 p422), etc.).
  - Cardiologist (congenital heart lesions, pulmonary hypertension, etc.).
  - Psychiatry (behavioural disorders, ADHD (see 📖 p126), ODD (see 📖 p334), OCD, etc.).
  - Dietician (dietetic evaluation, feeding problems (see 📖 p82 and p88), recommend balanced diet).
  - Geneticist (genetic counselling).
  - Audiologist (annual checks).
  - Ophthalmologist (annual).
  - Dentist (annual).
  - Dermatologist.
  - Endocrinologist (for thyroid disorders, diabetes, growth faltering).

Educational habilitation
EPs advice on special educational needs (see 📖 p533 and p534). Emphasize learning PSHE, dealing with money, self care, employment/career counselling. Supervised employment possible for many.

Social care
information on allowances, benefits, leisure, long-term living arrangements, respite care, (see 📖 p514) etc.

Prognosis
- The life expectancy for DS has increased 6-fold in the past 80 years.
- The average life expectancy now is into 5th/6th decade.
- Mortality is increased by severe intellectual disability (see 📖 p117), institutionalization, dementia, mobility restrictions, epilepsy, cardiac disease, etc.

Edwards syndrome or trisomy 18
- Caused by the presence of 3 copies of chromosome 18.
- High rate of spontaneous pregnancy loss or a poor outcome in surviving infants is seen.

Clinical features
- IUGR—a consistent feature.
- Small placenta.
- Facial features: microcephaly, microphthalmia, small pointed chin.
- Limbs: overlapping fingers, rocker-bottom feet and short hallux.
- Chest: short sternum.
- Congenital heart disease is common (in 90%).
- Other structural abnormalities: oro-facial cleft, radial ray defects, kidney and brain abnormalities.
- Survival rates are reported to be: 45% at 1 week, 9% at 6 months, and 5% at 1 year.
- Central apnoea and cardiopulmonary arrest are the causes of death.

Inheritance

In about 94% of cases this is caused due to *de novo* meiotic non-disjunction and is hence associated with a low recurrence risk (0.5%). In the remaining, it is caused by a mosaic trisomy 18 or a partial 18q trisomy.

Patau syndrome or trisomy 13

- Caused by the presence of 3 copies of chromosome 13.
- Associated with a high rate of spontaneous pregnancy loss or poor outcome in surviving infants.

Clinical features

- IUGR.
- Holoprosencephaly.
- Microphthalmia/anophthalmia.
- Scalp defects (cutis aplasia).
- Oro-facial clefts (may be midline).
- Congenital heart defects.
- Postaxial polydactyly.
- Omphalocoele.
- Kidney abnormalities.
- Severe developmental delay in survivors.
- Median age of survival is 7–10 days and survival rate at 12 months is 5–10%.
- Central apnoea and cardiopulmonary arrest are the common causes of death.

Inheritance

About 90% are caused by maternal meiotic non-disjunction, which results in a complete trisomy 13; the recurrence risk is low (0.5%). In the remaining 10%, a translocation (usually unbalanced Robertsonian translocation 13;14), mosaic trisomy 13 or partial trisomy 13, may cause Patau syndrome and the recurrence risk may vary accordingly.

Further resources

Down Syndrome Association: ☎ 0845 230 0372 ⚲ http://www.downs-syndrome.org.uk

Down Syndrome Education International: ☎ 02392 855330 ⚲ http://www.downsed.org

Down Syndrome Medical Interest Group: ☎ 0115 883 1158 ⚲ http://www.dsmig.org.uk

Common chromosomal syndromes: sex chromosome anomalies

Are abnormalities affecting the X or Y chromosome. Some common examples are discussed as follows:

Turner syndrome (TS)

- Is caused by the absence of 1 copy of the X chromosome in girls.
- It affects 1 in 2500 live female births.
- The majority of TS pregnancies are, however, lost spontaneously.

Clinical features

- Short stature (mean adult height of 147cm but may be increased by growth hormone treatment in childhood).
- Short webbed neck, low hairline.
- Oedema of hands and feet (in newborn).
- Heart defects: coarctation, bicuspid aortic valve and ventricular septal defect.
- Renal anomalies: horse-shoe kidneys, renal agenesis.
- Glue ears and hearing problems are common childhood problems (see 🕮 p306).
- Delayed or absent puberty and premature menopause are associated with the presence of streak ovaries and the majority of women are infertile.
- Intelligence is usually normal, but IQ may be 10–15 points lower than siblings.
- Social adjustment problems and subtle perceptual difficulties.
- Autoimmune diseases such as hypothyroidism and diabetes mellitus.
- Osteoporosis (see 🕮 p99) and obesity are more common.

Inheritance

In a study by Birkebaek et al. (2002) it was noted that: 49% of TS was caused by 45X, 9% by a structural abnormality of 1 X chromosome, 19% had mosaicism with 45X/46XX and 23% had mosaicism with structural abnormality of one X. The majority of TS karyotypes are thought to result from parental meiotic errors generating abnormal sex chromosomes.

Klinefelter syndrome

- Is caused by the presence of an extra X chromosome in males (47XXY).
- It has a prevalence of 1 in 600–800 with a significant maternal age effect.
- It is usually diagnosed prenatally as an unexpected finding on amniocentesis or CVS. In adult males it may be diagnosed during investigations for infertility.

Clinical features

- Facial dysmorphism is not present.
- Tall stature (final adult height 187cm).
- Transient gynaecomastia.

- Breast cancer risk (3%) is increased compared to men in the general population, but usually occurs later on in life (mean age at diagnosis 72 years).
- Boys enter puberty normally but develop low testosterone levels.
- Testes are small in adult life.
- Usually infertile due to low sperm counts.
- Decrease of 10–15 points in IQ compared to siblings and about 2/3 have additional educational needs (usually extra help in mainstream school) (see 📖 p533).
- Passive and unassertive behaviour has been frequently noted.
- Boys should be referred to paediatric endocrinologist before the age of 10 for monitoring of growth and hormonal levels.
- Testosterone supplementation may be needed to help with self-esteem, facial hair growth, and libido.
- Referral to a reproductive specialist is recommended in adult life to consider assisted conception or AID (artificial insemination using donor sperm). A slight increase in aneuploidy (sex chromosome abnormalities and trisomy 21) has been noted in the offspring of these men.

Recurrence risk

Is low (<1%) for parents of boys with 47XXY.

Triple X syndrome

- Is caused by the presence of an extra X chromosome in a female (47XXX).
- It is usually picked up as an incidental finding at amniocentesis or CVS and has an incidence of 1in 1000 live births.
- It is also associated with a significant maternal age effect.

Clinical features

- Tall stature with relatively small head size.
- No facial dysmorphism seen.
- Frequency of urogenital abnormalities is slightly increased.
- Puberty and fertility are usually normal, although there is a slight increased risk of premature ovarian failure.
- A 10–15 points decrease in IQ compared to siblings is noted. Speech and language delay (see 📖 p202 and p205) and the need for additional educational needs (see 📖 p524 and p531) have been seen in some individuals.

Recurrence risk

Is low for offspring and for siblings of affected females.

Further resource

Klinefelter Organisation: ☎ 01206 870430 🖰 http://www.klinefelter.org.uk

Common chromosomal syndromes: translocations

Reciprocal translocation

- Occurs when 2 or more separate chromosomes exchange pieces of chromosomes between themselves. This is termed 'balanced translocation' when the translocated chromosomes have not lost or gained any chromosomal material; this is not usually associated with a phenotype.
- An 'unbalanced translocation' occurs when chromosomal material is gained (duplication) or lost (deletion) and is often associated with a phenotype which is dependent on the genes affected and the size of the deletion or duplication.
- A parent with a balanced translocation has a risk of having children with an unbalanced translocation. The risk of having a live-born affected child is dependent on the size and content of the translocation, as large deletions or duplications may result in a miscarriage.

Robertsonian translocation

- Is the result of fusion of acrocentric chromosomes (those with a very short 'p' arm), e.g. chromosomes 13, 14, 15, 21, and 22.
- Some common robertsonian translocations are rob(13q14q) and rob(14q21q).
- The translocated chromosome may act as a single chromosome during meiosis and may be passed on together with a copy of the normal chromosome to the offspring resulting in disease, e.g. when a parent has a rob(14q21q), they may pass on this translocated chromosome along with a normal chromosome 21, resulting in DS (see 📖 p387) in the child.

Common chromosomal syndromes: microdeletion syndromes

- These are syndromes associated with deletion of parts of chromosomes, which cannot be identified on conventional karyotype. Specific FISH tests have to be done in order to confirm a clinical suspicion of the diagnosis.
- More recently with the use of array CGH several new microdeletion syndromes have been described.
- Many microdeletion syndromes have reciprocal microduplication syndromes. Some common examples of microdeletion syndromes are discussed as follows.

DiGeorge or velocardiofacial syndrome

This is caused by a microdeletion of the long arm of 1 copy of chromosome 22 (22q11 deletion).

Clinical features

- Facial features: short palpebral fissures, prominent nasal bridge and root with a pinched appearance to tip of nose, rounded ears with deficient upper helices.
- Cardiac defects: in ~75%. They could be tetralogy of Fallot, ventral septal defect, interrupted aortic arch, right-sided aortic arch, ASD, etc. Conversely ~10% of individuals with congenital heart disease have 22q11 deletion.
- Oropharyneal abnormalities: cleft palate, submucous cleft palate, velopharyngeal insufficiency.
- Genitourinary abnormalities: renal agenesis, multicystic dysplastic kidneys, hydronephrosis.
- Endocrine function: hypocalcemia (due to decreased parathyroid function), hypothyroidism.
- Immune function: recurrent minor infections may occur; in 1% abnormalities of T cell numbers and function may be seen (due to effects on thymus).
- Brain abnormalities: polymicrogyria (bilateral perisylvian) and pachygria.
- Development and learning: speech and language delay (see 📖 p200–5) is common. Learning difficulties (see 📖 p117) are reported in 68% of individuals and are often in the mild–moderate range. They often require special educational support (see 📖 p524 and p531).
- Psychiatric disorders: bipolar affective disorder and schizophrenia are described in 18% of adults.

Management

- Echocardiogram.
- Renal ultrasound scan.
- Audiometry.
- Plasma calcium: check at least once during infancy, childhood, adolescence and pregnancy.
- Immunology: T cell, B cell and NK (natural killer) lymphocyte subsets. Refer to immunologist if abnormal. Live vaccines (e.g. oral polio and BCG) should be avoided until immune function has been checked.
- Referral to speech therapy (see 📖 p88) and cleft team for palatal assessment.

Inheritance
Autosomal dominant (see 📖 p381). An affected person has a 50% chance of passing on the deletion in every pregnancy. Parental chromosome tests should be offered. If both parents do not have the deletion, the recurrence risk in their offspring is low, e.g. <1% due to gonadal mosaicism (when some cells in the gonads carry the mutation but the other cells are normal). Prenatal testing is available. Marked inter and intrafamilial variability is seen.

Williams syndrome
Is caused by the deletion of a small piece of the long arm of 1 copy of chromosome 7 (7q11.23 deletion). The elastin (*ELN*) gene is deleted.

Clinical features
- Facial features: characteristic appearance with periorbital fullness, bulbous nasal tip, long philtrum, wide mouth, full lips, full cheeks, lacy or stellate iris.
- Failure to thrive with feeding difficulties (see 📖 p88).
- Congenital heart disease: supravalvular aortic stenosis, peripheral pulmonary stenosis; other arteries may also be involved.
- Renal abnormalities: renal artery stenosis causing hypertension; nephrocalcinosis due to hypercalcaemia; renal cysts.
- Hypercalcaemia: ~15%; disappears in second year of life but may recur later. When present, it can cause constipation, failure to thrive and nephrocalcinosis.
- Development: variable (see 📖 Chapter 3: Development). Ranging from mild to moderate mental retardation (see 📖 p117); strength in language skills (but words may be used inappropriately); poor visuospatial skills (see 📖 p213).
- Behaviour: overfriendly personality; short attention span; (see 📖 p214) anxiety (see 📖 p354).

Management
- Monitoring of BP in both arms annually.
- Measurement of calcium/creatine ratio in a random spot urine and urinalysis annually.
- Serum calcium levels every 2 years.
- Thyroid function and TSH level every 3 years.
- Audiological examination every 5 years (see 📖 p300).
- Renal and bladder ultrasound every 10 years.
- Avoid multivitamins as they contain Vitamin D.
- The frequency of monitoring should be increased and appropriate treatment instituted in case of abnormal results.

Inheritance
Autosomal dominant, although in reality few patients with William syndrome go on to have children. If parents do not carry the deletion, gonadal mosaicism risk of <1% applies.

Further resources
22q11 Deletion Syndromes Max Appeal: ☎ 0800 389 1049 🖥 http://www.maxappeal.org.uk
William Syndrome Foundation: ☎ 01732 365 152 🖥 http://www.williams-syndrome.org.uk

Single gene disorders

Are caused by mutations or deletions in a single gene. Some common examples of single gene disorders seen in paediatric clinics are described.

Marfan syndrome

Is a connective tissue disorder caused by a mutation or deletion of the fibrillin 1 (*FBN1*) gene, present on chromosome 15q21.

Clinical features

- Build: tall stature, slim build, long arm span, arachnodactyly.
- Skeletal: pectus carinatum or excavatum, scoliosis (see 📖 p416), pes planus.
- Cardiac: aortic dilatation, regurgitation or dissection, mitral valve prolapse.
- Ophthalmological: ectopia lentis, abnormally flat cornea, increased axial length of globe.
- Pulmonary: spontaneous pneumothorax, apical blebs.
- Skin: striae atrophicae (stretch marks), recurrent or incisional hernia.
- Spine: scoliosis, lumbosacral dural ectasia.
- Clinical diagnosis is based on the *Ghent criteria*. Clinical diagnosis may be confirmed by genetic testing of the *FBN1* gene.

Management

Patients should be under the care of the specialist multidisciplinary Marfan syndrome clinic, if possible.

- Annual echocardiogram.
- Periodic ophthalmic review in childhood (see 📖 p271).
- Growth monitoring.
- Spine monitoring for scoliosis (see 📖 p416).

Inheritance

- Autosomal dominant with 50% risk to offspring; high new mutation rate of ~30%.
- Prenatal diagnosis is possible if mutation in family is known.

Ehlers–Danlos syndrome

- Is a connective tissue disorder caused by mutation or deletion in the collagen genes. Depending on the clinical features, EDS has been classified into several types.
- The classical forms of EDS are EDS type I and II and are caused by mutations in the *COL5A1* and *COL5A2* genes.

Clinical features

- Soft, hyperextensible skin.
- Easy bruising.
- Thin, atrophic, cigarette-paper scars.
- Joint hypermobility (see 📖 p178 and p180).
- Risk of prematurity in affected fetuses.

EDS type III

Is the hypermobility type EDS. This is a common but usually mild disorder, associated with soft skin and hypermobility of joints. Sometimes, joint dislocations may occur.

Vascular EDS or EDS type IV
Is an uncommon but serious type of EDS. It is caused by mutations in the *COL3A1* gene.

Clinical features
- Characteristic facial features of prominent eyes, hollow cheeks and pinched nose caused by decreased adipose tissue.
- Thin, translucent skin with visible veins.
- Easy bruising.
- Arterial rupture.
- Rupture of bowel, bladder or uterus.

Other types of EDS are less common and may be associated with kypho-scoliosis, rupture of optic globe, premature ageing, etc.

Inheritance
Predominantly autosomal dominant with 50% risk to offspring. Some inter and intrafamilial variability is seen. Genetic testing is recommended mainly for the 'Vascular type of EDS' or those that are associated with serious life-threatening complications.

Stickler syndrome or hereditary arthro-ophthalmopathy
Is caused by mutations in the collagen genes, *COL2A1* or *COL11A1* genes.

Clinical features
- Facial features: flat midface with depressed nasal bridge, short nose with anteverted nares and micrognathia. The facial gestalt is more distinctive in early childhood.
- Opthalmological: ~in 95% some involvement of eye. High myopia, cataract, retinal detachment (60%), blindness (4%) (see 📖 p275).
- Oropharyngeal: cleft palate (including submucous cleft palate) or Pierre Robin sequence (triad of wide U-shaped cleft palate, small chin and glossoptosis).
- Joints: hypermobility in childhood, may be associated with hip and other joint pains. In adulthood premature osteoarthritis may occur.
- Hearing loss: may be conductive due to glue ears (see 📖 p306) especially in those with a cleft palate; sensorineural deafness (see 📖 p307) is more diagnostic.

Management
- Ophthalmological assessment (see 📖 p271) by vitreo-retinal specialist- prophylactic retinopexy is offered to individuals at risk of detaching the retina.
- Audiometry (see 📖 p300).
- Referral to speech therapy (see 📖 p202) and cleft team for assessment.

Inheritance
Autosomal dominant with a 50% risk to each offspring. Prenatal testing is possible if mutation is known in family.

Neurofibromatosis type 1 or NF1
- Is caused by a mutation or deletion of the NF1 or neurofibromin gene.

Clinical features

Having 2 or more of the following features is sufficient to make a diagnosis of NF1:

- 6 or more café-au-lait patches. >1.5 cm in postpubertal individuals, >0.5cm in prepubertal individuals.
- Freckling in the axilla, groin, or neck.
- 2 or more neurofibromas.
- One or more plexiform neurofibroma.
- Optic glioma: more common in children below the age of 6 years.
- 2 or more Lisch nodules (benign iris hamartomas).
- Distinctive bony lesion, e.g. sphenoid wing dysplasia; pseudarthrosis of long bones.
- Family history of NF1.

Additional clinical features consist of:

- Short stature.
- Macrocephaly (see 📖 p231).
- Scoliosis (see 📖 p416).
- Learning difficulties needing extra help at school (see 📖 p117).
- Symptoms from internal neurofibromas.
- Phaeochromocytoma causing raised BP.
- Renal artery stenosis also causes raised BP but more common in those less than 20 years of age.
- Precocious puberty: related to chiasmal optic glioma.
- Malignant peripheral nerve sheath tumours or MPNST: originate in existing plexiform neurofibromas or from deep-seated nerves. They present with pain or rapid growth. Risk of MPNST is increased following radiation and hence it should be avoided whenever possible.

Investigations and management

- Skin examination: using a Wood's light to check for the presence of 6 or more cafe au lait patches, assessment of existing neurofibromas.
- Ophthalmological referral: to look for Lisch nodules using slit-lamp examination. Annual ophthalmic surveillance is recommended, for children <6 years of age, for optic glioma (see 📖 p271).
- Annual BP monitoring.
- Monitoring of growth parameters (see 📖 pp602–9 and pp616–19).
- Developmental assessment (see 📖 p36).
- Clinical assessment of spine (see 📖 p416).
- MRI brain scan: is not routinely recommended. But should be considered in those with:
  - Rapidly increasing HC to exclude acqueduct stenosis.
  - Epilepsy (see 📖 p240).
  - Acute onset of headaches (see 📖 p235), visual disturbances or vomiting.
  - Focal neurological signs.
  - Precocious puberty.

Inheritance

Autosomal dominant: 50% risk to each offspring of being affected. Prenatal testing is available if the familial mutation is known. However, due to the wide inter- and intrafamilial variability, the phenotype cannot be predicted.

Segmental NF1

- This is the mosaic form of NF1 affecting only one part of the body (varying from a narrow strip to a whole quadrant of the body).
- Distribution of features may be unilateral or bilateral.
- It is caused by a postzygotic mutation in the NF1 gene. The risk of a parent with segmental NF1 having an offspring with NF1 ranges from <1% to 50% depending on how many germline cells carry the mutation. An empiric risk figure of 5% is quoted.
- An affected offspring would have features of NF1 but not in a segmental form as all the cells would carry the mutation.

Tuberous sclerosis or TS

Is caused by mutations in the *TSC1* or *TSC2* gene.

Clinical features

- CNS: cortical tubers, subependymal nodules, subependymal giant cell astrocytoma (SEGAs) may manifest as seizures, e.g. infantile spasms (see 📖 p240).
- Skin: facial angiofibromata, fibrous plaques, subungual fibromas, hypomelanotic ash-leaf macules, Shagreen patch, 'confetti' skin lesions.
- Ocular: retinal nodular hamartoma (tend to be asymptomatic), retinal achromic patch.
- Cardiac: rhabdomyoma (may present antenatally).
- Renal: angiomyolipoma, multiple renal cysts.
- Respiratory: pulmonary lymphangiomyomatosis (usually presents in adult life).
- Skeletal: bone cysts.
- Oral: pits in dental enamel, gingival fibromas.
- Gastrointestinal: hamartomatous rectal polyps.
- Learning disability (see 📖 p117): about 50% of individuals with TS have a normal IQ. Learning difficulties are linked to seizures and may range from mild to moderate. Children who present with infantile spasms in the first 2 years of life are more likely to have learning disability.
- Behavioural problems : autism (in 25–61%). Risk is higher if tuber in temporal lobe (see 📖 p107), hyperactivity, attention deficit (see 📖 p126), sleep disturbance (see 📖 p168).

Investigations and management

- Ophthalmological assessment (see 📖 p271): for retinal hamartomas.
- Cranial imaging: CT scan. To look for cortical tubers, subependymal nodules and SEGAs.
- Renal ultrasound scan to look for angiomyolipomas and renal cysts.
- Echocardiogram in infants to look for rhabdomyomas.
- Mutation analysis of *TSC1* and *TSC2* genes.
- Refer family to clinical genetics for examination, investigation and counselling of at-risk relatives (see 📖 p380).

Inheritance

Autosomal dominant with 50% risk to each offspring if a parent carries the mutation. About 60% of cases arise as a result of a new mutation in the family. If neither parent is affected there is a 2% risk of recurrence due to gonadal mosaicism. Prenatal testing is on offer if the mutation in the family is known.

Approach to evaluation of a child with learning difficulties ± behavioural problems

- Cognitive difficulties occur in 2–3% of the population.
- They are often multifactorial.
- It can be difficult to differentiate the contribution of genetic susceptibility factors from that of environmental factors especially in children with mild learning difficulties without any other associated features.
- In children with moderate to severe learning difficulties (see 📖 p117), after a careful personal and family history and a detailed clinical examination the following baseline investigations should be carried out: Chromosomes, Fragile X, TFTs, urine: amino acids, organic acids, and mucoploysaccharides (see 📖 p123).

Common syndromes associated with learning difficulties

Several genetic syndromes are associated with developmental delay and learning difficulties (see 📖 p117). Some of the more common ones likely to be seen in a paediatric clinic are discussed:

Fragile X syndrome (FRAXA)

- Is the most common genetic cause of mental retardation in boys, with approximately 1 in 5500 males carrying the full mutation.
- The *FMR1* gene is on the X chromosome and contains trinucleotide repeats (TNR) of CGG.
- These repeats are likely to expand when passed on to their offspring, particularly when inherited from the mother. This is called *anticipation*. The box below shows the classification of different TNR sizes in FRAXA.

Box 10.1 Allele sizes in FRAXA

- Normal: <45 repeats.
- Intermediate allele: 45-54 repeats.
- Premutation carriers: 55–200 repeats.
- Full mutation: >200 repeats.

Full mutation

Males with full mutation present with features of FRAXA. These include:
- Physical features: long face, large prominent ears with cupping of pinnae, joint hypermobility (see 📖 p180), large testes post-puberty.
- Developmental delay (see 📖 p36 and p57): hypotonia, mild motor delay, speech and language problems ranging from no speech to mild delay.
- Learning difficulties (see 📖 p117): most boys have additional educational needs. IQ is reduced but may range from 41–88 (the latter is seen in mosaics). A degree of supported living as adults is required in most full mutation carriers.
- Behavioural problems (see 📖 p340): overactivity, poor concentration, impulsivity (see 📖 p126), autistic spectrum disorder (see 📖 p107), echolalia.

Female full mutation carriers are less affected, as they have a normal X which produces variable amounts of the protein. Up to 50% of females will show learning difficulties and behavioural problems, but are less severely affected compared to males. Those with skewed X-inactivation are more likely to show symptoms.

Premutation

- Those with premutations are less likely to present with developmental delay (see 📖 Chapter 3: Development), learning difficulties, and behavioural problems (see 📖 p340). Hence in a child with neurodevelopmental problems, in whom a premutation allele is identified, further investigations should be done to find out the cause.
- Premutations are likely to expand into a full mutation when passed on from a premutation carrier mother to her children. Fathers that carry a premutation, pass it on to all their daughters, but these are less likely

to expand. They cannot pass it to their sons, as the sons will inherit the Y chromosome from them.

- Adult female premutation carriers are at risk of premature menopause and adult male premutation carriers are thought to be at a risk of FRAXTAS (fragile X tremor ataxia syndrome).

Intermediate alleles

These may represent precursors of a premutation in a successive generation. They do not have a phenotypic effect on the individuals that carry them.

Inheritance

X-linked inheritance with carrier mothers being at a 50% risk of having an affected son and a 50% risk of having a carrier daughter (who may be affected). Prenatal testing is available and consists of maternal blood sampling for fetal sexing at 9 weeks, followed by chorionic villus sampling to test the mutation (usually in case of a male pregnancy).

Angelman syndrome

Is a neurobehavioural disorder caused by a disturbance in the maternally imprinted region of chromosome 15q11.13, which includes the *UBE3A* gene.

Clinical features

- Severe developmental delay (see 📖 p57): speech is particularly poor or even absent.
- Wide-based ataxic gait.
- Characteristic EEG (2–3Hz large-amplitude slow-wave bursts) with or without seizures.
- Microcephaly (see 📖 p231).
- Excitable, happy personality (the syndrome was previously termed 'Happy Puppet syndrome' due to the happy affect with the wide-based gait.
- Love of water and fascination with reflections.
- Facial features: deep set eyes, wide smiling mouth and prominent chin.
- Hypopigmentation in some patients (blonde and blue-eyed).

Inheritance

The recurrence risk depends on the mechanism by which the Angelman syndrome has been caused.

- In 70% of individuals it is caused by a deletion of maternal chromosome 15q11–13; identified using a FISH test or routine karyotyping. The recurrence risk is low (<1%), if parental testing is normal.
- In 20% a mutation in the imprinted *UBE3A* gene is the cause; women carrying a *UBE3A* mutation are at a 50% risk of passing on Angelman syndrome in each pregnancy. If men carry the mutation, their children are not affected as the gene is silenced.
- In 2–5% it results from paternal uniparental disomy of chromosome 15; recurrence risks are low (0.5%)
- In 2–5% an imprinting defect is the cause; recurrence risk may be as high as 50% if due to an imprinting centre mutation.

Prader–Willi syndrome (PWS)

The most common genetic syndrome associated with obesity and neurodevelopmental problems is PWS.

Clinical features
- Neonatal central hypotonia (see 📖 p233).
- Feeding difficulties (see 📖 p88) and failure to thrive in infancy.
- Rapid weight gain between 1–6 years of age.
- Facial features: almond-shaped eyes, V-shaped mouth may be present in young children.
- Truncal obesity.
- Small hands and feet.
- Small genitalia, hypogonadotrophic hypogonadism, fertility is rare.
- Short stature.
- Behaviour: insatiable appetite and food-seeking behaviour, ritualistic behaviour, insensitivity to pain.
- Developmental delay and learning difficulties are present (see 📖 p117): mean IQ of 60. Adults may be able to live independently but need some degree of support and supervision.

Inheritance
- In 75% of individuals PWS is caused by a deletion of paternal chromosome 15q11–13. The recurrence risk is low at <1% if neither parent has the deletion.
- If a father has the deletion there is a 50% risk of PWS but this is rare due to decreased fertility; if a mother has the deletion she is at a 50% risk of having a child with Angelman syndrome this too is rare but has been reported.
- In 24% it is due to maternal uniparental disomy of chromosome 15, recurrence risk is low. 1% have an imprinting centre mutation with recurrence risk of 50%.

Rett syndrome

This is a severe X-linked dominant neurodevelopmental disorder that affects females and is caused by mutations in the *MECP2* gene.

Clinical features
- Normal prenatal and perinatal development.
- Loss of acquired skills: speech, communication and hand skills.
- Postnatal microcephaly (see 📖 p231).
- Stereotypic hand movements (see 📖 p238).
- Seizures and abnormal EEG (see 📖 p240).
- Episodes of hyperventilation and breath-holding.
- Bruxism.
- Cold feet.
- Scoliosis (see 📖 p416).
- Spontaneous outbursts of laughter/crying.
- Autistic features (see 📖 p107).
- Severe developmental delay (see 📖 p57 and p117).

Inheritance
The majority have a new mutation, which is not inherited. The mutation is usually on the paternal X chromosome. There is a small risk of gonadal mosaicism. Affected girls do not reproduce due to severe mental disability and hence familial cases are rare. It is lethal in males, unless it occurs as a

result of somatic mosaicism or occurs in a male with Klinefelter syndrome (47XXY) (see 📖 p393).

X-linked mental retardation syndromes (XLMR)

• This should be suspected in boys with mental retardation (see 📖 p117) where other X-linked causes, e.g. fragile X syndrome has been ruled out. A family history (see 📖 p6) of brothers of the proband being affected and/or maternal uncles being affected strongly point to this diagnosis.

• Several genes on the X-chromosome are expressed in the brain and are important for normal neurodevelopment. Several XLMR genes have been identified so far, e.g. *CUL4B*, *OPHN1*, etc., but individually these are a rare cause of mental retardation.

• Due to the significant recurrence risks involved it is important that these individuals are referred to the genetics service (see 📖 p380).

Further resources

Angelman Syndrome: ☎ 0300 999 0102 🖰 http://www.angelmanuk.org
Fragile X Society: ☎ 01371 875100 🖰 http://www.fragilex.org.uk
Prader–Willi Syndrome Association (UK): ☎ 01332 365676 🖰 http://www.pwsa.org.uk
Rett UK: ☎ 01582 798 911 🖰 http://www.rettuk.org

Other common genetic referrals

Congenital anomalies

- Several patients with isolated congenital anomalies are referred to the genetics service.
- The presence of >1 structural abnormality or the accompaniment of other problems such as dysmorphism (see ☐ p384), developmental delay (see ☐ Chapter 3: Develpment), behavioural problems may indicate a syndromic diagnosis which may be associated with a significant recurrence risk.
- However, some isolated congenital anomalies may be associated with a recurrence risk, e.g. cleft lip and palate, cleft palate, spina bifida, congenital heart disease, craniosynostosis (Table 10.1).

Table 10.1 Recurrence risks of common isolated congenital anomalies

Anomaly	Sibling risk in %	Offspring risk in %
Cleft lip and palate	4	4.3
Cleft palate	1.8	3
Congenital heart disease	2–3	3–5
Neural tube defects	3	4
Craniosynostosis		
Coronal	5	–
Sagittal	1	–

This risk is in addition to the 2–3% risk in the general population of having a baby with a congenital anomaly in any pregnancy.

- Isolated congenital anomalies are often multifactorial in inheritance. Some non-syndromic isolated congenital anomalies may be inherited often in an autosomal dominant manner and may show reduced penetrance, e.g. cleft lip and palate.

Sensorineural hearing loss (SNHL)

- Severe deafness affects 1 in 1000 children between infancy and early childhood (prelingual years).
- ~60% of SNHL is genetic in origin.
- For causes of SNHL, see ☐ Audiology p307.
- The most common gene accounting for recessive form of SNHL (in about 50%) is the connexin 26 gene. The carrier frequency of this gene in European, North American, and Mediterranean populations is 1 in 50. Pendred syndrome is another common recessive form of SNHL and accounts for 5% of severe deafness (see ☐ pp307–10).
- For investigations of SNHL, see ☐ Audiology p304.

Autism

- The cause is unknown in the majority of patients (~90%) and is multifactorial in aetiology.
- The genetic causes that should be considered are:
  - Chromosomal abnormalities.
  - Fragile X syndrome (see 📖 p403).
  - Rett syndrome (see 📖 p405).
  - Tuberous sclerosis (see 📖 p401).
  - Mutations in neuroligin3 and neuroligin4 (X-linked autism).
- Siblings of individuals with autism are at a 3–5% risk of developing the disorder with an additional 5–7% risk of having a milder communication disorder. In those patients with a family history of autism, the risk will vary depending on the type of inheritance suspected.
- For further details on autism and ASD (see 📖 p107).

Further resources

Bardet–Biedl syndrome: ☎ 01633 718415 🖲 http://www.lmbbs.org.uk

Beckwith–Wiedemann syndrome: ☎ 07889 211000 🖲 http://www.bws-support.org.uk

Cleft Lip &/or Palate CLAPA: ☎ 020 7833 4884 🖲 http://www.clapa.com

Contact a Family (UK) 🖲 http://www.cafamily.org.uk

Deaf Education through Listening & Talking (DELTA): ☎ 0845 108 1437 🖲 http://www.deafeducation.org.uk

Geneclinics: 🖲 http://www.geneclinics.org

Genetic Alliance UK: ☎ 020 7704 3141 🖲 http://www.geneticalliance.org.uk

National Deaf Children's Society (NDCS): ☎ 0808 800 8880 🖲 http://www.ndcs.org.uk

National Organisation for Rare Disorders (US): 🖲 http://www.raredisease.org

Online Mendelian Inheritance in Man (OMIM): 🖲 http://www.ncbi.nlm.nih.gov

Pubmed: 🖲 http://www.ncbi.nlm.nih.gov/PubMed

Restricted Growth: Child Growth Foundation: ☎ 020 8994 7625 🖲 http://www.childgrowthfoundation.org

Restricted Growth Association: ☎ 0300 111 1970 🖲 http://www.restrictedgrowth.co.uk

RNID: ☎ 0808 808 0123 🖲 http://www.rnid.org.uk

Unique: ☎ 01883 330766 🖲 http://www.rarechromo.org

Undiagnosed Children (any disorder/syndrome): 🖲 http://www.makingcontact.org

Orthopaedics

Nothing ventured, nothing gained.

Japanese proverb

Orthopaedic assessment

The orthopaedic examination is tailored to the patient's age, compliance, and presenting complaint. A full description of the numerous musculoskeletal examinations is beyond the scope of this book, but a general orthopaedic examination must be performed to avoid missing additional pathologies.

Head

- Examine the head from above for evidence of plagiocephaly (see 📖 p231).
- Observe how the head is held (?torticollis).
- Observe the face for dysmorphic features (see 📖 p384).

Spine

- Assess the range of cervical spine movement, active and passive.
- Look for spinal deformities in the coronal and sagittal planes. A better impression may be gained by running a finger down the spinous processes (also see 📖 p416 and p436).
- Look for sacral pits, hairy patches, appendages (see 📖 p261).
- Asses spine ROM and observe for a rib hump on forward flexion.
- Check that a clavicle is present both sides and look for chest wall asymmetry.

Upper limbs

- Fully expose the limbs and observe any asymmetry and abnormal posturing.
- Ask about limitations in function and sensation (age appropriate).
- Assess passive and active ROM of shoulder, elbow, forearm, wrist, and hand.

Lower limbs

Standing

- Check for leg-length inequality.
- Look for deformity, e.g. genu varum or valgum (see 📖 p415).
- Check the feet are plantigrade and assess arch height (see 📖 p415).
- Observe the gait (see 📖 p433) noting: any asymmetry in stance time; foot progression angle, and the progression of heel strike, foot flat, and toe-off.

On the couch

- Check for leg-length inequality.
- Examine the ROM of the hips and note any discomfort (also see 📖 p419).
- Assess knee ROM and palpate the joint lines for tenderness.
- Assess ankle ROM especially dorsiflexion range with the heel in neutral alignment. An increased range may be possible with the knee flexed due to release of tension in gastrocnemius.
- Note the foot shape and observe for callosities on the sole of the foot (also see 📖 p422).

The examiner may then move on to a specific and targeted examination and neurological examination (see 📖 p228) if required.

Orthopaedic assessment in cerebral palsy

Sensation

- May be affected in all modalities.
- Is predictive of spontaneous use of the limb.
- Correlates with limb size.

Tone

- Resting posture gives an indication of tone.
- Stretching the affected muscles will give an idea of whether this is dystonia (see 📖 p238) or velocity dependent.
- The degree of spasticity can be assessed with the modified Ashworth scale.

The Modified Ashworth Scale

- 0: no increase in muscle tone.
- 1: slight increase in muscle tone manifested by a catch and release or minimal resistance at the end range of motion.
- 1a: slight increase in muscle tone manifested by a catch followed by minimal resistance through the remainder of the range of motion.
- 2: more marked increase in muscle tone through most of the ROM.
- 3: considerable increase in muscle tone, passive movement difficult.
- 4: affected part is in rigid flexion or extension.

Strength

- Spastic muscles are usually weak.
- Spasticity may need to be reduced (e.g. with botulinum toxin or nerve blocks) in order to determine the strength of the antagonist muscles.
- Strength of individual muscles or muscle groups is measured using the Medical Research Council (MRC) grading.
- Determination of strength will give an indication of function, but will also inform decision making particularly with regard to surgery.

The Medical Research Council strength grading

- Grade 5: muscle contracts normally against full resistance.
- Grade 4: muscle strength is reduced but muscle contraction can still move joint against resistance.
- Grade 3: muscle strength is further reduced such that the joint can be moved only against gravity with the examiner's resistance completely removed.
- Grade 2: muscle can move only if the resistance of gravity is removed.
- Grade 1: only a trace or flicker of movement is seen or felt in the muscle or fasciculation's are observed in the muscle.
- Grade 0: no movement is observed.

Contractures

- Initially muscles show a dynamic increase in tone, i.e. they can be stretched out to their full length.
- Over time the muscles become shortened. This can be distinguished from joint contractures by altering joint positions when testing muscles that cross >1 joint. For example, finger extension may be possible with wrist flexion but not with the wrist in neutral, illustrating shortening of the finger flexor muscles. Also, limited dorsiflexion at the ankle may be improved by flexing the knee thus slackening off the gastrocnemius muscle. If there is no improvement then shortening of soleus is responsible (the Silverskjold test).

Torsional profile

Bones grow and remodel in response to the forces acting on them. Children with CP often have abnormal torsion of the long bones, particularly increased femoral anteversion which often produces an intoeing gait. The child will have more internal than external rotation at the hips.

Function

If ambulatory, an assessment is made of the child's ability to walk. 3-dimensional gait analysis may be helpful in treatment planning.

Upper limb function is assessed by asking about age appropriate activities such as ability to dress, cut up food, do up buttons etc. Validated assessments of the child's function such as the Assisting Hand Assessment (AHA) or Shriners Hospital Upper Extremity Evaluation (SHUEE) give an objective measure of function and are useful in planning treatment and as an outcome measure.

The AHA measures how the affected arm and hand are used in bimanual performance by observing the child's spontaneous handling of certain toys. It is validated for children aged between 18 months and 12 years with hemiplegic CP, obstetric brachial plexus palsy, and upper limb reduction deficiency. After obtaining video of the 'play session' the accredited assessor then scores the movement and use of the limb.

The SHUEE analyses the spontaneous use and the positioning of the upper limb during defined tasks. Again the assessment is videoed and scored afterwards. The SHUEE is validated and used for children aged between 7–18 years with hemiplegic CP.

Normal variants

- Normal variants are common.
- They do not require intervention, just parental reassurance.
- Most resolve over time.
- Careful examination is required to exclude pathology.

Intoeing gait (Fig. 11.1)

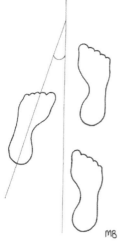

MB

Fig. 11.1 Foot progression angle. Drawing by Meg Buckingham.

Foot progression angle describes the angle between the longitudinal axis of the foot and the direction of walking. 'Normal' is between 20 external and 5 internal.

'Intoeing' describes an internal foot progression angle. This may be due to:
- Persistent femoral anteversion.
- Internal tibial torsion.
- Metatarsus adductus.

Persistent femoral anteversion (Fig. 11.2)
- Seen most commonly in girls with ligamentous laxity.
- For the femoral head to sit comfortably in the acetabulum during walking, the whole leg is rotated internally.
- Examination reveals more internal than external rotation at the hips in extension (Fig. 11.3).
- Improves over the first decade of life.
- Tripping improves by age 4 as coordination develops. Running may look awkward but is functional.

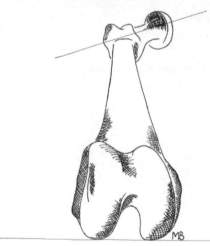

Fig. 11.2 Femoral anteversion—the angle between the longitudinal axis of the femoral neck and the femoral condyles. Drawing by Meg Buckingham.

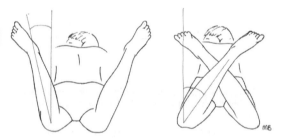

Fig. 11.3 Clinical measurement of internal (left) and external (right) hip rotation. Drawing by Meg Buckingham.

Internal tibial torsion
- The angle between the transcondylar axis of the upper tibia and the transmalleolar axis at the ankle is usually 15 degrees external.
- If <5 this is internal tibial torsion.
- This can also be assessed using the foot thigh angle (Fig 11.4).
- Internal tibial torsion can be due to moulding *in utero* and improves by ~8 years.

Metatarsus adductus
- This is a bean-shaped foot with curved lateral border.
- Due to moulding *in utero*.
- If flexible it will resolve spontaneously.

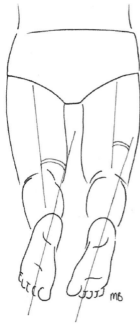

Fig. 11.4 Measurement of tibial torsion—the foot thigh angle. Drawing by Meg Buckingham.

• If stiff it will require treatment with casting and rarely surgery.
• NB *It must be distinguished carefully from congenital talipes equinovarus.*
• NB *Associated with hip dysplasia. Examine the hips!*

Genu varum, genu valgum

• Physiological bowing occurs around age 18 months and is commoner in heavier children and early walkers.
• Physiological 'knock knees' occurs around aged 3.
• In both genu valgum and genu varum: unilateral involvement, severe deformity, or failure to improve over 2 years requires investigation.

Planovalgus feet

• Assess for flexibility (the arch should reconstitute when standing on tiptoe or on passive dorsiflexion of the big toe).
• Flexible flat feet are due to ligamentous laxity or a tight Achilles tendon (refer to PT for stretches).
• Arch supports have not been shown to affect arch development in flexible flat feet.
• Stiff flat feet require orthopaedic referral and further investigation.

The spine

Scoliosis

Scoliosis describes a spinal curve in the coronal plane but is usually associated with extension in the sagittal plane and rotation in the axial plane (Fig. 11.5).

Causes of scoliosis

- Idiopathic (80% of all cases):
  - Infantile (<3 years).
  - Juvenile (3–10 years).
  - Adolescent (>10 years).
- Congenital.
- Neurofibromatosis (see 📖 p399):
  - Dystrophic.
  - Non-dystrophic.
- Marfan syndrome (see 📖 p398).
- Congenital heart disease.
- Post laminectomy.
- Irradiation.

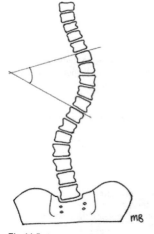

Fig 11.5 Cobb angle. Drawing by Meg Buckingham.

Examination of scoliosis

With the patient standing

Allow for leg length discrepancy by standing shorter leg on blocks to level the pelvis.

Look for:
- Shoulder asymmetry.
- Asymmetric scapular prominence.
- Asymmetric hip prominence.
- Asymmetry of space between arm and waist.
- Is the head centred over the pelvis?
- Rib hump prominence as the patient bends forwards (the Adams forward bend test).
- Trace out the curve following the spinous processes with a finger.

With the patient supine:
- Perform a full neurological examination (see 📖 p228) including abdominal reflexes (asymmetry may be a sign of syringomyelia).

Adolescent idiopathic scoliosis
- Most are convex right thoracic curves. Curves may be double or single with or without a compensatory curve.

Risk of curve progression is determined by:
- Gender (increased risk in females).
- Remaining growth—assessed by:
  - Menarchal status.
  - Risser grade.
  - Peak height velocity.
- Curve magnitude (greater progression with larger curves).
- Curve pattern (greater risk in double and thoracic curves).

Investigate with PA and lateral standing films. Consider MRI if neurological examination is abnormal and in convex left thoracic curves.

Treatment: curves of 30–45°—consider bracing (controversial), curves of >45°—surgery is recommended. (Thoracic scoliosis of >50° in adulthood will progress and reduce pulmonary function. A lumbar curve of >50° in adulthood will progress and develop osteoarthritis.)

Juvenile idiopathic scoliosis

Most curves are convex to the right. *Treatment* is similar to adolescent curves.

Infantile idiopathic scoliosis

Most are left-sided curves. Many resolve spontaneously. The angle between the ribs and the vertebrae on radiographs can help predict progression. Progressive curves are treated with bracing until surgery at aged 7–8 years.

Congenital spine abnormalities

May be due to:

- Defects of formation:
  - Hemivertebra.
  - Wedged vertebra.
- Defects of segmentation:
  - Block vertebrae.
  - Bars.
- May be associated with neural axis abnormalities:
  - Diastomatomyelia (see 🕮 p261).
  - Syringomyelia.
  - Diplomyelia.
  - Arnold–Chiari malformation (see 🕮 p263).
  - Intraspinal tumours (see 🕮 p264).
  - And with cardiac anomalies, DDH, club foot (see 🕮 p422).

Spondylolysis/spondylolisthesis

Spondylolisthesis is forward slippage of one vertebra upon another. It may be asymptomatic or present with severe low back and leg pain, neurological involvement, hamstring spasm, and gait disturbance. The forward slip may be due to anatomical abnormality of the L5–S1 articulation or a stress fracture of the pars intra-articularis. Stress fracture may occur without forward slip and is termed spondylolysis. This has an incidence of ~6%.

Examination should assess for a hyperlordosis, step-off at the lumbosacral junction, flexed knees and hips when standing, and hamstring tightness. Neurological examination is mandatory (see 🕮 p228).

Patients should be referred to an orthopaedic surgeon and will require close follow-up if <10 years old or symptomatic. If slippage continues, neurological signs develop or pain persists then stabilization surgery is performed.

Vertebral disc herniation

The true incidence in the skeletally immature is unknown. There is likely to be a genetic predisposition and frequently there is association with congenital spinal anomalies. It is associated with repetitive trauma, i.e. certain sports such as gymnastics. Usually presents with back pain. Neurological symptoms are relatively uncommon compared to the adult presentation. May be associated with a slipped vertebral apophysis. MRI is the investigation of choice. Surgery is indicated if there is a large central herniation with neurological signs, progressive worsening of neurology, or persistence of symptoms after 1 month of conservative treatment including rest, analgesia, and lumbar orthoses (see 🕮 p220).

Further resource

Scoliosis Association (UK): ☎ 020 8964 1166 ✆ http://www.sauk.org.uk

The hip

Developmental dysplasia of the hip (Fig. 11.6)

This is a spectrum of conditions. The hip may be stable and in joint but with poor acetabular coverage, it may be unstable such that the femoral head is subluxable or dislocatable from the socket, or the femoral head may be displaced—either subluxed or frankly dislocated. It is commoner in first borns and in females.

- Incidence of dislocation 1:1000.
- Incidence of all forms of dysplasia up to 1:50.

Risk factors

- FHx.
- Cramped position *in utero*:
  - Oligohydramnios.
  - Twin pregnancy.
- Breech presentation.
- Ligamentous laxity (see 🕮 p176 and p180).

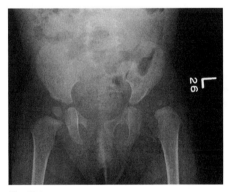

Fig. 11.6 Developmental dysplasia of the hip.

Examination

Careful examination of all babies is essential soon after birth and at the 6-week check. Failure to detect DDH results in much litigation!

Look for:

- Other signs of intrauterine moulding: torticolis, plagiocephaly (see 🕮 p231), metatarsus adductus.
- Spinal anomalies (see 🕮 p261).
- Leg-length difference. With the child supine, flex the hips and knees to 90° and look for a difference in knee height (Galeazi test).

- Asymmetry of perineal creases.
- Reduced range of abduction in flexion (may be noticed by parents when changing nappies).
- The Barl**O**w manoeuvre gently manipulates the femoral head **O**ut of joint by applying downwards, axial pressure on the adducted flexed thigh.
- The Ortolan**I** manoeuvre puts it **I**n joint. Holding the thigh with the thumb on the inner aspect and fingers over the greater trochanter, the femoral head is lifted into the actabulum by upward pressure on the greater trochanter and abduction of the hip. A clunk is felt as the hip relocates.

▶NB Beware the child with bilateral dislocations as the examination will give symmetrical findings.

▶NB Hip dislocation may be a result of other conditions such as spina bifida (see 🕮 p261), arthrogryposis (see 🕮 p427), and these must be excluded.

Investigations

Some centres perform ultrasound scans on *all* newborns, others just those with risk factors or positive examination findings. Ultrasound is used up to 4 months of age while the femoral head is still cartilaginous and X-ray thereafter.

Treatment

Up to 6 months of age a pavlic harness is trialled. If the hip does not relocate within 2 weeks it is removed due to the risk of avascular necrosis.

If irreducible or after 6 months a closed reduction is attempted with the aid of an arthrogram under general anaesthetic, and the hip held in joint with a spica cast for 12 weeks.

If this fails, then open operation to relocate the hip is performed, and again a spica cast is used for 12 weeks. In the older age group additional procedures such as femoral or acetabular osteotomies may be required.

Legg–Calve–Perthes disease
(See Fig. 11.7)
This is an idiopathic avascular necrosis of the femoral head. During the avascular period the femoral head is soft and may become deformed.

Occurs in:
- 1 in 9000.
- 4–10 year-olds (boys>girls).
- 10% bilateral.

Presents with:
- Pain (often only in the knee).
- Fatigue.
- Irritable hip with reduced range.

The disease process lasts ~2 years. Sphericity of the femoral head at the end of the remodelling phase is predictive of the risk of secondary osteoarthritis.

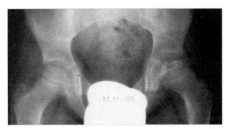

Fig 11.7 Perthes disease left hip.

Slipped upper femoral epiphysis

This rare but important condition requires immediate diagnosis and treatment to prevent worsening deformity and long-term disability. Displacement occurs between the femoral neck and head due to shear forces through the physis which has become weakened under hormonal influences during adolescence.

Incidence and aetiology
- 1:100,000.
- Boys >girls.
- 40–60% bilateral.
- Average age at diagnosis: boys=13.5, girls=12.
- Obese, hypogonadism.
- Hypothyroidism.
- Growth hormone treatment.

Presentation
Patients may present with knee pain only.

Investigations
- X-ray: AP pelvis and frog leg lateral.
- Those presenting <10 years of age should be investigated for underlying endocrine pathology.

Treatment
Less severe slips are pinned *in situ* with a single screw passing across the physis into the epiphysis. In the more severe slips an osteotomy may be indicated to shorten the femoral neck, reduce tension on the posterior vessels and reduce the head, thereby limiting deformity.

Further resources

Perthes Association: ♒ http://www.perthes.org.uk
STEPS: ♒ http://www.steps-charity.org.uk

The foot

Metatarsus adductus

See 📖 Normal variants p413.

Flexible flat foot

See 📖 Normal variants p415.

Congenital talipes equino varus (club foot) (Fig. 11.8)

- Most cases are idiopathic:
  - Incidence 2 per 1000 live births.
  - Twice as common in boys than girls.
  - 40% bilateral.
- But it may also be associated with syndromes such as spina bifida (see 📖 p261) and arthrogryposis (see 📖 p427).
- Often detected on the 20-week scan and consultation with a paediatric orthopaedic surgeon at that stage is helpful to talk through treatment.

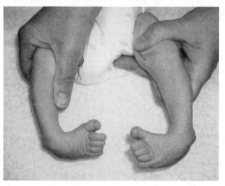

Fig. 11.8 Congenital talipes equino varus.

Deformity components

- The first metatarsal is plantar flexed in relation to the lesser metatarsals.
- The forefoot is adducted.
- The heel is in varus.
- The heel is plantar flexed (in equinus).

Treatment—the Ponseti regime

Beginning at ~10 days after birth the foot is manipulated raising the first ray and abducting the foot using the talar head as a fulcrum, and serially casting above knee to address each component of the deformity in turn. The final component of the deformity—the equinus, usually requires a full tenotomy of the Achilles tendon which can be performed under local anaesthetic in the clinic followed by casting for a further 3 weeks. Relapse is prevented by the wearing of boots attached to a bar and set at 70° external rotation full time for 3 months then night time and naps for 4 years. This is a vital part of the treatment. Surgery is required for the rare resistant case.

Stiff flat foot

The arch is dropped and does not form when standing on tiptoe or on passive dorsiflexion of the big toe. Likely causes are:
- Tarsal coalition.
- Vertical talus.
- Pain e.g. JIA, Koehler's disease.
- Paralytic.

Tarsal coalition

2 or more tarsal bones are joined with either fibrous tissue or bone. The commonest are calcaneonavicular and talocalcaneal coalitions. Incidence is <1 %.

Patients present usually after the age of 10 with pain, often on the lateral border of the foot. Diagnosis may be obvious on plane oblique radiographs if a bony bar is present. Fibrous unions are best seen on an MRI scan. Patients may have more than one coalition.

Treatment is with orthotics (see 🔲 p220) initially then surgery to take down the coalition if unresponsive to conservative treatment.

Vertical talus

The foot may have a rocker-bottom appearance. This is caused by a vertically oriented talus with dorsal subluxation of the navicula. Lateral radiographs taken in dorsi- and plantar-flexion reveal that the talus is not in line with the metatarsals. It is often associated with syndromes (see 🔲 p391). Treatment is with manipulation and serial casting but surgical treatment is often required.

Cavus foot

There may be an underlying neurological cause for the high-arched foot and so full neurological and spinal examination should be performed (see 🔲 p228).

The first ray is often plantar-flexed to a greater extent than the other lesser metatarsals and this drives the heel into varus when weight bearing. Eventually this may become fixed. Patients may present with progressive deformity, a tendency to inversion injuries, or neurological symptoms from the underlying condition.

Treatment is usually surgical with release and rebalancing of soft tissues to prevent deterioration and bony procedures to address fixed deformities.

Hallux valgus

The first metatarsal is in varus with an increased angle between the 1st and 2nd metatarsals. The great toe is in valgus and may under-ride the 2nd toe. This is usually painless in adolescence but may progress and eventually cause pain over the prominent 1st metatarsal head or rubbing of the over-riding 2nd toe on shoewear. The bigger issue for most adolescents is cosmesis. Conservative treatment is unsuccessful. Recurrence rate after surgery is high in adolescence but surgery may be justified if pain does not respond to alteration of footwear (see 🕮 p220).

Further resource

STEPS: 🕂 http://www.steps-charity.org.uk

Orthopaedic aspects of ...

Orthopaedic aspects of non-accidental injury

The incidence of child abuse is difficult to determine but is thought to be ~1% of children each year. Some will present with bony injury. *Of all patients <3 years who present with a fracture, 1/3 will have been a victim of child abuse* (see 🕮 Chapter 12: Child Abuse). These fractures rarely occur in isolation but are often accompanied by soft tissue injuries (see 🕮 p444). The child must be seen by the relevant specialists.

Certain types of fractures should raise alarm bells (also see 🕮 p446):
- Multiple fractures of different ages.
- Rib fractures.
- Femoral and humeral fractures in children <2 years.
- Metaphyseal, corner, or bucket handle fractures.
- Skull fractures (see 🕮 p447).
- Abundant callus formation due to lack of fracture immobilization and delayed presentation.

A careful history (see 🕮 p455) should be taken from the carer and the child. It is worth writing down *verbatim* their description of the mechanism of injury. Note any discrepancies and obtain expert opinion as to whether the reported mechanism fits with the injury.

Thorough examination (see 🕮 p455) of the child is mandatory and meticulous detailed note keeping is vital, as are photographs (see 🕮 p456) of any lesions and adequate radiographic views of fractures (you may be required to give evidence in court!).

Orthopaedic aspects of Down syndrome

Children with DS (see 🕮 p387) tend to have very lax ligaments which accounts for most of the orthopaedic conditions they present with.

Atlanto-axial instability
- Occurs in ~15% of patients but <2% show neurological symptoms.
- Is due to laxity of the transverse ligament of C1.
- Investigate with a lateral cervical spine radiograph in flexion and extension. An atlanto-dens interval of >5mm is abnormal.
- There is lack of evidence for screening programmes to prevent sport related spinal cord injury.
- Prophylactic stabilization to prevent onset of symptoms has not been substantiated.
- Surgical stabilization is recommended if neurological symptoms are present to prevent deterioration.
- Atlanto-occipital instability may coexist.

Hip disorders
Hip dislocations
- Can occur despite surprisingly normal looking joints.
- Incidence: 5%.
- This is not congenital but begins between the ages of 2–10 years and is initially painless.
- The situation tends to deteriorate with time.

- Conservative treatment entails long periods of bracing and often fails.
- Surgical treatment consists of varus derotation femoral osteotomy, capsular plication ± acetabular osteotomy.

Other hip disorders

Slipped upper femoral epiphysis and avascular necrosis have a higher incidence in those with DS.

Patellofemoral instability

This can be quite disabling and is difficult to treat due to the laxity. Quadriceps strengthening (see 📖 p179) and bracing can be tried in the first instance but surgical stabilization may be required.

Flat feet and hallux valgus

These are rarely symptomatic and do not require treatment other than accommodating shoe wear (see 📖 p220).

Orthopaedic aspects of spina bifida

(Also see 📖 p261)

Orthopaedic input for these children aims to maximize function and minimize disability and discomfort.

Spinal deformity

Scoliosis (see 📖 p416) and kyphosis are more severe in those with more proximal spinal cord lesions. Generally deformity is progressive and is not effectively treated by bracing. Surgery should be considered for curves of 50° or more and is typically required by ~8–9 years of age. This helps to maintain sitting balance especially in the non-ambulant patient.

Hips

Hips are prone to contractures (especially flexion) and dislocation in all levels of spina bifida. Controversy remains about undertaking surgery to relocate the hips in those with higher level lesions, but those with lesions of L5 and below should have bony surgery to reconstruct their hips, as should any patient with a painful dislocation.

Knees

Surgery may be required to manage knee flexion or extension contractures that do not respond to stretches (also see 📖 p179).

Feet

A variety of foot deformities occur including club foot, vertical talus, and cavovarus feet (see 📖 p422). A progressive cavovarus deformity may be due to a tethered cord requiring referral to a neurosurgeon. In the non-ambulant child it is important to have feet that rest comfortably on the foot plate of the wheelchair (see 📖 p183). In walkers, a supple, pain free, plantar grade foot is the aim.

Management ranges from the use of custom made orthoses (see 📖 p220), to serial casting or surgery, including soft tissue and bony procedures. Lack of sensation and the risk of pressure sores are important considerations.

Fractures

Patients with spina bifida are prone to pathological fractures (see 📖 p99) which tend to heal with abundant callus formation.

Orthopaedic aspects of neurofibromatosis type 1

NF1 is the result of a single gene mutation. Incidence is 1 in 3000 (also see 📖 p399). Orthopaedic manifestations include:

- Scoliosis.
- Spinal tumours.
- Pseudarthrosis of long bones.
- Pectus excavatum.
- Limb hypertrophy.
- Plexiform neurofibromas.

Other manifestations:

- Café au lait spots (>6).
- Axillary freckles (begin developing around aged 5).
- Lisch nodules.
- Neurofibromas.
- Patients may also have or develop brain tumours, leukaemia, phaeochromocytoma, learning disability.

Scoliosis (see 📖 p416) may be non-dystrophic and behave in a similar way to an idiopathic curve, or may be dystrophic with a short sharp progressive curve that can lead to neurological defect, sometimes associated with spinal tumours. Surgical intervention is required. Pseudarthrosis is difficult to manage and usually requires surgery. The tibia is most commonly affected producing an anterolateral bow. Focal gigantism requires combined orthopaedic and plastic reconstruction. Plexiform neurofibromas have extensive bone and muscle involvement and are often impossible to resect but need monitoring with MRI or PET scans because of the risk of malignant transformation.

Orthopaedic aspects of arthrogryposis

This is a group of conditions that can affect joints alone (classical arthrogryposis or the distal form); or in addition can affect other body systems (e.g. Freeman–Sheldon syndrome); or have central nervous system involvement. Joint contractures occur due to lack of fetal movement, and deformities can be severe at birth. Many contractures respond well to early splintage and serial casting but recurrences are common (see 📖 p179). The classic form shows symmetrical limb involvement with tubular featureless limbs. Typically shoulders are internally rotated and elbows extended. Muscle transfers can be performed to improve elbow flexion but not at the expense of extension which is needed for walking with crutches, and rising from a chair. In the classic and distal forms wrists tend to be flexed with ulna deviation; fingers curved; and thumb in palm. Surgery may be required to improve wrist and thumb position. Hip dislocation (see 📖 p419) occurs in around half of patients and requires open surgical reduction. Knees may be flexed or extended. Flexion can be gained with a quadriceps plasty unless severe weakness is likely to affect walking. Extension may be gained with soft tissue releases, femoral osteotomy or gradual correction with a ring fixator. Typically feet show either a rigid club foot deformity (see 📖 p422) or vertical talus. Treatment is likely to be a combination of serial casting started soon after birth and surgery to achieve plantar grade feet. Scoliosis occurs in ~30% and requires surgery for curves >50° (see 📖 p416).

Orthopaedic aspects of Marfan syndrome

This is a dominantly inherited condition causing an increase in height with disproportionately long limbs (see 📖 p398). It is caused by a defect in fibrilin—a component of elastic tissues. Features include joint laxity, arachnodactyly, pectus carinatum or excavatum, lens dislocation, aortic dilatation, spontaneous pneumothorax, scoliosis.

Scoliosis (also see 📖 p416) often requires orthopaedic intervention and patients may request epiphyseodesis during growth to reduce ultimate height.

Orthopaedic aspects of osteogenesis imperfecta

This is a disorder of type 1 collagen. A number of varieties exist with different inheritance patterns. Overall incidence is 1 in 20,000. In addition to multiple fractures, patients may display thin sclerae (giving a bluish tinge), ligamentous laxity, skin hyperextensibility, heart valve incompetence. The most severe forms are lethal. The commonest forms are the least severe. Fracture rate is reduced by bisphosphonates (also see 📖 p99). Fractures are treated as required. More severe types may need prophylactic intramedullary rodding of long bones to prevent fractures and manage deformity. It is important to distinguish between osteogenesis imperfecta and NAI (see 📖 p444). The 2 may coexist.

Further resources

Association for Spina Bifida and Hydrocephalus: ℬ http://www.asbah.org
Brittle Bone Society: ☎ 0800 028 2459 ℬ http://www.brittlebone.org
Down's Syndrome Association: ℬ http://www.downs-syndrome.org.uk
Osteogenesis Imperfecta Foundation: ℬ http://www.oif.org
The Neuro Foundation: ℬ http://www.nfauk.org
The Arthrogryposis Group: ℬ http://www.tagonline.org.uk

Skeletal dysplasias

This is a group of conditions that affect skeletal development. Together they account for 1% of short stature cases (>2 sd below the mean) and the incidence is 1 per 2000–5000. Skeletal survey may help in the diagnosis. Assess which region of the bone is involved—metaphyseal or epiphyseal—and whether the spine is affected. In general, the orthopaedic problems encountered are spinal instability and deformity, limb deformity, and joint degeneration.

Orthopaedic aspects of achondroplasia

Abnormality in the fibroblast growth factor receptor 3 gene affects chondroblast function in the physis resulting in rhisomelic short-limbed disproportionate short stature. Inherited as autosomal dominant, though most cases are spontaneous mutations. Features are noticeable from birth. Characteristic mid-face hypoplasia. Patients may suffer from hydrocephalus (see 📖 p264) (NB ventricle size is reduced in achondroplasia), spinal stenosis, increased lumbar lordosis causing back pain, bowing of the legs, etc. Patients may request leg lengthening procedures.

Orthopaedic aspects of epiphyseal dysplasia

There is failure of formation of secondary centres of ossification leading to an appearance of fragmented epiphyses on X-ray. In spondylo-epiphyseal dysplasia the spine is also involved and there may be odontoid hypoplasia causing atlanto-axial instability (see 📖 p425). Scoliosis may develop (see 📖 p416). Angular knee deformities may occur. Patients often need early joint replacements.

Orthopaedic aspects of hereditary multiple exostosis

Mutation in the *EXT1* or *EXT2* genes cause multiple cartilage capped exostoses to arise adjacent to the physes of long bones. This autosomal dominant condition often results in short stature. Lesions require surgical removal if causing mechanical symptoms or angular deformity of a limb. There is a 1% lifetime risk of malignant transformation. Lesions that grow after skeletal maturity require investigation. A cartilage cap of >1cm thickness as seen on MRI or ultrasound scan is suggestive of malignancy.

Orthopaedic aspects of mucopolysaccharidoses

(Also see 📖 p155 for mucopolysaccharidoses)
Failure of breakdown of glycosaminoglycans causes accumulation in tissues. Chondroblast function in the physis is affected resulting in abnormal skeletal growth. Hurler and Hunter syndromes are less likely to present with orthopaedic problems than Morquio syndrome which may have odontoid hypoplasia resulting in atlanto-axial instability. Severe genu valgum may also require limb realignment.

Orthopaedic aspects of cerebral palsy

Introduction

CP is a motor impairment resulting from a non-progressive brain lesion (see 🕮 p67).

Physiologic classification

Describes the type of movement disorder present:

- Spasticity: results from damage to the pyramidal system. Increased muscle tone is proportional to velocity of stretch. Loss of inhibition of reflex arcs means that muscles may contract out of phase, i.e. when it is not desirable for them to do so. This is particularly true of muscles that cross >1 joint, e.g. hamstrings, rectus femoris, gastrocnemius. Spastic muscles and their antagonists show varying degrees of weakness. This is the commonest form of CP and the one most amenable to orthopaedic intervention.
- Dystonia/rigidity: increased tone which is not velocity dependant (see 🕮 p238).
- Athetosis: abnormal writhing movements caused by damage to the basal ganglia.
- Ataxia: disturbed balance caused by a cerebellar lesion (see 🕮 p247).

Geographic classification

Explains which region of the body is involved:

- Hemiplegia (ipsilateral upper and lower limbs and trunk).
- Diplegia (bilateral lower limbs, minimal upper limb involvement).
- Total body involvement.

As part of the multidisciplinary team approach (see 🕮 p20 and p23) for these patients, *orthopaedic input* is important for the following:

- To help with spasticity management and posture control (see 🕮 p183).
- To prevent or treat contractures of muscles and joints.
- To prevent or treat hip dislocations.
- To improve gait (see 🕮 p433) and upper limb function (see 🕮 p193) where possible.

(For orthopaedic examination in CP see 🕮 p410.)

Management of spasticity

Physiotherapy
A stretching program encourages muscle growth; adding sarcomeres to the muscle length (see 📖 pp176–80).

Orthotics
These may be used to provide passive stretching. They can also aid function, prevent deformity, and provide stability either by local control or on more proximal joints by the effect on the ground reaction force (see 📖 p220).

Baclofen
This is a gamma amino butyric acid (GABA) agonist. GABA is an inhibitive neurotransmitter in the brain and spinal cord. Baclofen may be given orally or intrathecally. The intrathecal route has the advantage that larger doses reach the target tissue—the spinal cord—thus reducing side effects seen with the high doses given orally. It is used for patients with predominant lower limb spasticity but there are no strict indications as yet. After a test dose to ensure efficacy, a pump containing the baclofen is inserted, usually into the abdominal wall and the drug is administered via a catheter into the intrathecal space. The dose is titrated according to need.

Complications include:
• Cerebrospinal fluid leak.
• Infection.
• Catheter migration.
• Overdose causing hypotonia and respiratory depression (see 📖 p90).

Patients may still need orthopaedic intervention for hip subluxation and joint contractures.

Botulinum toxin
Having determined which muscles are spastic, these can be injected with botulinum toxin at the neuromuscular junction under ultrasound or electrostimulator guidance. The toxin blocks the release of acetyl choline at the neuromuscular junction thus reducing tone and relaxing the muscles until new nerve endings sprout at ~3–6 months.

Important considerations when administering botulinum toxin

• Botulinum toxin is useful for dynamic shortening but will not affect fixed muscle contractures.
• If weakness is a major factor, botulinum toxin may be disadvantageous as it will further weaken the muscle.
• Sedation or general anaesthetic is helpful if multiple muscles are to be injected.
• Dose is calculated according to the size of the muscle and the weight of the patient. NB several preparations are available and their concentrations differ.

- Accurate placement is important and after insertion of the needle and confirmation of position with stimulator or ultrasound, the syringe plunger should be pulled back to ensure the needle is not in a blood vessel.
- Injections must be followed by a course of intensive physiotherapy plus or minus splinting to obtain the maximum benefit.
- Effects are temporary (3–6 months) but repeat doses can be given after 6 months.

Selective dorsal rhizotomy

Public interest in this treatment is growing. This is a neurosurgical technique that sections a proportion of the dorsal sensory rootlets (between L1 and S1) found on electrical stimulation to be most responsible for the abnormal reflex arc that causes spasticity. It produces a permanent decrease in muscle tone. Ambulatory spastic diplegic patients are the most likely to benefit.

NICE guidelines from 2010 state that patients should be selected and treated by a multidisciplinary team (see 📖 p20 and p23); however, criteria for treatment are still evolving. Patients require prolonged postoperative physiotherapy (see 📖 p179). Complications include decreased walking ability due to the unmasking of muscle weakness; reduced bladder function, and spinal deformity. It should be performed before the development of significant contractures.

Orthopaedic surgery

- Surgical lengthening of a musculotendinous unit will decrease spasticity.
- Muscles firing out of phase can be transferred to become an antagonist (see 📖 p433).

Further resource

NICE: 🖰 www.nice.org.uk/guidance/IPG373/publicinfo

Orthopaedic surgery

Surgery is performed to:
- Lengthen musculotendinous units: at the origin, at the musculotendinous portion (fractional lengthening) or within the tendon (z lengthening or tenotomy).
- Transfer tendons: the tendon of a muscle which is firing out of phase is transferred, usually to become an antagonist to the function it originally performed. This reduces its deforming force and enhances the action of the weak antagonists.
- Cut and re-orientate deformed bones (osteotomies).
- Relocate subluxed or dislocated joints (usually hips).
- Fuse joints (rarely).

Gait (Fig. 11.9)
- Careful evaluation of the gait is required to understand the causes of abnormalities. Some abnormal features of the gait may be compensatory and disappear once the primary problems are addressed.
- 3-dimensional gait analysis may be helpful for treatment planning and evaluation.
- 3-dimensional gait analysis consists of:
  - Clinical examination.
  - Video.
  - Kinematics (a measure of joint angles during the gait cycle).
  - Kinetics (assessment of the forces involved to produce movement).
  - EMG.
  - Plantar pressures.

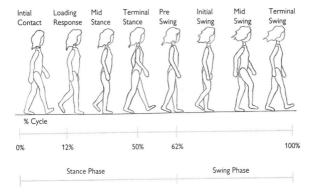

Fig. 11.9 The gait cycle. Drawing by Meg Buckingham.

- *Kinematics* assesses the movement of the pelvis, hips, knees and ankles during a gait cycle in the sagittal, coronal, and transverse planes. These values can then be compared to an able bodied population.
- Information is gathered by infrared cameras which detect reflected light from appropriately placed markers on the lower limbs.
- *Kinetics* uses force plate data to calculate the ground reaction force during the gait cycle, and consequently the forces acting at the different joints.
- Patients are often assessed at age 5 or 6 for a baseline measure. They should be reassessed if gait deteriorates or to assess treatments such as orthotics (see 🕮 p220) (particularly to measure effects at distant joints) and botulinum toxin (see 🕮 p431). They are also assessed prior to surgical intervention to guide treatment planning, and postoperatively as an outcome measure.

Every child is different but there are certain typical gait patterns:
- *Intoeing:* in CP this usually is due to excessive femoral anteversion. It can be treated with derotational osteotomies.
- *Vaulting:* there is difficulty in clearing the foot from the ground during swing and so the foot in stance phase has an early heel raise to allow the opposite leg to swing through without hitting the ground.
- *Short leg gait:* the pelvis dips on the affected side during stance.
- *Scissoring:* spasticity in the hip adductors means the legs tend to cross over each other in the coronal plane during walking and it can be difficult to get one leg past the other.
- *Toe-toe gait:* this may be due to spasticity in the calf muscles preventing dorsiflexion at the ankles which consequently remain in equinus throughout the gait cycle and the heel does not reach the ground. Alternatively, there may be adequate dorsiflexion at the ankle but flexion of the knee throughout stance makes it impossible for the heal to reach the ground.
- *Crouch gait:* there is flexion of the knee >30° throughout the gait cycle. Excessive dorsiflexion at the ankle (which can cause a crouched gait) may allow the heel to contact the ground.
- *Stiff knee gait:* the knee has a reduced range of motion through the gait cycle. It may be due to spasticity of rectus femoris reducing the range of flexion during swing.

Typical foot deformities include:
- Planovalgus foot with equinus hind foot and mid-foot break (commonest in diplegics).
- Equinus/equinovarus foot (commonest in hemiplegics).

After around the age of 9 or 10 years a patient may be considered for *SEMLS* (single event multilevel surgery). This includes a variety of procedures, often bony and soft tissue, tailored to the individual patient and aiming to address all gait abnormalities simultaneously with a single period of rehabilitation.

Hips

Due to muscle imbalance, hips are prone to subluxation and dislocation. This is silent in the early phase and only detectable with radiographs. If left untreated, dislocations can cause problems with sitting imbalance, pain and difficulties with perineal hygiene due to restricted movement.

Displacement occurs in up to 75% in those with spastic quadriplegia.

Hip surveillance

Children with bilateral CP should have a radiograph by the time they are 18 months old and then 6–12-monthly thereafter.

Assessments are made of the *Reimer's migration index* and *acetabular index*. A horizontal reference line is drawn through the triradiate cartilage of the acetabulae (Hilgenreiner's line). A line perpendicular to this is drawn at the edge of the acetabulum (Perkin's line). The Reimer's migration index is the percentage of the femoral head lying lateral to Perkin's line. The acetabular index is the angle that the roof of the socket makes with Hilgenreiner's line (Fig. 11.10).

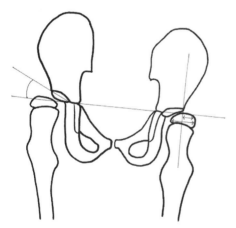

Fig. 11.10 Reimer's migration percentage (left hip) and acetabular index (right hip). Drawing by Meg Buckingham.

Many children become 'windswept' i.e. one hip lies in adduction and is at risk of posterior dislocation; the other in abduction is at risk of anterior dislocation. Therapy aims at trying to retain as symmetrical a ROM as possible although evidence that therapy and positioning of the child reduces the dislocation rate is lacking.

Surgery is performed to prevent dislocation. If a hip is allowed to dislocate and becomes painful then this is a difficult situation to remedy.

Preventative surgery (soft tissue releases) are indicated where:
• Migration index is >40%.
• Increase in migration index is >10%.
• Acetabular index >27%.

Reconstructive surgery is indicated if:
• Migration index >50% despite soft tissue releases.

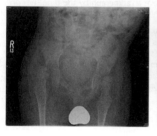 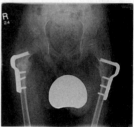

Fig. 11.11 Pre- and post-treatment for hip subluxation in cerebral palsy.

Reconstructive surgery usually consists of femoral and pelvic osteotomies ± open reduction of the hip.

Hips must then be monitored until skeletal maturity as there is a risk of recurrent subluxation with growth.

Spine
• Scoliosis is most common in non-ambulatory patients. Those with spasticity are at highest risk. Unlike idiopathic scoliosis, the curves tend to be long 'c' shaped curves down to the pelvis with an apex at the thoracolumbar junction.
• Bracing does not affect curve progression but may improve sitting comfort.
• Indications for surgery:
  • Progressive deformity.
  • Sitting imbalance.
  • Pelvic obliquity.
  • Curves over 50° in ambulatory patients (these will progress).

Upper limb
In addition to spasticity; weakness, altered sensation, dystonia, and poor selective control are all a problem for the involved upper limb. For the hemiplegic patient, tasks are more easily performed with the 'good' hand and so the affected hand may become neglected and pattern of 'learned non-use' develops.

Goals of treatment need to be carefully agreed with the patient and carers (also see 🕮 p188 and p193).

- The aims for those with total body involvement are usually to improve ease of care, including dressing and hygiene.
- Those with diplegia have little upper limb involvement.
- Hemiplegic patients are the most likely to be helped in terms of cosmesis and function.

Assessment
- Should focus on measuring:
  - Sensation (which is predictive of spontaneous use of the limb).
  - Spasticity.
  - Strength.
  - Contractures of both muscles and joints, e.g. it may be possible to fully extend the fingers with the wrist flexed but not with the wrist in neutral due to shortened length of the finger flexor musculotendinous unit.
- An idea of function and how the 2 hands are used together needs to be gained (see the AHA and the SHUEE functional tests 📖 p412).

Treatment
- The involvement of the multidisciplinary team (including PT, OT, and surgeon) is vital for treatment planning and implementation (see 📖 Chapter 5: Consults with allied professionals).
- Goals must be clearly defined.
- Each patient should have a physiotherapy programme to stretch spastic muscles and strengthen weak ones in order to try and prevent contractures and maximize function (see 📖 p179).
- Constraint-induced movement therapy (CIMT) encourages use and awareness of the affected limb by restricting the 'good' hand. This reduces the pattern of 'learnt non-use' and has been shown to maintain long term improvements (see 📖 p193).
- Malposition of the wrist and thumb impact significantly on function (see 📖 p220).
- Surgery:
  - Usually in the form of musculotendinous releases and transfers, aims to improve positioning of the joints thereby improving function and cosmesis. It does not improve the fine dexterity of the digits.
  - Because most muscles cross >1 joint it is important to consider the limb as a whole when planning surgery. Just as with the lower limb, it is usual to perform several procedures in one sitting (multilevel surgery) (see 📖 p434).
  - It is important to note that no amount of surgery is going to improve the function of a neglected hand, and so there must be reasonable spontaneous use of the hand before surgery is considered for functional gain.
  - A literature review from 1966 to 2006 showed that surgery improves the position of the hand and is likely to improve function.
- Validated outcome measures must be used to demonstrate efficacy of treatments.

Further resource
Upper Limb Anomalies Reach Charity Limited: ☎ 0845 130 6225 🖰 http://www.reach.org.uk

Child abuse

Unless there is opposing wind, a kite cannot rise.

Chinese proverb

Definitions

- Child abuse and neglect are forms of maltreatment of a child.
- They are caused either by inflicting harm on the child or by failing to protect the child. There are 4 recognized categories of child abuse:

1. Physical abuse

- Also known as non-accidental injury (NAI).
- May involve the following acts resulting in injury: hitting, shaking, throwing, poisoning, burning, scalding, drowning, suffocating, or otherwise causing physical harm to a child.
- Fabrication or induction of illness in a child (FII) also falls into this category.
- Smacking a child is not currently illegal in the UK, but is now in some EU countries (Sweden).

2. Sexual abuse

- Involves the enticement or coercion of a child to take part in some form of sexual activity.
- This can range from viewing pornography or sexual acts (non-contact activity) to oral sex or full penetrative sexual intercourse (contact activity).
- Often there is a power/age difference between abuser and victim.

3. Neglect

- Is the persistent failure to provide for a child's basic psychological and physical needs, e.g. food, clothing, supervision, and access to medical care.
- This can result in failure of normal development of the child, both physically (growth) and in achieving normal developmental milestones.
- Neglect can occur in pregnancy through maternal substance misuse.

4. Emotional abuse

- Is the prolonged emotional maltreatment of a child causing long-term severe psychological effects to the child.
- It is often found in association with (1), (2), and (3), but can present in isolation.
- This category includes serious bullying and recently cyber-bullying.

Identification

All categories of child abuse may present in different ways and should always be considered/suspected on the list of differential diagnoses for a variety of conditions and presentations, especially the following:

- Injuries in a non-mobile child.
- Severe head injury.
- Unconscious child.
- Unexplained/unusual injuries, including burns, fractures, soft tissue, and major organ injuries.
- Frequent attendance at A&E/GP.
- FTT.
- Abdominal pain and headaches.
- Urinary symptoms.
- Psychological problems, e.g. self-harm, behavioural changes, eating disorders, secondary enuresis, encopresis.
- DNA medical appointments.
- Non-attendance at school.
- Delay in seeking medical attention for an injury.
- Explanation for injury not compatible with injury seen.
- Explanation for injury changes over time (detail is absent, as the account is fabricated and therefore alters with each telling).
- Previous NAI or child may have a child protection plan.
- Child may be known to social services.
- Parents affect may be flat, frightened (mother), or aggressive (father).
- The child may show frozen watchfulness (a sign seen in children who have been repeatedly physically abused, who learn to keep still in the presence of the abuser and are hypervigilant).

Abusers are most commonly adult males and often known to the child, but may also be female or children.

▶▶The child may disclose. Must ask them for their account.

Epidemiology

- ~1 in 4 (25.3%) 18–24-year-olds report experiencing severe physical abuse, sexual abuse or neglect in childhood.
- Both parents were equally likely to be involved in physical abuse, emotional abuse, and neglect.
- Child protection plan registrations do not give an incidence of the problem, but give an indication of the scale of the problem.
- In 2010 in England there were a total of 39,100 registrations (more boys than girls):
  - 17,200 for neglect
  - 11,400 for emotional abuse
  - 4700 for physical abuse
  - 2200 for sexual abuse
  - 3400 >1 category.

Neglect

~1 in 10 children experienced serious absence of care at home in childhood.

Emotional abuse

~5% of children experienced frequent severe emotional maltreatment.

Physical abuse

- ~7% of children experience serious physical abuse at hands of their parents/carers in their childhood.
- ~1–2 children die in the UK each week at the hands of their carers. 40% of these are <1 year of age.
- ~1/800 infants will suffer severe physical abuse requiring treatment, e.g. severe head injury or fracture.

Sexual abuse

- The exact prevalence of child sexual abuse (CSA) is unknown, but the incidence appears to be decreasing.
- A retrospective survey of 18–24-year-olds found 11% reported sexual abuse aged 12 years or below.
- 1% of children <16 years will have experienced sexual abuse by a parent or carer usually father or stepfather. A further 3% by another relative during childhood.
- Only 5% of children will have been sexually abused by an adult stranger or someone that they have just met.

▶▶Disabled children are 3 times more likely to experience abuse and neglect than their non-disabled peers.

Predisposing factors for child abuse

Child
- Non-mobile child, especially <1 year.
- First-born child.
- Boys >girls for physical abuse.
- Girls >boys for sexual abuse.
- Number of children in the household (larger the number, higher the risk).
- Disability, especially speech and language disorder.
- Attachment disorder (can also occur when premature baby has been in SCBU).
- Chronic medical problems (can lead to parental exhaustion).
- Behaviour problems/screaming baby/feeding difficulties.
- Trafficked child.

Parent/carer
- Young immature parent(s).
- Mental health problems, including postnatal depression.
- Domestic violence (DV).
- Drug and alcohol misuse (parent 'unavailable' for child).
- Learning difficulties (unable to meet the child's needs, lack coping strategies).
- Abused themselves as children (cycle of deprivation).
- Lack of support network.
- Social mobility.

General
- Social deprivation (poor housing, poverty).
- Previous history of child abuse (check for a child protection plan for index child and siblings).

Physical abuse or non-accidental injury

- Suspicion of NAI arises when child presents with soft tissue injury, e.g. a bruise, burn, bite mark, laceration or a fracture, not adequately explained by parent/carer/child.
- In the history there may be *certain pointers to NAI* (📖 Identification pointers and/or pre-disposing factors p441 and p443).

Bruises

▶'Those who don't cruise rarely bruise.'
- Bruises are the commonest abusive injury.
- Non-mobile children <1 year do not get bruises, prevalence of <1% for accidental injury. Unless there is a witnessed, clear explanation, do not accept as accidental injury.
- Undertake a careful assessment and perform appropriate investigations, especially if bruising is around the face, as this is the most commonly bruised site in fatal NAI (see 📖 Medical assessment p455).

Accidental bruises
- Usually over bony prominences, on front of body when children start to be mobile, increasing as they start walking.
- Commonest sites are knees, shins, and forehead, nose, upper lip, and chin (T shape). Also back of the head (see Appendix: Accidental bruising patterns 📖 p632).

Non-accidental bruises
(See Appendix: Abusive bruising patterns 📖 p632)
- Occur over soft tissue areas and unusual places, often on head and neck, over cheeks, below jaw line, and over ears.
- Presence of petechiae in bruising is strong predictor for NAI.
- Bruises over the upper limbs and outer thighs may indicate 'defensive' bruises where child has tried to protect themselves from assault.
- Certain *patterns of bruising* may suggest NAI, e.g.
  - 'Finger tip' bruises on upper arms/trunk from grip marks.
  - Petechial bruising around the ear, cheek and neck from a slap mark (try placing your own hand over the mark and see if it fits).
  - Petechial bruising on the lower part of the face and upper neck from near strangulation.
- Bruises in suprapubic area and 'finger tip' bruises on thighs suggest possible sexual abuse and warrant specialist examination of genital/anal area with colposcope.
- Two black eyes from a forehead injury with bruising tracking down around the eyes, raises suspicion of NAI, unless history of memorable accident, e.g. thrown forward in car accident and hit head.
- Marks from implements may leave clear imprints, e.g. a pattern from belt buckle and may help to corroborate the child's allegation.

Differential diagnosis
- Mongolian blue spots: don't fade over time, if any doubts review after 4–5 weeks, when a bruise will have disappeared.
- Bleeding disorders need to be excluded with appropriate blood tests and an extended clotting screen may be necessary.

- Drugs can cause petechial rash, e.g. aspirin.
- Some marks self inflicted by child, e.g. sucking or bite marks. Dental impressions from child can exclude self-biting (need forensic dental opinion).
- Infection-viral /meningococcal.

❶ Do not attempt to age bruises by colour, as they can change colour at different rates even on same child.

Bite marks

- Can be human or animal (often puncture skin). The teeth in human dental arches usually leave 2 distinct semi-circular arcade marks on the skin, forming a circle or oval shaped mark, with individual teeth marks in some cases, called a 'smoke ring'.
- Abusive bite marks tend to be found on the back, legs, and face.
- Any bite leaving a mark will have caused significant pain and is abusive.
- Always document the mark and get a series of photos with a rigid right angled measure in the photo. Include a 'distant' photo of whole child, to orientate the mark anatomically.
- Consider taking a wet and dry forensic swab for DNA evidence. Remember chain of evidence (📖 Forensic sampling p461).
- Involve a forensic dentist to aid identification of perpetrator through dental impressions (🕸 http://www.bafo.org.uk).

Oral injuries

In children, particularly <1 year of age, e.g. torn frenulum, lacerations to lip or broken teeth, without adequate explanation highly suggestive of abuse and warrant thorough assessment for NAI.

Thermal injuries

- Burns and scalds to children are common, most result from accidents and majority seen in children <5 years.
- Boys >girls 2:1.
- Usually present to A&E.
- Often associated with neglect.
- Some are, however, inflicted deliberately.
- Prevalence of 10–12% of abused children.
- 95% of thermal injuries occur at home. >50% of all severe burns or scalds happen in the kitchen.
- Most thermal injuries are due to scalds from hot liquid, usually drinks. Also from kettle steam, hot tap water, hot oil or fat.
- Contact burns from fires, heaters/radiators, matches, lighters, candle, irons, chemicals etc. are common, may leave specific patterns on child's skin, e.g. grid pattern from electric fire cover.
- Burns from neglect outnumber those inflicted deliberately by 9:1.

Accidental scalds

- Usually from pulling over hot liquid, this pours down front of the child over face, neck, upper limbs, and trunk with an asymmetric irregular edge and irregular depth.
- May also have splash marks.

Non-accidental scalds

(See Appendix: Abusive scald patterns 📖 p633)

- Often due to immersion of child in hot water, involves lower limbs/ buttocks/perineum. Also 'glove and stocking' burns to hands and feet.
- The burn has a clearly defined regular edge from the waterline and is of consistent depth and symmetry.
- There may be associated finger tip bruises where the child has been gripped and held.
- Also other injuries, previous burns, blaming a sibling, family known to social services.

Thermal burns

From contact with hot surface.

Accidental burns

Usually on palm of hand, occasionally on dorsum of hand or foot from heated hair tongs etc.

Non-accidental burns

- Tend to be full thickness and on the back or neck, with a clear edge.
- It may be possible to match the injury with the object used, e.g. an iron.
- Can occur at all ages.
- Need to obtain a good history and if necessary a home visit by the police, to check water temperature, electrical devices etc.

Cigarette burns

- From *accidental* brushing against tip of a cigarette, tend to cause a more superficial burn, with a tail to one side from the ash.
- A *deliberate* 'stubbing' burn on the child is often full thickness, circular and with a slightly raised edge, approx 1cm in diameter (may vary if roll ups) and found on exposed body parts.
- Multiple burns high chance of NAI.
- Can be confused with impetigo.
- Take swab and ask for plastic surgery opinion if any doubt.

Differential diagnosis

- Includes impetigo, photo-dermatitis, scalded skin syndrome.
- Take good photos.
- Get an opinion from plastic surgeon even if not severe enough to require treatment from them.

Fractures

- Are common injuries in children, most are related to falls, RTA, or sport.
- All fractures must be explained and be consistent with child's developmental age.
- The younger the child the greater likelihood of a NAI. 80% of abusive fractures occur <18 months age.
- 85% of accidental fractures occur >5 years of age.

- It is estimated that 1/3 of abused children have fractures.
- Infants <1 year with fractures are more likely to have been abused.
- Remember osteogenesis imperfecta (rare), child will continue to fracture even when in care.

The following fractures are suspicious of abuse:
- Spiral fractures of the humerus (and any fracture of the humerus in a non-mobile infant).
- Fractures of ribs (high specificity for abuse) often associated with squeezing/shaking injury in an infant. Usually posterior and anterior rib fractures but can also be lateral. Rarely anterior rib fractures (not posterior) have been reported following resuscitation.
  - Need to look for rib #s on skeletal survey and if necessary repeat CXR 10 days later to look again for recent/healing fractures.
  - Multiple fractures commoner in NAI.
- Old fractures may be found on skeletal survey, which were never presented for treatment.
- Fractures of the femur in young children <1 year. As the child starts to walk they can sustain both spiral and transverse femoral fractures accidentally.
- Metaphyseal fractures of the lower limbs are most commonly due to abuse.

Skull fractures
- Linear, parietal fracture of the skull is common in both abusive and non-abusive injuries.
- Skull fractures of concern for NAI include:
  - Occipital.
  - Depressed.
  - Growing, complex, or multiple.
  - Wide (3.0mm or more on X-ray).
  - Crossing suture line.
  - Associated with intracranial injury.
- Most abusive skull fractures occur <1 year of age.
- Need to determine and document the height and force of the fall and note the surface the child landed on.

Investigations
- Full skeletal survey in all children <2 years of age (need to get consent for this from parent and explain purpose of the X-rays),
- CT head (<2 years of age), possible radionucleide bone scan, Ca/PO$_4$, ALP, FBC, vitamin D level.
- If concerns, consider assessing bone density in discussion with paediatric radiologist.
- Eye examination (see 🕮 p288) for retinal haemorrhage (<2 years of age).

Non-accidental head injury (NAHI)
- Is the commonest cause of death in cases of physical abuse.
- 95% of severe head injuries <1 year are abusive.
- Most common under 6 months of age, with a mortality up to 30%.
- Often a surviving child is left with disability.

- May present acutely fitting or unconscious, or with breathing difficulties and lethargy.
- Those with subdural may present less acutely, with enlarging head.
- Mechanisms may be direct blow to head or repetitive injury from shaking, or combination.
- There may be obvious external injury, skull fracture, intracranial bleeding, retinal haemorrhage, brain injury (hypoxic/ischaemic) or other injuries (bruises or fractures).

▶Need low threshold to consider this as diagnosis.

Investigations

Include skeletal survey, ophthalmological examination of retina (also see 📖 p288) and CT scan of head, followed by MRI. Coagulation screen.

Differential diagnosis

Includes birth trauma, severe RTA and bleeding disorders. Glutaric aciduria in cases of subdural haematoma (check organic acids)

Intra-abdominal injury

- Uncommon, occurring usually in children <3 years.
- High mortality rate.
- Difficult to diagnose with no history and often delay in presentation.
- Involves small bowel tears, rupture of liver/spleen.
- Abusive injuries often associated with abdominal bruising (60%).
- Presents with collapse/abdominal pain/sepsis.
- Examine abdomen for:
  - Pain/distension/absent bowel sounds.
  - NGT may get blood back.
  - Examine anus for injury as CSA can perforate rectum.

▶Accidental injury is rare.

Investigations

CT abdomen. FBC, LFT (hepatic trauma), serum amylase (pancreatic/splenic injury), urinalysis (haematuria) and X-ray chest and abdomen (looking for free air).

Further resources

Accident prevention: 🖰 http://www.capt.org.uk
Bruises/fractures: 🖰 http://www.core-info.cardiff.ac.uk

Emotional abuse and neglect

- Emotional abuse seldom occurs in isolation and is usually associated with other aspects of abuse, most often neglect.
- Emotional abuse and neglect is usually a chronic condition with 3 areas of concern:

1. Problems with parenting

Drug/alcohol abuse, learning difficulties, domestic violence, mental health problems, unemployment, chronic illness or young age, may result in the parent being physically or emotionally 'unavailable' and predispose child to poor care and neglect.

2. Harmful interactions between parent and child

- The child may be subjected to emotional coldness and rejection or harsh criticism.
- The child may have developmentally inappropriate expectations placed upon them (parent may treat child as a 'friend' not as a child).
- The child may be overprotected and not allowed to play with their peer group.
- The child may witness inappropriate behaviour between adults, e.g. domestic violence or sexual activities.
- The child may be exploited in sexual or criminal activities.
- Such emotionally abusive behaviours can be hard to recognize but early recognition and management is essential for a good outcome. (Refer to CAMHS or clinical psychologist.)

3. Impairment in the child due to failure to meet their physical needs

- The child may be unkempt and dirty with dirt under fingernails.
- The child may have untreated medical conditions, e.g. head lice, eczema and asthma.
- The child may show poor growth/FTT due to lack of nutrition. It is essential therefore to chart their growth on each occasion they are seen to monitor growth trajectory.
- The child may show 'catch up' growth when in hospital or in care, only for growth to falter when they return home (step pattern on growth chart). Rule out medical causes.
- The child may also be overweight from eating only high calorie 'junk' food.

Clinical evidence of emotional abuse and neglect

Often the child shows:
- Developmental delay in early milestones due to lack of stimulation and play. Speech and language often the key area of delay.
- When child starts nursery/school they lack social skills.
- Self-care skills delay, e.g. not toilet trained, unable to dress/feed themselves etc.
- Social isolation and lack of interpersonal skills needed for play.

- Poor educational attainment, behaviour problems and often have special educational needs. Poor school attendance.
- Clothes are often dirty, ill fitting and inappropriate for weather, e.g. no socks in winter, no underwear etc.
- Young infants may be left in wet clothes in a cold room and suffer from 'cold injury' or redness and swelling of the hands and feet.
- Lack of emotional warmth and affection may result in attachment disorder (leading to poor social skills, emotional and behavioural difficulties in the child).
- Lack of supervision of the child can lead to increased chance of accidents within the home, e.g. falls and scalds. Outside the home such children may wander off and be involved in road accidents or stranger abuse.

Investigations

- Often need to gather information and monitor health over a period of time to provide evidence of significant harm.
- Children need to have growth charted.
- Baseline investigations if concerns, for anaemia and rickets (FBC, iron and ferritin, vitamin D level, and wrist X-ray).
- They should be subjected to a full multiagency assessment with a *section 47* investigation if needed (see 📖 p471).
- Involve all agencies i.e. GP, HV, education and social services.

▶▶Remember extreme case of neglect can be fatal due to severe malnutrition with multiorgan failure.

Fabricated or induced illness

Definition
A condition whereby a child suffers harm through deliberate action of her/his main carer and which is attributed by the adult to another cause.

It may involve:
- Fabrication of signs and symptoms, including fabrication of past medical history (seizures—common).
- Falsification of hospital charts, records, letters and documents and specimens of bodily fluids.
- Induction of illness by a variety of means, e.g. by smothering
- Harm from unnecessary or invasive medical investigations and treatment, which are performed because of above points.
- Typically presents to health professionals.
- Identification is challenging (need to distinguish between abnormally anxious parents, parents exaggerating symptoms and FII).
- Rare 1/100,000. More in <1 year olds.
- Significant morbidity and occasional mortality.

When to consider FII
- Symptoms and signs are not explained.
- Investigation results don't tally with Hx.
- Inexplicably poor response to treatment.
- New symptoms are reported on resolution of previous ones.
- Reported symptoms and found signs are not observed in the absence of the carer.
- Child is repeatedly presented with a range of symptoms to different professionals in a variety of settings.
- Child's normal/daily life activities curtailed beyond that expected.
- Carer or relatives expressing concern about FII.

Other factors
Mother most commonly perpetrator, parent often has healthcare background, parent often has history of somatisation.

Common presenting features
- Fits, acute life-threatening event, drowsy/coma.
- Blood in vomit/per rectum/urine/haemoptysis.
- FTT, feeding difficulty, vomiting/GOR, bowel disturbance.
- Asthma, skin lesions.
- Fabricated disability.
- False allegations of abuse or disclosure accidental overdose.

Management
- One consultant must assume responsible role.
- Discuss with named and designated professionals.
- Document concerns (may need confidential notes—restrict access).
- Obtain chronology, including information from other hospitals and primary care.

- Assess risk of harm (?child needs supervision).
- Consider further opinion/investigations to help with diagnosis.
- Stop harmful procedure/treatments unless clearly needed (may need admission).
- Say 'no explanation found, needs further assessment'—to parents.
- Refer to SS and ask for strategy meeting.
- Confrontation only in a planned and controlled way, with arrangements to ensure that child is safe.
- Trail of separation.

▶▶Do not share concern about FII with parents in initial stages.

Sexual abuse

- Often a secretive activity by someone known to child, much CSA goes unreported.
- May be intra or extrafamilial.
- Institutional or stranger abuse.
- 'Grooming of child' and coercion are important features.
- Girls 80%: boys 20%.

The 'diagnostic jigsaw' of sexual abuse (SA) needs to be pieced together and includes:

- Disclosure from child: present in around 70 % cases.
- ▶ Most useful part of 'jigsaw' child seldom lies.
- History from parent/carer/child.
- Sexual abuse may have been witnessed.
- Inappropriate sexualized behaviour for developmental level.
- Injuries found including bruising/bleeding, in genital/anal area.
- Medical concerns: recurrent dysuria (with no infection)/vaginal discharge/secondary enuresis/encopresis ~7.6%.
- Evidence from police video interview.
- Assessment of child by social worker.
- STIs/positive forensic evidence.
- Contact with known sex offender.

Keep SA on list of differential diagnoses for:

- Genital bleeding: could also be straddle injury/lichen sclerosus et atrophicus/early puberty.
- Rectal bleeding: could also be fissures from constipation.
- Vulvo-vaginitis: could also be due to poor hygiene/eczema/allergies/ *Candida*/foreign body/strep A and Hib infection/threadworms.

Referrals usually from:

- Police/SS following a strategy meeting.
- Primary health care team.
- School.
- Other paediatrician, often from A&E.

Who examines child

- Often a joint examination, usually 2 paediatricians (best practice for pre-pubertal child) or paediatrician + forensic physician (for forensic samples).
- Usually in paediatric department or Sexual Assault Referral Centre (SARC).

Timing of examination

- Acute case, abuse within previous 72 hours, consider collection of forensic samples and see child on day of referral.
- If child is bleeding from genital/anal area, needs to be assessed urgently, usually in A&E.

- Historic allegations (most common presentation) do not require urgent assessment. A planned approach is best but without too much delay.

Competencies required for CSA examinations
- Able to take informed consent.
- Able to undertake paediatric history and examination.
- Need to understand child's developmental level and emotional needs.
- Recognize normal and abnormal genital and anal anatomy.
- Use the colposcope and photo-document findings.
- Recognize when additional help is required, e.g. for STI tests/PEP for HIV/postcoital contraception/forensic sampling.

Further resource

Oxford Child Sexual Abuse Examination Skills Training model and DVD: ℜ http://www.pharm-abotics.co.uk

Medical assessment and investigation

The investigation and management of a case of possible deliberate harm to a child should be approached in the same systematic and rigorous manner as would be appropriate to the investigation and management of any other potentially fatal disease.
Lord Laming (2003). Victoria Climbié inquiry.

History
- A detailed history should be obtained (consider any need for an interpreter) from several sources if possible (referrer/parent/child).
- Establish if any need for immediate medical treatment.
- Document *verbatim* replies and who from.
- Record date/time of examination, who is present and who gave Hx.
- Document a full medical history using any local proforma available. Include antenatal and neonatal information, attendances at A&E/OPD. Remember to gather information from secondary sources i.e. GP, HV.
- Check if child has a *child protection plan* (on a register).
- Document a full FHx with genogram.
- Always ask about drug/alcohol use, mental health, and any domestic violence (when partner not present).
- Record developmental history and school progress also any emotional/behavioural difficulties.
- Take a *sexual health* history from adolescents, including menstrual history.
- For CSA examinations ask specifically for child's terminology for genital and anal anatomy.
- Record details of alleged perpetrator, time of last incident and post incident activity, e.g. washing, clothing change, toileting.

Consent
- *Written consent* for examination from adult with parental responsibility is best practice.
- Consider consent from child if appropriate.
- Use a standard consent form if available locally (see 📖 p634 Sample consent form).
- Remember to consent for special investigations i.e. X-rays, swabs and blood tests, for photography (of injuries or for CSA using a colposcope).
- Take separate consent for photographs to be used for teaching and training and for peer review.
- Consent also for sharing of information and with whom.

Examination
- Examine child thoroughly completely undressed, do not forget hidden areas, mouth (frenulum), eyes, ears and genitalia/buttocks/anus (unless child refuses, give older child informed choices).
- Measure height, weight, and head circumference and plot on growth chart.

- Look for signs of neglect i.e. dirty clothes/hair, head lice, dirt under nails, severe nappy rash and dental decay.
- Note child's demeanour, frightened or withdrawn?
- Record all information onto the proforma, use body maps to document injuries (see 📖 p635 and p636, Appendix).
- Get photographs (medical or forensic photographer). Include a right angled measure on all photos.
- Remember to sign notes and record time examination completed.

Investigations

- Baseline investigations when needed.
- Physical abuse:
  - FBC, clotting studies, Ca/PO4, ALP, vitamin D.
  - If <2 years skeletal survey, CT head. Repeat CXR after 10–12 days to look for rib fractures. Ophthalmology to examine for retinal haemorrhages.
- Sexual abuse:
  - Forensic Tests (see 📖 p461).
  - STI tests (📖 p462).
  - Consider pregnancy test and urine for chlamydia PCR.
- Neglect:
  - Photographs.
  - If FTT standard bloods + iron/ferritin.

❶ Discuss cases with a senior colleague.

Management

- If needed refer on for *second opinion* and further investigation and management.
- In some CSA cases refer to dermatology (e.g. lichen sclerosus et atrophicus).
- To genito-urinary medicine (GUM) clinic for STI investigation.
- To family planning clinic for postcoital contraception.
- Radiology opinion on X-ray findings in some cases of physical abuse.
- To growth clinic if FTT.
- To plastic surgery for burns.
- Consider need for counselling/therapeutic support from CAMHS.
- Plan *follow-up* appointment and write prompt reports (see 📖 Writing a report p464).
- Always write letter to GP.
- Continue to liaise with police/social services (responsible for investigation). If not already involved, refer to them.

❶ Consider safety and examination of *siblings* if concerns.

Examination of alleged sexual abuse

Purpose of examination

- Assess need for treatment.
- Provide information/evidence for court proceedings.
- Begin the therapeutic process for the child/reassurance for family.

Before starting

- *Who does it?* Ensure examiner has necessary core skills, a forensic physician can assist if forensic samples needed.
- Good *preparation* of child/parent with explanation of process.
- Consider timing and place of examination (child-friendly room).
- Allow child to have a trusted adult present.
- Set up colposcope with DVD ready to record/forensic kit available.
- Check written (best practice) consent obtained from person with PR.
- If child refuses examination consider offering a further appointment.

At examination

- Show child the colposcope.
- Assess best way to examine child, on couch/parent's knee.
- Full physical examination, then genital/anal examination. Record to DVD.
- Note child's demeanour and record anything child says verbatim in notes.

Genital examination (female)

- Examine in *supine frog-leg position* hips flexed, soles of feet together.
- Note Tanner staging if pubertal.
- Inspect external genitalia (labia majora) for abnormalities.
- Use labial separation to view hymen configuration/fossa navicularis/urethral meatus/labia minora and posterior fourchette (see 📖 p637, Appendix).
- Apply labial traction to aid visualization of hymenal margin and vagina (see 📖 p638, Appendix)
- Use *clock face* to record any abnormal findings on body map in notes (see 📖 p639, Appendix)
- *Confirm* any abnormal findings of posterior hymen by examining in different position, e.g. prone knee chest or by another technique, e.g. flooding vestibule with sterile water (pre-pubertal)/using moist cotton bud to tease out hymenal edge (post-pubertal).
- Consider using a Foley catheter in post-pubertal girl, insert into vagina, inflate balloon then gently pull back. Aids examination of hymenal edge.
- Take any forensic and infection screening swabs needed.

Anal examination (boys and girls)

- Examine in *left lateral position* legs flexed at hips and knees.
- Inspect perianal skin/rugae (perianal folds).
- Separate buttocks for ~30 seconds, look at anal margin, assess anal sphincter tone/any reflex anal dilatation constipation/skin tags, etc.
- Take any forensic and infection screening swabs needed.

End of examination

- Remember any further tests (HIV/Hep B/Hep C, pregnancy tests).
- Explain findings and reassure child.
- Give any treatment necessary.
- Line drawings on body maps to supplement photo-documentation.
- Review DVD and write reports.
- Referrals on and follow-up arrangements.
- ▶ Peer review of cases both normal and abnormal findings is good practice.

Normal and abnormal genital and anal findings

(See 🕮 p637 and p640, Appendix)

- Become familiar with 'normal' anatomy during your routine examination of children.
- Findings can vary with examination technique, position, and degree of relaxation of child.
- Confirm abnormalities in a different position.
- There is variation of normal anatomy depending on age of child and stage of puberty. Hymen not damaged by tampon use or masturbation.
- In infants the hymen is often fleshy and redundant due to maternal hormonal influence, the hymen then tends to become a thin elastic membrane with a central orifice during childhood, becoming fleshy and fimbriated as child enters puberty.
- Normal variations of hymen configuration in pre-pubertal child include annular (53%), crescentic (29%), septate (2%), sleeve-like (15%). Imperforate hymen is uncommon.
- Describe location of your findings using *clock face* notation with 12 o'clock at symphysis pubis (see 🕮 p639).

Congenital findings

- Hymen notches between 9 and 3 o'clock anteriorly, particularly anterior 'cleft' in a crescentic-shaped hymen.
- 'Bumps' on hymenal edge, a bump at 6 o'clock is often due to the posterior intravaginal ridge.
- Small tags on edge of hymen.
- Failure of midline fusion.

Significance of findings for diagnosis of CSA

Low significance—genital findings (girls)
- Labial adhesions/fusion found in ~16% infants.
- Erythema of genitalia especially labia majora. Friability of skin.
- Vulvo-vaginitis.

Low significance—anal findings
- Single anal fissure (constipation).
- Perianal venous congestion.
- Anal dilatation with stool visible in rectum.

Medium significance—genital finding
- Genital warts/herpes.
- Cleft or notch (V or U shape) of posterior hymen between 3 and 9 o'clock, which is >50% of hymenal depth.

Medium significance—anal findings
- Several anal fissures. Anal scars and skin tags outside midline.
- Loss of normal rugae (perianal skin folds) with smooth shiny skin.

High significance—genital findings
- Need to see in acute period.
- Positive forensic evidence of semen/sperm.

- Pregnancy.
- STI screen positive for gonorrhoea or chlamydia (when no reported consensual activity). Remember vertical transmission.
- Acute injury-transection of hymen to its base, tears of vagina and posterior fourchette (exclude straddle injury). Bruising/abrasions.
- Absent posterior hymen (hymen depth of <1 mm).

High significance—anal findings
- Acute anal tear/injury.
- Circular oedematous swelling around anal margin (Tyre sign).

❶ In some areas of the UK female genital mutilation (FGM) may need to be considered if abnormalities of external female genitalia involving labia majora/labia minora or clitoris are found. FGM is an illegal practice in the UK (FGM Act 2003).

Further resource

FORWARD (Foundation for Women's Health Research and Development): ℘ http://www.for-warduk.org.uk

The colposcope in CSA examinations

- The colposcope is a non-invasive, powerful magnifying light source.
- Provides ability to *photo-document* genital and anal examination to DVD or video for future reference, preventing unnecessary repeat examination of child. (Now considered best practice.)
- The use of the colposcope is a specialist examination undertaken by a person with necessary competence/experience.
- Variation in models, therefore need to be familiar with local equipment.

Photo-documentation

- Written informed consent from adult with PR is good practice and from child if appropriate.
- Consent also for sharing images for peer review/second opinions/teaching/training (see 📖 Consent p455).
- Clear explanation of procedure to carer/child. **Never** attach photos to reports or take DVD/photos to court unless ordered to do so by Judge.
- Continue to use line drawings of findings on body maps as these can be shown in court (see 📖 Body maps pp635–40, Appendix).

DVD

- Anonymised with child's details/date recorded and by whom.
- No pictures taken of child's face.
- If consent refused for photo-documentation, record reasons in notes and use body maps.
- When recording is finished, DVD can also be marked with anonymised details using permanent marker pen.
- Must be securely stored, separately from clinical notes in a locked cabinet, in a locked room, with any photos which are printed.
- Forms a part of clinical record and must be retained until child reaches age of 26 years (or 8 years after death of child), before it can be destroyed.
- Is a useful reference when writing your report/for review before attending court.
- Never store any images on memory stick/Flash media.
- May be requested to share photo-documentation with an expert for court case. Advisable to ask them to view in your department, (many DVDs will only play back on the machine on which they were recorded).

Forensic sampling in CSA cases

- Health needs of the child are paramount.
- Consider following any allegation of recent sexual assault.
- Think about timing of forensic sampling and examination/sooner the better (best within 72 hours). Photo-document examination (use colposcope).
- May be undertaken in a SARC.
- Ensure informed consent taken in writing (see 📖 Consent p455):
  - Forensic sampling is a specialist activity; need to have necessary skills and competencies. If do not have these skills, offer to undertake a general paediatric examination and request from police a forensic physician, to take forensic samples (joint examination).
  - Take forensic samples before swabs for infection screen.
  - Forensic samples, usually swabs/cut hair/nail clippings/blood/urine etc. are taken and labelled with child's name/description (e.g. anal swab)/Dr's ID and number, e.g. (SK1)/date and time taken.
  - Remember to ensure that underwear/clothes are seized and sent for forensic examination.
  - Each swab placed in individual *evidence bag* and sealed.
  - The bag is then labelled with same information as above and signed by the doctor who took the sample.
  - The bag is handed to a police officer (usually) who signs it and afterwards it is signed by anyone else who handles it.

❶ *Chain of evidence:* keep a list of all specimens taken in clinical notes and the order taken with ID numbers. Put this information into any reports you write.

Sexually transmitted infections: investigations/referrals and management

❶ Presence of STI in a child must always raise concern of CSA.
- Children alleging SA if in 'risk' group need screening for STIs.
- 'Risk' depends on type of abuse/age of perpetrator and risk factors in perpetrator, e.g. IV drug user/ethnicity (for HIV) and local prevalence of STIs. See Fig 12.1.
- Consider timing for screening, e.g. too soon may give negative results due to incubation period.
- Mode of transmission: vertical transmission from mother to child at birth or direct sexual contact.
  - Currently no accurate information available for upper age limits for vertical transmission therefore difficult to be categorical but consider up to age of 3 years.
  - Blood-borne infections include hepatitis B and C, and HIV.
  - Viral infections include genital herpes and ano-genital warts.
  - Bacterial infections include chlamydia, gonorrhoea, syphilis, *Mycoplasma* and bacterial vaginosis.

Commonest STIs seen in CSA cases:

- *Chlamydia*: often asymptomatic and often associated with penetrative abuse. Ascending infection more likely in post-pubertal child. Chlamydia can also be transmitted vertically at birth.
- *Ano-genital warts* (HPV virus): can also be from auto-inoculation and vertical transmission. Typing of virus is not helpful. HPV vaccination of girls may decrease this infection in the future.
- *Genital herpes:* painful ulcerative STI caused by HSV type 1 or 2. Typing not helpful in aiding diagnosis of CSA.
- *Gonorrhoea*: if found association with CSA is high, unless obvious vertical transmission.

Investigation

- Consider referral to local GUM consultant.
- If undertaking tests review classification of 'risk' to decide on appropriate tests and know about local prevalence (see Fig, 12.1).
- Remember 'chain of evidence' for any swabs, bloods, if criminal proceedings likely (See Forensic sampling 🕮 p461).
- Some tests will need repeating at a later date, e.g. HIV.

Treatment

- Consider postexposure prophylaxis (PEP) for HIV, and 1st Hep B immunisation.
- See Fig. 12.1 for management of STI/consult with local GUM or infectious disease team for up-to-date treatment.
- Prophylaxis occasionally indicated if child unlikely to return for treatment, e.g. for chlamydia, but not routinely recommended.

Further resource

British Association for Sexual Health and HIV: ℘ http://http://www.bashh.org/

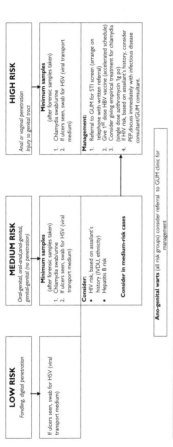

Fig. 12.1 Management of suspected STIs in sexually abused young people.

Writing a report

- These reports may well be used as *medical evidence in court* and therefore should be carefully written with this in mind.
- A separate letter will also be written on all occasions to the GP with an outline of findings, any treatment required and follow-up plans.
- A confidential report for social workers will vary from that required for a witness statement for the police (this is usually a special format).
- Social work report may include a large amount of detail about child's background and 'second-hand' or hearsay evidence which is not included in a witness statement.
- It is helpful to discuss your reports with another suitably qualified person, e.g. named/designated person in your Trust, before sending report.

❶ All of these reports may be used in court and therefore need to be consistent.

Report for the court

- Set out in clear paragraphs which can be numbered.
- Use non-medical language where possible, explain medical terms.
- Start with your *name* and *qualifications* then outline your experience including relevant child protection training/roles undertaken.
- State the name/DOB of the child, why you were asked to examine child, by whom and date, time, and place of examination. List who was present for examination.

Then give details of:
- *Consent* taken (written or verbal).
- Relevant *history* relating to child, details of current complaints.
- Record *verbatim* any spontaneous pertinent information which child gives you, as this is not hearsay evidence.
- List *findings* of medical examination and state time you finished examination. Include body maps.
- List any *investigations* carried out, specimens taken and results if available.
- Record if colposcope used for CSA examination and if photos taken.
- Detail any *treatment* and advice given and *follow-up* arrangements.
- In *conclusion* state important findings, positive and negative.
- **❶** A normal examination does not rule out abuse.
- Abnormal signs may have resolved if there is delay from the time of abuse to time of examination. This can be stated in your summary. The *child's disclosure* is the most important piece of evidence where there are no abnormal findings.
- List your *differential diagnosis* and your *professional opinion* of most likely diagnosis. Give any references which are mainstream to support your opinion.
- **❶** Do not be tempted to stray outside your areas of expertise.
- Sign and date each page of the report (see 📖 p465).
- Following peer review with colleagues you may wish to change the opinion in your report. It is good practice to do so if there are evidence-based reasons for your new opinion. Write a further report stating why you have changed your opinion and citing new evidence.

Sample report for court

Confidential medical report

Introduction and Hx

I am Dr...my qualifications are.... I have been a paediatrician for...years. I work for...NHS Trust. I am on the hospital child protection rota once a week, seeing children with a wide range of child protection concerns, including sexual abuse. I have attended regular child protection peer review sessions and a level 3 course on recognition of child abuse.

I was asked to examine X on (date) at (time) by [name person requesting]. This followed an allegation by X to his teacher that he had been hit by his father the previous evening. I recorded the details of this incident given to me by X and his mother and by the social worker (name) in the clinical notes.

PMHx

Family/social history/behaviour.

Developmental milestones/school progress.

With written consent from (mother of X) I examined X at (time) in (Department) with his mother present, and with assistance from Dr... (ST4 community paediatrics).

Examination

X was noted to be rather withdrawn. He was pale with dirty clothing.

Ht...and Wt...(centiles). General examination (list all).

Genital and anal examination.

X had the following injuries:
1) Red/purple coloured petechial bruising on the left side of his face and ear as documented on the attached body map.
2) 4 small faded brown bruises on both shins (see attached body map). There were no other injuries noted.

Blood samples were taken to exclude a bleeding/clotting disorder. These were all normal. Clinical photographs were taken of X's bruises in the department of medical illustration [hospital name].

Following my examination, I discussed my findings with X's mother and social worker. An initial case conference was recommended. No follow-up has been arranged in our department.

Opinion

The petechial bruising (small spots of bruising) on X's face and ear had the appearance of a slap mark and is consistent with the allegation that X has made that his father hit him on the face. The bruises on his legs are not significant and are likely to have occurred during normal play activities.

Signed —— Date ——

Giving evidence in court

▶*Try to attend a course on giving evidence in court (www.rcpch.ac.uk).*

Before the day

- Ensure you have written instructions and know why you are attending, e.g. finding of fact/criminal proceedings.
- Give your availability early in writing to witness warning officer from the court.
- If never been to court, you can ask witness support team for a visit.
- Get a copy of your written report, read it and discuss with a senior colleague any potential questions.
- Assemble clinical notes and copies of any references given (take originals if possible)
- Consider taking anatomical model to demonstrate anatomical findings to judge/jury in CSA cases.

On the day

- Dress in professional attire.
- Have all your papers with you.
- Allow time, arrive early. You may need to speak with lawyers/ barristers.
- Make yourself known to the court usher when you arrive. Ask who the judge/magistrate is and how to address them, e.g. Your Honour.
- Take a book to read, you may have a long wait.

In court

- When court is ready, the usher will lead you to the witness box.
- You will be asked to either take an oath on the bible/holy books or affirm (your choice).
- Then you will be asked your name/address/qualifications.
- The prosecution will commence questions/then defence/then any others barristers/then ending with any further questions from prosecution.
- Look at the person asking the questions then turn toward judge to give response, addressing appropriately 'Your Honour…' etc.
- Use non-medical language when possible or explain terminology.
- Do not hurry your answer. Consider the question before replying.
- Beware of adversarial style of questioning by barristers.
- ▶▶Do not be tempted to stray outside your area of expertise.
- If you don't know the answer, say so.
- If you don't understand the question or want it repeated, say so.
- When questions are finished the judge will tell you that you may leave the court.
- On leaving the court room, turn to face the judge and bow your head briefly.

Afterwards

- Claim any expenses owed.
- Ask for the outcome of the case. Can also ask for feedback about your performance.
- Consider a *mini-pupillage* with a local judge by arrangement.

The assessment framework

See Fig. 12.2.

Initial assessment

- The initial assessment is undertaken by the LA children's social care, in accordance with statutory guidance.
- This determines whether the child is in need, is suffering or likely to suffer *significant harm* defined as the threshold of ill treatment or impairment of health (physical or mental) or development, which justifies compulsory intervention in family life. This is usually established by the courts.
- Such assessments might look at situations involving domestic violence, mental ill health, drug and alcohol abuse and learning disabilities in the parent or carer.
- Other situations might involve children in care, those in secure accommodation, asylum seekers, children with LD, and those living in poverty.

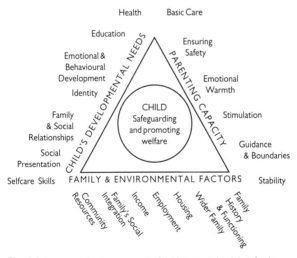

Fig 12.2 Framework for the assessment of children in need and their families. Contains public sector information licensed under the Open Government Licence v1.0. Reproduced from *The Framework for the Assessment of Children in Need and their Families*. London: Department of Health/Department of Education & Employment/Home Office, 2000.

Referral

- If there are concerns about significant harm a telephone referral for an assessment can be made to SS, always followed by a *written referral* within 48 hours.
- Record details of any phone conversations.
- Using a *multiagency* approach to share responsibility and promote working together a *strategy meeting* involving police, health, and social care is then convened to gather information and plan an appropriate coordinated course of action.
- This may involve a *medical assessment* if this has not already occurred. (see 📖 Medical assessment p455). It is likely also to involve a video-interview of the child undertaken by police/social worker with appropriate training.
- The initial assessment should be completed within 10 working days of the date of referral (under section 47 of Children Act).

Outcomes of referral

- 'Child in need' that justifies an initial assessment, but no present concerns about significant harm.
- 'Child in need' and concerns about actual or potential significant harm which justify an initial assessment, which will probably lead to a strategy discussion and may be a child protection assessment.
- Emergency immediate protective action—usually determined by strategy discussion (between SS and police and other agencies as appropriate) with legal advice leading to:
  - Alleged abuser agreeing to leave house.
  - Voluntary agreement for child to move to safer place.
  - Application for Emergency Protection Order (EPO) decided by court lasts initially 7 days.
  - Removal of child on Police Protection Order (PPO) used by police, when child is in danger and not enough time to get EPO.
  - Removal of alleged abuser through exclusion requirement attached to EPO or Interim Care Order (ICO) decided by court lasts initially 8 weeks.
  - Child Protection assessment leading to case conference.

The 3 domains of the assessment framework look at:
- The child's developmental needs.
- The capacity of the parent/carer to respond to those needs.
- The wider family and environmental factors.

Child protection case conference

Should be held within 15 days of start of child protection assessment. Meeting involves family, the child (where appropriate) and professionals involved with the child and family (including adult workers, e.g. drug and mental health).

- Aims to share/evaluate information, assess risks, and formulate an agreed plan.
- Chaired by an independent chairperson.
- Parents generally present, may be excluded under exceptional circumstances.
- Social worker presents details of initial assessment and all professionals share their findings.
- Paediatrician involved should attend, if not possible then deputy should be sent.
  - Medical report for conference sent beforehand, and take report and notes to conference.
  - Inform chairperson in advance if there are issues.
  - Paediatrician presents medical details in layman's terms.
- After all information presented professionals are asked to give opinion whether child is at risk of significant harm and needs:
  - A 'child protection plan' and if so in what category (physical/sexual/ emotional abuse or neglect).
  - A 'child in need' plan, if child protection plan not recommended. Child will be supported by a team around the child and progress monitored by TAC meetings (see below).
- *Pre-birth case conferences* held when assessment leads to concerns that an unborn child may be at risk of significant harm (e.g. previous child removed, other children in family have child protection plan, Hx of parental mental health problem, LD, substance misuse or domestic violence, etc.).
- *Review conferences* are held to collate information, ensure interagency coordination, review the level of risk, and if a child protection plan still needed.

Child protection plan

- A multiagency plan.
- Initially formulated at case conference to ensure child and family are appropriately supported/monitored by all agencies and that expectation of the family is made clear.
- *Core group* (appointed at case conference) including a lead social worker is responsible for keeping plan up to date and coordinating interagency activities.
- LA keeps record of all children with child protection plans in their area, which is accessible to other agencies if they have a concern about a child.

Children in need plan
- Aims:
  - Identify child's additional needs by common assessment framework (CAF) process.
  - To share this information between organisations and
  - To coordinate service provision.
- With consent of child or parents/carers, practitioners undertake a common assessment in accordance with nationally agreed framework to assess the needs and to decide how best to support them.
- Findings from CAF may identify concerns about child's safety and welfare. These should be used to support a referral to social services.
- Children in Need are then supported by TAC.

Team around the child (TAC)
- Multidisciplinary team of practitioners established on case-by-case basis to support a child, young person, or family in need.
- Includes joined-up working, information sharing, and early intervention with a lead professional.
- Child/young person and family at the centre of the process.
- A virtual or flexible multiagency team that changes as needs change.
- A TAC support plan is produced to meet the needs of the child/young person, regular meetings held.

Legal aspects

- The *Children Act 1989* introduced 'significant harm' as threshold that justifies compulsory intervention in best interests of child.
- Harm is defined as ill treatment or impairment of health and development.

The following sections of Children Act 1989 are relevant to safeguarding:

Section 17

- Places obligation on LA to safeguard and promote welfare of 'children in need' which includes:
  - Looked-after children (LAC) in care of local authority
  - Those in secure accommodation and
- By promoting their up-bringing within their families if possible by providing support.

Section 20

- Places duty on LA to provide accommodation for a child in need if:
  - No one has parental responsibility.
  - Child is lost or abandoned.
  - Person caring for child is prevented from providing suitable accommodation or care.
- It is done with consent of parent/carer who maintains parental responsibility.

Section 47

If child is suffering or is likely to suffer significant harm the LA has a duty to investigate whether any action is necessary to safeguard a child.

Care proceedings

(Covered by Section 31 of Children Act.)

- Are applications for a care or supervision order when the LA considers that parent/carer cannot or is unlikely to be able to provide safe or appropriate care for a child.
- Heard in *Family Proceedings Court*.
- Children's guardian appointed to represent child and any necessary expert assessments commissioned.
- '*Finding of fact*' hearing is often held at beginning of proceedings to establish what has actually happened to child.
- Decisions are made on principle of 'the balance of probabilities'. After deliberations the Family Proceedings Court could issue interim care order (ICO).

Interim care order

- LA shares parental responsibility, whilst LA completes full assessment for proceedings and child may remain at home.
- After assessment completed the LA will make recommendation to court for one of the following, which will be decided in court at the Final Hearing:

Full care order
- LA acquires parental responsibility, and makes plan for child to be placed for long-term fostering or adoption.

Residence order or Special Guardianship Order
- Child placed with extended family.

Supervision order
- Child remains at home with supervision from LA to monitor and support family.

Criminal proceedings
- If it is thought that a parent/carer has committed a crime, separate criminal proceedings will be initiated by Crown Prosecution Service. Heard in the Crown Court.
- Decisions are made on principle of 'beyond all reasonable doubt'.

Working with the police

- Police have a specialist team who are involved with child protection work—Child Abuse Investigation Unit (CAIU).
- However 'out-of-hours' and when potential crimes have occurred uniformed police will be involved.
- Their prime duty is to establish if crime has occurred by collecting evidence and then pressing charges (at times can conflict with health and social services assessment and case management).
- It is vital teams work together and understand each other's roles to ensure correct procedures are followed and best outcomes are achieved.
- Following referral multiagency *strategy meeting* ensures case is managed in cohesive way that does not compromise evidence or the child's safety.

National and local safeguarding procedures

- *Working Together 2010* is a key government document that describes how organisations/individuals should work together to safeguard and promote the welfare of children.
- The statutory framework for it is *Children Act 2004* (sections 10, 11, and 12) and the *Education Act 2002* (section 175).
  - Emphasises need for shared responsibility and effective joint working between agencies and professionals.
  - Requires constructive relationships between frontline practitioners, but also between operational and senior managers of services.
- It provides guidance on the following:
  - Roles and responsibilities.
  - Local Safeguarding Children Boards (LSCB).
  - Interagency training and development.
  - Managing individual cases.
  - Child death review (CDR) processes.
  - Serious case reviews (SCR)
- Each NHS Trust has a *named doctor* and *named nurse for child protection* responsible within that trust for taking the lead on child protection matters.
  - They can be consulted with any child protection concerns.
- Each PCT also has a *designated doctor* and *nurse for child protection* who work with the named professionals within each trust.
  - Often sit on the Local Safeguarding Children Board (LSCB).

LSCB

- Is a key statutory mechanism for agreeing how organisations will work together to ensure their effectiveness.
- This includes:
  - Engaging in activities to safeguard and promote welfare of all children.
  - Leading and coordinating proactive work that targets particular groups and arrangements for responsive work to protect children who are suffering or at risk of suffering maltreatment.
- Membership includes:
  - Senior managers from different services, e.g. police, ambulance, education, social services, etc.
  - Agencies including voluntary sector.
  - Experts, e.g. designated doctor and nurse for child protection.
  - Lay members.
- Functions:
  - To produce policies/procedures for effective safeguarding.
  - Raise awareness.
  - Monitor/evaluate aims and effectiveness.
  - Participate in planning/commissioning.
  - Review deaths of children and undertake SCRs.

- Managing individual cases:
  - LSCB has local procedures in place to ensure information is shared.
  - Appropriate referrals are made and assessed.
  - Child protection investigations are conducted jointly between SS and police.
- Procedures:
  - Include detailed information on when and how to refer.
  - Timing and type of assessment.
  - Outcomes of referrals.
  - Emergency protective action including strategy discussions/meetings.
  - Case conferences.
  - Child protection plans.
- Information sharing:
  - When there is a clear risk of significant harm, safety and welfare of a child is paramount and overrides confidentiality, hence information must be shared.
  - It is best practice to share information with consent of parent/carer or child/young person.
  - If not possible to gain consent or actively withheld, information can be disclosed in order to protect a child/young person and, or to protect the public interest.
  - Where it is not so clear about risk of harm, professional is justified in sharing some (relevant and proportionate) confidential information as part of consultation with others, to enable them to make a decision.

❶ Overriding consideration must be the *best interests of the child* and absolute confidentiality cannot and should not be promised to anyone.

Child death review processes

- Involves rapid response by team of key professionals looking into and evaluating each unexpected death of a child.
- Undertake review of all child deaths (birth to 18 years) in local area by Child Death Overview Panel (CDOP)—is a subcommittee of the LSCB with representatives from key organisations.
- On-call rapid response team is coordinated by designated doctor for child deaths. The team is available to support family and visit home where necessary soon after death.
- Professionals must notify designated doctor of an unexpected death, who will discuss case with key professionals and decide whether a *strategy meeting* is indicated following the initial postmortem findings.
- Multiagency strategy meeting is held within 3–7 working days of child's death:
  - To share information about events leading to the child's death.
  - To provide background history for the pathologist.
  - To ensure a coordinated bereavement plan for the family.
  - Consider any child protection risks.
- Following staff could be invited to the strategy meeting: pathologist, consultant paediatrician, GP, HV, SS manager, senior police officer, coroner's officer, specialist HV, school staff and ambulance staff and is chaired by the designated paediatrician.
- *Case discussion* is held 8–12 weeks after death with final postmortem results.
- Report goes to CDOP.

CDOP

- Undertakes an overview of all child deaths within a locality.
- Collects standard minimum dataset as agreed nationally.
- Reviews and evaluates information collected.
- Identifies lessons to be learnt, issues of concerns, and common themes emerging.
- Considers whether death was avoidable and whether there may be grounds for SCR. Informs chair of LSCB.
- Monitors support and assessment service offered to families of children who have died.
- Produces annual report, shares with LSCB among others.
- Cooperates with regional and national initiatives.

Sudden unexpected death in infancy

- Definition: sudden death of an infant <1 year of age which remains unexplained after:
  - A thorough case investigation including postmortem.
  - Examination of death scene.
  - Review of clinical history.
  - Death occurs unobserved during sleep, with no obvious signs of major illness.
- Incidence 0.4/1000 live births in UK.
- Epidemiological evidence in 1980s suggested it was related to sleep position.
- *'Back to sleep campaign'* informed mothers to place babies on their back when they are put to sleep. This led to a 70% reduction in SUDI.
- Other factors associated with increased risk: overheating, parental smoking, soft sleep surface, deprived families and co-sleeping (especially when parent has used alcohol or illegal drugs).

Serious case reviews

LSCB is required to undertake a SCR when a child dies and abuse or neglect is known or suspected to be a factor in the death.

Consider SCR:

- When child sustains life-threatening injury or serious and permanent impairment through abuse or neglect.
- Or child subjected to particularly serious SA.
- Or parent has been murdered and homicide review is initiated.
- Or child killed by parent with mental illness.

and a case gives rise to concern about interagency working to protect children.

Purpose of SCR

- Establish whether lessons are to be learnt about how local professionals and agencies work together to safeguard and promote welfare of children.
- Identify clearly what the lessons are, how they will be acted on and what is expected to change.
- Improve interagency working and better safeguard children.

How is SCR done?

- LSCB determines scope of the review.
- Timing: decision within 1 month, completed within 6 months (unless criminal proceedings hold up review).
- Each relevant service undertakes separate individual management review which should look openly and critically at individual and organisational practice and whether changes could be made.
- *Overview report* commissioned from a person who is independent of all agencies, which includes:
  - Introduction: summary of circumstances.
  - Terms of reference.
  - List of contributors.
  - The facts: genogram, integrated chronology and an overview.
  - Analysis: how and why, whether different decisions and actions could have led to different outcome.
  - Highlight good practice.
  - Conclusion and recommendations: focused, specific, and capable of being implemented.

Learning the lessons locally and nationally

- Review should be a learning process.
- Findings should be disseminated and recommendations implemented.
- LSCB audit 'action plan' and 'outcomes'.
- Ofsted review the SCR reports:
  - Child deaths and SCRs important source of information.
  - National overview of reports—key findings and implications.

Themes from national overview reports
- About 150–200 SCR reviewed/done per year.
- Most commonly conducted in those <1 year—who are most likely to die.
- 2/3 children known to SS at time of death.
- Family circumstances are common factors, e.g. domestic violence, drug/alcohol misuse, mental illness, neglect.

Nature of incidents
- <1 year commonest:
  - Physical abuse (parent or parent's partner).
  - Others, e.g. SUDI (with neglect, drugs, and alcohol).
  - Death after teenage mothers concealed pregnancy.
  - Babies overlain by parents (alcohol).
- Children 1–5 years:
  - Commonest: physical injury (parent or parent's partner).
  - Neglect (including methadone ingestion).
  - Witnessed murder/attempted murder/suicide of parent.
- Children aged 6–10 years: less of a pattern:
  - Murdered/attempted murder by mother or father (mental health problems).
  - Witnessed murder of mother.
  - Sexual abuse and neglect.
- Children 11 years plus:
  - Commonest suicide.
  - Murder (shooting and stabbing).
  - Sexual assault (including sexual exploitation).

Adoption, fostering, and looked-after children

An optimist sees an opportunity in every calamity. A pessimist sees a calamity in every opportunity.

Anon

Adoption, fostering, and looked-after children statistics in UK

The Office for National Statistics keeps data on these issues in the United Kingdom (℘ http://www.statistics.gov.uk/default.asp).

In England, for the year ending 31 March 2010:
- There were 64,400 looked-after children (LAC)—an increase of 7% since 2006 and up from 50,700 in 1996.
- 27,800 children started to be looked after and 25,100 children ceased to be looked after during the year.
- Maltreatment was the main reason why social care services first engaged with children who became looked after during the year.
- 73% of children were in a foster placement.
- There were 2300 children placed for adoption.
- There were 3400 unaccompanied asylum seeking children.
- There were 350 looked-after girls aged 12 or over who became mothers.

The following data shows the trends in adoption over the longer term:
- In 1930 there were 4000 adoptions
- By 1950 there were 14,500 adoptions
- 1968 was the year with the greatest number of adoptions with 27,000.
- In the 1970s, following the legalization of abortion (Abortion Act 1967) and the implementation of the Children Act 1975, there was a rapid decline in the number of adoptions from 22,502 in 1974 falling to 10,870 in 1979.
- The number of adoptions continued to fall steadily over the 1980s and 1990s; there were 1800 in 1997
- Adoptions have increased since then with 3800 in 2004 and 2005.

In Scotland, 15,892 children were in the care of LAs on 31 July 2010 and 455 adoptions took place in 2009. In Wales 5162 children were in the care of LAs on 31 March 2010 and 229 children were adopted from care during the year ending 31 March 2010. In Northern Ireland 2606 children were looked after on 31 March 2010 and 50 LAC were adopted in the year ending 31 March 2010.

Further resources
℘ http://www.baaf.org.uk/res/statengland
℘ http://www.baaf.org.uk/res/statscotland
℘ http://www.baaf.org.uk/res/statwales
℘ http://www.baaf.org.uk/res/statni

Adoption and fostering legislation

Adoption means the permanent transfer of parental responsibility for a child from birth parents (who cease to have any parental responsibility when the adoption order is granted) to adoptive parents. It is a legal term.

Adoption was first introduced into the UK under the terms of the Adoption of Children Act. The initial emphasis was on the needs of adults; adoption providing relief for unmarried mothers and meeting the desire to parent for couples unable to conceive themselves.

The Adoption Act 1976 is the main legislation governing the process of adoption in the UK but it has been updated with the Adoption and Children Act 2002. Key features of this act are:
- Paramouncy of the child's welfare over other issues.
- Preventing delay.
- Promoting permanence by extending residence orders to 18 year olds and creating special guardianship.
- Widening access to adoption by allowing unmarried couples, single people, and same-sex couples.
- Improving support for long-term impact of adoption by requiring adoption agencies to assess the support needs of those who are affected by adoption and setting out a more consistent approach to the release of sensitive and identifying information held in adoption records.

In Scotland the Adoption and Children (Scotland) Act 2007 replaced the Adoption (Scotland) Act 1978 in 2008. The current legislation in Northern Ireland is the Adoption (Northern Ireland) Order 1987.

In England, Wales, and Scotland there are national standards for the level of service adoption agencies must provide for all involved in the adoption process, including birth parents.

Adoption is solely administered through adoption services and agencies approved by the secretary of state. Therefore, private adoption is prohibited in the UK.

An extensive revision of adoption and fostering regulations, guidance and national minimum standards came into force in 2011. Further details can be found at: ℰ http://www.baaf.org.uk/newadoptionregulation

Further resources
ℰ http://www.legislation.gov.uk/ukpga/1976/36/contents
ℰ http://www.legislation.gov.uk/ukpga/2002/38/contents
ℰ http://www.legislation.gov.uk/asp/2007/4/contents
ℰ http://www.legislation.gov.uk/ukpga/1978/28/contents
ℰ http://www.legislation.gov.uk/nisr/1989/253/contents/made

The adoption process in the UK

Adoption provides a new legal family to children who cannot be brought up by birth parents. Deciding to become an adoptive parent is a major decision and there are a series of processes before a child can join a new family.

- *Register with an adoption agency*: LAs have adoption agencies within Children's Services (England and Wales) or Social Services (Scotland) or there are independent adoption agencies run by charities. A full list of adoption agencies is available from Adoption UK.
- Prospective adopters are invited to an information meeting and can then complete a formal application. Once accepted by the agency, a social worker is allocated and from this point the agency has a maximum of 8 months to make a decision on the application.
- Training is offered to groups of prospective adopters. The challenges of parenting any child are discussed as well as the additional complexities that children for adoption may present (because, for example, of experiences of maltreatment and attachment difficulties). Many other issues such as contact with birth families are considered.
- The assessment involves the social worker visiting the prospective adopters at home over a period of time and completing a Prospective Adopters Report (PAR). This comprehensive report explores the applicants' ability to adopt. It includes information on motivation to adopt, family background, childhood experiences, current relationships, financial circumstances, the safety and suitability of the home and neighbourhood for a child. A health assessment, LA, and police checks are required and at least 3 referees are interviewed face to face.
- The assessment allows prospective adopters to understand the challenges to adopting a child and the social worker to make an informed assessment of the adopter/s strengths and weaknesses. The adopters have 10 days to review the completed PAR and comment.
- The application is then considered by the agency's adoption panel. Prospective adopters are invited to part of the panel meeting to answer questions. The panel makes a recommendation to the agency's decision maker. If approved, the process of finding a suitable child begins. If not approved in England or Wales, the prospective adopters can involve the Independent Review Mechanism.
- When approved, a suitable child may come from the approving agency or elsewhere. Prospective adopters can use resources such as those available through *Be My Parent* or *Adoption UK*.
- When a suitable child is found, his/her agency arranges a meeting with the agency of the prospective adopters to look at the child's needs and the ability of the prospective adopters to meet these needs. If the match meets the child's needs, an Adoption Placement Report is written and presented to the child's adoption panel to recommend, and the agency decision-maker to approve, the match.
- If approved, an adoption placement plan is written detailing how introductions of the child to the family and vice versa will take place, what the contact plan will be and what post adoption support is needed and how this will be provided.

- Providing introductions go well, the child moves to the adopter/s home. The adopter/s, at this point share parental responsibility with the LA; the child is only legally adopted after an adoption order is granted by court. This order can be applied for after a minimum of 10 weeks. When it is granted, the child is legally part of the new family and can take their surname.

Further resources

🔊 http://www.adoptionuk.org/area_search/100172/100262/102988/find_an_agency/
🔊 http://www.adoptionuk.org/information/103163/ab_cwwmag/
🔊 http://www.bemyparent.org.uk/

Siblings in adoption and public care

- Many children are part of complex family structures. This is particularly the case for LAC, 80% of whom will have siblings, though not necessarily in LA care.
- When siblings enter public care, Section 23, part 7 of the Children's Act 1989 (England and Wales) puts a duty on the local authority to accommodate siblings together. The guidance in Scotland promotes placement together 'except where this would not be in one or more of the children's best interests' Children (Scotland) Act 1995.
- The term 'sibling' is not legally defined. It can include step-siblings, half-siblings, or unrelated children who have been brought up together.
- Research into siblings' placements has received less attention than other aspects of permanent placement.
- Social workers have to make decisions about separation or maintenance of sibling groups. Placing siblings together is often the best option with fewer problems for the siblings. However, sometimes the needs of siblings are so different (one having special needs, for instance) that social workers decide that separating the sibship is the best option.
- However, siblings are often placed separately for logistical reasons: many children enter the care system at different times to their brothers and sisters, and are placed individually. Older children can be resistant to permanent placements or adoption, whereas younger children are more likely to find, and want, a long-term placement.
- Contact between separated siblings placed for permanence has been low, but there are charities working to promote contact for siblings: 'Siblings Together' works to promote positive contact between siblings separated by care

Further resource

℘ http://www.siblingstogether.org.uk/index.php

Assessment of prospective adoptive parents or foster carers

- Prospective adoptive parents and foster carers go through an assessment process—such an assessment has a number of functions:
  - Describe the needs of children who are in public care.
  - Explore the impact of maltreatment before entering public care.
  - Discuss strategies for dealing with vulnerable children.
  - Reflect on their formal and informal support networks.
  - Consider the impact on the child of separation from birth family.
  - Look at contact with birth family.
  - Explain the legal framework of accommodation, care orders, special guardianship, adoption orders.
- Social services provide formal support mechanisms with social workers for the adoptive parents and foster carers. In addition there is often support available from other families at the same training course and local foster care organizations or postadoption support groups.
- Medical issues in adoptive parents are rarely an absolute contra-indication to adopting but there are important issues that do need debate and discussion at the adoption panel. Examples include:
  - Life-limiting condition.
  - Disability.
  - Significant mental illness.
  - Smoking.
- Medical issues in foster carers are similar.
- The health group in British Agencies for Adoption and Fostering provides a source of advice on particular health dilemmas and published *The Adoption and Fostering* journal and *Practice Notes* on specific issues published in the *Adoption and Fostering Journal*.

Further resources

℞ http://www.adoptionuk.org/
℞ http://www.baaf.org.uk/info/adoption
℞ http://www.baaf.org.uk/catalog/2223

Health needs of looked-after children

Looked-after children and young people have higher levels of physical, mental, and health promotion needs than other children of the same age.

The evidence for looked-after young people's significant mental health needs and risk-taking behaviours is presented in 📖 Adolescents in public care p.000).

There are patterns to the health needs of LAC though, of course, individual children may have none of these issues:

- Intrauterine exposure to *alcohol*—consider fetal alcohol syndrome or fetal alcohol effects.
- Intrauterine exposure to *drugs*—can lead to neonatal drug withdrawal symptoms and the need for morphine in the neonatal period. There can also be a longer term impact on behaviour.
- There is a risk of exposure to *vertically transmitted infections* such as syphilis, gonorrhoea, hepatitis B, C, and HIV. Mothers of LAC are more likely not to have accessed antenatal care and therefore may not have been tested in pregnancy
- *Neglect* of children's healthcare is a common prepublic care experience and so common problems such as squint, undescended testes, asthma, and chronic secretory otitis media may not have been addressed satisfactorily.
- *Immunisations* are commonly not up to date at entry to public care.
- *Developmental delay*, particularly in speech and language, is common in children entering public care.
- Some children enter public care because their parents have learning difficulties that impact on their parenting capacity. Sometimes the learning difficulties can have a genetic aetiology (e.g. fragile X syndrome) and genetic testing may be warranted

See 📖 p346 for attachment difficulties.

Looked-after children routine care and health assessments

- Children in care are almost unique as they may be seen by doctors without their birth parents.
- Birth parents have important and detailed health information and many parents want to communicate this face-to-face with the doctor. Therefore, provided it is appropriate, social workers should encourage the birth parents to attend health assessments.
- Children in care are a vulnerable group. The *Healthy Child Programme* identifies these children as a group for targeted health visiting and school nursing.
- From 1 April 2008 the Strengths and Difficulties Questionnaire (see 📖 p.000) must be completed to provide information on the emotional and behavioural well-being of children in care for children over the age of 4 years. This questionnaire should be completed by the child/young person's carer, and discussed and validated at the health assessment appointment. Young people should be encouraged and supported to complete their own version of this questionnaire.
- Information from the Health Care Plan should be incorporated into the Statutory Review minutes and the Care Plan. Independent Reviewing Officers should ask specifically for the Health Care Plan and clarify that all actions have been completed. If these have not been followed they should be identified as recommendations from the statutory review and stated as specified in the minutes.
- It is the social workers responsibility to provide information for an effective health assessment including:
  - Care Plan.
  - Essential Information Part 1.
  - Placement Plan 1.
  - Essential Information Part 2.
  - Placement Plan Part 2.
  - BAAF PH Forms.
  - BAAF Consent to Share Information Forms.
  - 'Red Book' to be brought by carers, if available.
  - SDQ completed by carer
- Looked-after children and young people are required to have health assessments, every 6 months for children under the age of 5 and every year over that age. The current guidance on the service looked after children should receive is *Promoting the Health and Wellbeing of Looked after Children* published by the Department of Health in 2009.
- Every looked-after child should have a lead health professional to coordinate the actions from the healthcare plan.

Further resources

1. *Healthy Child Programme: Pregnancy and the first five years of life.* Department of Health. Oct 2009. ℳ www.dh.gov.uk/publications
2. *Promoting the Health and Wellbeing of Looked After Children*—Revised Statutory Guidance Department of Health, Nov 2009. ℳ www.dh.gov.uk/publications

Looked-after children health assessment case vignettes

Vignette 1

Two siblings placed out of area for 3 years in a short-term foster care placement were invited to health assessment because the social worker was concerned that they were 'ruminating on their food'.

The head teacher of their school wrote a letter saying 'I am concerned that their emotional and psychological needs are not being met. They have many physical and medical problems, but the outstanding problem is their obsessive need for food (and drink). They steal, lie, and manipulate to obtain food and have to be constantly supervised'.

On examination both siblings were stunted with a height velocity of <1cm in the previous 12 months. After extensive investigations in hospital a diagnosis on hyperphagic psychosocial short stature was made and the children moved to a different foster placement. In the next 12 months both children demonstrated catch-up growth, one growing 17cm in that year!

Vignette 2

A looked-after child living with an extended family member was brought to her health assessment by the family and a social worker. The social worker reported that 'There is something wrong with her eyes, something wrong with her ears and she isn't doing very well at school'.

On examination there was hypertelorism and her nose was of an unusual shape. Audiology testing revealed a 50dB hearing loss. On direct questioning there was a family history of premature greying of hair in mother and grandfather. A diagnosis of Waardenburg syndrome was made.

Adoption medical assessments

Children under the age of 5 years need to see a doctor every 6 months to ensure the medical information for the adoption process is current. Children over the age of 5 years with an adoption plan are seen at least every 12 months.

It is important that social care information is sent to the doctor to enable a comprehensive Adoption Health Report to be written. In many areas the information forms developed by the Health Group at BAAF are used to ensure that the required information as follows is obtained:

- The initial or review health assessment form (child or young person) signed by whoever has parental responsibility.
- The Care Plan and Review Minutes.
- Child's Permanence Report.
- BAAF forms M & B, which contain useful information on the obstetric and neonatal histories respectively.
- Form PH for both parents. These are an opportunity for parents to explain any health issues they have and sometimes these are directly relevant to the ongoing health of the child.
- BAAF Consent Forms which address the issues of consent for treatment and for access to medical information on the child and also has a section to allow the parents to give consent for the doctor to access information on the birth parent.
- BAAF Carer report which provides detailed information on the behaviour of the child.
- School/nursery/child development centre/other relevant reports.

A comprehensive Adoption Health Report is required for the purposes of Adoption Panel, adoption court reports, and for the child's new GP when adopted.

It needs to include:
- Name, date of birth, sex.
- Neonatal history including:
  - Details of the birth and any complications.
  - The results of a physical examination and screening tests including blood-borne infections (hepatitis B, C, HIV, and syphilis).
  - Details of any problems in management and feeding.
- A full health history including:
  - Details of any serious illness, disability, accident, hospital admission or attendance at an out-patient department, and in each case any treatment given.
  - Details and dates of immunisations.
  - A physical and developmental assessment according to age, including an assessment of vision and hearing and of neurological, speech and language development, and any evidence of emotional disorder.
  - For a child >5 years of age, a report on learning and behaviour at school.
  - A description of how the child's physical and mental health and medical history have affected his/her physical, intellectual, emotional, social, or behavioural development.

• A full examination including height, weight, and head circumference. Comments on any dysmorphology if noted and a full systems examination including cardiovascular, respiratory, abdominal, and neurological systems.

Adoption health assessment case vignette

A 27-month-infant presented for an adoption health assessment. She was well but presented with some speech and language delay. She was in foster care because her mother had learning difficulties. There was a family history of significant learning difficulties with maternal uncle and maternal great uncle both attending special school.

Mother was invited to the health assessment and explained about possible genetic causes of learning disability. With her permission, genetic testing of her daughter was arranged. The results revealed that she was a carrier of fragile X syndrome. Further testing in the birth family confirmed that this was the cause of the significant learning disabilities seen in the male members of the family.

Contributing to an adoption panel

Purpose

An adoption panel makes recommendations on 3 issues:

- Should a child/sibship have a plan for adoption?
- Should prospective adopters be approved to adopt?
- Should a potential link between a child/sibship and approved adopters progress?

Membership

- An adoption panel requires a medical advisor by law. In most cases this is a community paediatrician, but other doctors such as GPs can provide good advice to panel.
- Other members include an independent chair, a panel advisor from the adoption service, members with experience of the care system such as foster carers, people who were adopted as children or have adopted children

Medical role

- The medical advisor is a full member of the panel, reading all the papers for the panel meeting and contributes equally in the general panel discussion.
- In addition the medical advisor provides specialist advice to the panel on:
  - The health and development needs of the child/sibship.
  - The health of the adopters.
- The medical advice forms part of the child's permanence report.
- The medical advisor is responsible for identifying health issues in the birth family that could be significant for the child.
- Potential adopters should have this information as they decide about whether to adopt a child. Important issues include:
  - Risk of vertical infections from an infected mother (hepatitis B, C, HIV, syphilis, gonorrhoea, chlamydia).
  - Investigation of learning difficulties in the birth family. Some of these causes can be inherited (e.g. fragile X).
  - FHx of inheritable conditions. An example is a birth grandparent with Huntington's chorea whose child (the parent of the child for adoption) has refused to be tested. In this situation the child with a plan for adoption has a 1:4 risk of developing Huntington's chorea. The ethical advice in this scenario is not to test the child until they have reached the age of majority and can make the decision themselves, but potential adoptive parents need the opportunity to discuss this dilemma.
  - FHx of mental illness. There is an inheritable component to a number of mental illnesses. This is highest in schizophrenia and so clarity on the specific diagnosis is important in order to counsel the potential adopters on the level of risk to the child.
- The medical advisor also guides the adoption panel on health issues in the prospective adoptive parents that may be relevant to caring for a child.

- These are rarely absolute but debates arise on the impact of mental illness, chronic disease, life-limiting conditions, and disabilities.
- The key issue is to focus the discussion on what is in the best interests of the child.

Further resources

The British Association for Adoption and Fostering (BAAF) provides extensive information on all aspects of adoption, including adoption panel. It has a specific text called *Effective Panels*. BAAF runs a health group for doctors and nurses working in this field and holds an annual conference. See ✆ www.baaf.org.uk

BAAF also published *Adoption and Fostering*, a journal that has articles on the medical issues in Adoption. There are also relevant *Practice Notes* published by BAAF including 'Reducing the risks of environmental tobacco smoke for looked after children and their carers', 'Guidelines for the testing of looked after children who are at risk of a blood-borne infection' and 'Genetic testing and adoption'.

Adolescents in public care

Adolescents are the most common group of LAC. These young people have the same issues that all adolescents face. But mental health issues and risk taking behaviours are more common in looked-after young people than other adolescents. Figs. 13.1–13.3 are taken from 2 surveys of mental health in the general population of young people and looked after young people and published by the Office of National Statistics.

Mental health issues

Fig. 13.1 shows that looked-after young people commonly experience mental health problems, particularly conduct disorders and that the prevalence rates are considerably higher than in children not looked after.

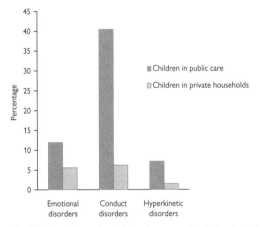

Fig. 13.1 Prevalence of mental disorders among 480 children in public care and 4609 private household children aged 11–15 years, Meltzer H, Corbin T, Gatward R, Goodman R, Ford T. *The mental health of young people looked after by local authorities in England*. London: The Stationery Office, 2003. Contains public sector information licensed under the Open Government Licence v1.0.

Young people in public care are more commonly involved in risk-taking behaviours such as smoking (Fig. 13.2), alcohol (Fig. 13.3), drug use and early sexual activity than their peers:

• In Sweden 15–20% of girls who were involved with social services as teenagers became teenage mothers compared with <3% of the general population.
• Every 3rd girl placed in a secure residential unit and every 4th girl placed in other residential homes because of behavioural problems became mothers as teenagers
• 5–6% of boys involved with social services as teenagers became teenage fathers compared to 0.7% of the general population.
• Almost 1 in 5 of all Swedish teenage parents in the cohort had been involved with social services.

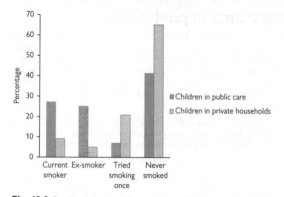

Fig. 13.2 Smoking behaviour of looked after and private household children 11–15 years. Meltzer H, Corbin T, Gatward R, Goodman R, Ford T. *The mental health of young people looked after by local authorities in England*. London: The Stationery Office, 2003. Contains public sector information licensed under the Open Government Licence v1.0.

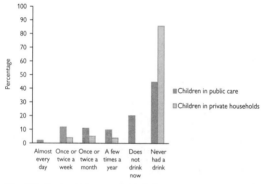

Fig. 13.3 Drinking behaviour of looked after and private household children 11–15 years. Meltzer H, Corbin T, Gatward R, Goodman R, Ford T. *The mental health of young people looked after by local authorities in England*. London: The Stationery Office, 2003. Contains public sector information licensed under the Open Government Licence v1.0.

These issues are present in many looked-after young people at entry to public care and the prevalence only drops slowly over time in public care. There are a wide range of sources of useful information available on line or from NICE, but further research is needed on effective strategies.

Further resources

℘ http://www.teenagehealthfreak.org/
℘ http://www.talktofrank.com/

Unaccompanied asylum seeking children

Introduction
The United Nations Convention on the Rights of the Child is a foundation document informing many issues in Paediatrics and Child Health (see 📖 p502). UNCRC Article 22 says 'children who come into a country as refugees should have the same rights as children born in that country'.

Definitions
'Refugee' is a legal term used to describe a person who fulfils the definition set out in the Geneva Convention of 1951. To be recognized as a refugee, the Convention says that a person has to show that:

'Owing to a well-founded fear of being persecuted for reasons of race, religion, nationality, membership of a particular social group or political opinion, is outside his country of nationality and is unable or, owing to such fear, is unwilling to avail himself of the protection of that country; or who, not having a nationality and being outside the country of his former habitual residence as a result of such events, is unable or, owing to such fear is unwilling to return to it.'

An asylum seeker is a person who has lodged an asylum claim with the Home Office and is waiting for a decision on the claim. A person with this status is not allowed to work, but is entitled for basic healthcare.

A child's circumstances mean they are a refugee then the Immigration and Nationality Directorate should be notified and an application for asylum made. The Home Office can make one of the following decisions:
1. To allow the asylum application and recognize the child as a refugee.
2. To refuse the asylum application, but allow the child to remain in the UK on Human Rights grounds.
3. To refuse the application and refuse any other kind of permission to remain in the UK.

The National Asylum Support Service, (NASS) will support persons above the age of 18. Unaccompanied minors do not receive any support from NASS. But become the responsibility of the Local Authority Children Services. If the asylum claim is refused for an unaccompanied child under the age of 18 years, discretionary leave may be granted until the child reaches 18 years of age.

Unaccompanied asylum seeking children and young people, irrespective of immigration status, are entitled to all public health services, including medical and dental treatment, vision testing, family, and mental health services.

This special group of looked-after children and young people should receive health assessments tailored to their particular needs. These needs include:
• Physical health including dental health.
• Evidence of previous trauma (e.g. fractured bones incorrectly set, perforated tympanic membranes following bomb blasts).

- PTSD (see 📖 p365) or other mental health issues.
- Evidence of infectious disease (e.g. cutaneous leishmaniasis, tuberculosis, hepatitis B).
- Health promotion needs (e.g. a basic understanding of puberty can be missing).
- Immunisation—Health Protection Agency advice is to assume that these children and young people are unimmunized and follow a catch-up schedule.

Further resources

The Department of Health has published an introduction to the NHS in 40 languages and provides hand-held health records for refugees and information on how professionals could use these in a clinical setting.

🔊 http://www.dh.gov.uk/en/Healthcare/Asylumseekersandrefugees/index.htm

🔊 http://www.dh.gov.uk/en/Publicationsandstatistics/Publications/PublicationsPolicyAndGuidance/DH_4122587

🔊 http://www.dh.gov.uk/prod_consum_dh/groups/dh_digitalassets/@dh/@en/documents/digita-lasset/ dh_079284.pdf

Leaving care

- Young people leaving care at 16–18 years of age will need accurate information about their medical history and health needs in order to take responsibility for their own health.
- The 2010 NICE/SCIE guidance on 'Promoting quality of life for looked after children and young people' recommends that young people leaving care are given this information in a letter (see below, An example of a leaving care letter).
- At the medical review the aim is to outline the discussion held at the last medical review, any medical advice given, and as complete a summary as possible of all health information to the young person.
- It is good practice to inform the young person about the information that would be in the letter so that he/she does not discover this information for the first time via the exit letter. This would allow any queries to be answered during the last medical review.
- The letter should be copied to the GP and social worker with the young person's consent.
- The following information should be included in the letter:
  - Birth Hx.
  - PMHx: any illnesses, hospital attendances/admissions, information from LAC reviews.
  - Immunisation Hx.
  - Developmental Hx.
  - Medication Hx.
  - History of allergies if any.
  - Relevant family medical Hx.
  - Ongoing health issues if any.
- There may be some leavers with complex medical needs where it may be more appropriate to provide a formal medical report for transfer to an adult service.

An example of a leaving care letter

Dear ——

When we met in September I said I would try to get together some of the health information on you in order to write you a summary. I am sorry it has taken so long to get the information together but I hope that you find this letter useful.

You were born at —— Hospital by a forceps delivery at 3.51 in the morning. You were born a week earlier than your mother was expecting and you weighed 2.96kg with a head circumference of 35cm. You were a healthy new born baby and did not require any special care and you had a normal neonatal examination.

As far as I can tell you have no family history of illness. You have in the past had a couple of admissions to the Accident & Emergency Department at —— Hospital. The first was on 3 August 2005 when your left foot was caught in the wheel of a bike the day before and X-ray showed you had an avulsion fracture at the base of your fifth metatarsal, that is a small bone in your foot, and that will have healed up without any long term effects. You then injured your left ankle in May 2007 and again was seen in the A&E Department but no significant injury was found.

You told me that you had been bitten by a dog and required sutures to your chest but I can't find any record of that in the notes that have been available to me.

You have seen Dr ——— Consultant Child and Adolescent Psychiatrist in recent years and a diagnosis of attention deficit hyperactivity disorder (ADHD) has been made. You are receiving treatment with methylphenidate and Equasym XL® (this is another methylphenidate preparation).

I have uncovered the details of most of your immunisations. You had diptheria, tetanus, whooping cough, polio and *Haemophilus influenzae* type B immunisations on 16/11/92, 1/01/93, and 12/04/93. You had a preschool booster on 02/05/96. You had two doses of measles, mumps, and rubella vaccine on 23/12/93 and 05/04/97. I informed you when we met about the need to arrange your school leaving booster vaccines and you gave me permission to write to your GP about whether you have had the meningitis C vaccine.

You need to organize a dental appointment to ensure that your teeth are healthy.

You had a normal Guthrie test in the newborn period that ensured that you didn't have neonatal hypothyroidism or a condition called phenylketonuria.

When we met on ——— you were 15 years 9 months old and you presented as a physically healthy boy. Your growth is normal with a height of 172cm between 25th and 50th centile, which means just below average for a boy of your age. Your weight of 68kg was on 75th to 91st centile which is above average for a boy of your age. Examination of your heart, lungs, and abdomen was normal.

You and your carer completed the Strengths and Difficulties questionnaires for me and those both produced relatively low scores; 6 from your carer and 9 from yourself.

To summarize, you are a physically healthy 15-year-old boy. You are up to date with your immunisations other than school leaving booster and meningitis C. You have had no significant past medical history other than a diagnosis of ADHD and a fracture of bone in your foot in 2005. You take methylphenidate as treatment for ADHD.

With kind regards.

Yours sincerely

——— ———

Community Paediatrician

Intercountry adoption

Intercountry adoption is governed (in those countries that are signatories) by the 1993 Hague Convention on Protection of Children and Co-operation in Respect of Intercountry Adoption. The Hague Convention aims to:

- Eliminate abuses associated with intercountry adoption such as profiteering and bribery, coercion of birth parents, and the sale and abduction of children.
- Develop a child-centred approach with the process being more about finding a suitable family for a child than a suitable child for a childless couple.
- Improve regulation and procedures to protect prospective adopters.
- Bring about automatic recognition of adoptions in all contracting states.

Intercountry adoption may mean:

- Placing a British child for adoption outside of the UK.
- A child from abroad being placed in the UK.

Around 300 children a year are adopted into the UK. Information on the background of children in this situation can be very limited indeed; they may have been abandoned or taken to institutions by parents who provide little or no medical information on themselves or the child.

In this situation prospective adopters need to know that there is considerable uncertainty about health issues:

- Genetic factors: a FHx of learning difficulties, mental illness, or genetic disease will not be clear
- Exposure to abuse and neglect: information on the early life experiences of children can be very limited and it is difficult to assess impact. The strongest predictor of continuing psychological deficits and impairments is overall duration of institutional privation.
- Developmental progress: at the point of assessment the developmental status will be clear but without a trajectory it can be problematic predicting the likelihood of developmental catch-up. Encouragingly, in the English and Romanian Adoptees Study there was considerable developmental catch-up so that all the children were functioning in the normal range by 4 years of age when half had profound developmental delay at entry to the UK.
- Risk of exposure to infectious diseases: such as tuberculosis, hepatitis B, C, or HIV.
- Immunisation: schedules vary by country and details of vaccinations received are lost. In this situation the Health Protection Agency advice is to treat the child as unimmunized and follow a catch-up immunisation schedule.

Overall the findings from the English and Romanian Adoptees Study give a complicated picture of real success and worrying sequelae and prospective intercountry adopters need to understand this complexity. For a child from another country to be legally adopted in the UK, the prospective adoptive parents have to be assessed in a similar way to other prospective adoptive parents and so training is an opportunity to discuss these issues.

Postadoption support

- Between 1926 and 1990 there were 876,601 recorded adoptions in England and Wales, so being adopted is a relatively common experience.
- Postadoption support has slowly developed to meet the needs of this population and others affected by adoption. Every LA has an Adoption Support Service Advisor (ASSA) who is the first point of contact for all post adoption queries.
- Adoption agencies have a duty to consider requests for postadoption support, to assess what is needed and if they are in a position to meet that need, e.g.
  - Adopted people over the age of 18 years who are seeking information about their origins through access to their birth records or adoption records.
  - Adopted people who are seeking or have made contact with their birth parents and other relatives and are seeking advice and support.
  - Birth parents and birth relatives seeking information or counselling service.
  - Financial support (means tested)
  - Support with parenting children.

Social paediatrics

Ability is of little account without opportunity.

Chinese proverb

The United Nations Convention on the Rights of the Child

The United Nations Convention on the Rights of the Child (UNCRC) is fundamental to a full understanding of the role of paediatricians. It is a legally binding set of non-negotiable promises (or standards and obligations) that governments make to their children.

Paediatricians have a role in advocating on behalf of children when these and other promises are not kept. UNCRC was adopted by the United Nations General Assembly in 1989. It is the most widely ratified UN convention, entering into law in all UN member states except Somalia and the USA. It was ratified by the United Kingdom of Great Britain and Northern Ireland on 16 December 1991.

What does the UNCRC say?
- UNCRC contains 42 articles grouped into 4 themes:
  - Guiding principles.
  - Survival & developmental rights.
  - Protection rights.
  - Participation rights.
- All 42 articles of the convention are important but key articles are described in Table 14.1.

Table 14.1 Key articles from the UNCRC

Articles	
	Rights to protection
Article 6	Right to life
Article 9	Right not to be separated from parents (unless this harms the child)
Article 19	Right to be protected from all forms of abuse
Article 20	Right to special attention (e.g. adoption and fostering if deprived of family)
Article 32	Right to be protected from economic exploitation
Article 33	Right to be protected from illicit drugs
Article 34	Right to be protected from all forms of sexual exploitation
	Rights of provision
Article 24	Right to the highest standard of healthcare
Article 27	Right to a standard of living adequate for the child's physical, mental, spiritual, moral and social development
	Rights of participation
Articles 7, 8	Right to an identity (name, family, nationality)
Articles 12, 13	Right to express views freely and be listened to

Table 14.1 (Continued.)	
Article 17	Right to access to information
Article 23	Right for disabled children to enjoy life and participate actively in society

Data from Goldhagen J. Children's Rights and the United Nations Convention on the Rights of the Child. Pediatrics 2003; 112(Suppl 3):742–5.

The Convention in practice

The UNCRC is a declaration of universally agreed and *non-negotiable* standards and obligations. It is therefore the basis of advocacy for children where rights have been infringed and has been described as 'among the most powerful tools available to respond to and increase the relevance of paediatrics to contemporary disparities and determinants of child health outcomes'.

The UNCRC can be used to provide:
- A framework for a redefinition of what constitutes child health.
- A template for child advocacy.
- A matrix for establishing new approaches in health services.
- A curriculum for professional education.
- Challenges for future child health outcomes and health service research.
- A framework to redefine the determinants of child health.
- Process and outcome measures for gauging our progress towards these goals.

It has also set in motion the movement for participation of children and young people in decisions made about them which has seen the establishing of Children's Commissioners in the 4 countries of the UK and policy documents such as *Not Just a Phase – a guide to the participation of children and young people in health services* published by the Royal College of Paediatrics and Child Health.

United Nations Convention on the Rights of People with Disabilities (UNCRPD)

In 2008 the UNCRPD came into force with a code of implementation. The UK is a signatory.

It is likely that it will take many years for the full impact of this convention to emerge but it builds on the social model of disability which moves away from seeing people with disabilities as objects for charity, medical intervention and social protection.

Instead UNCRPD conceptualizes people with disabilities as having rights that they should claim and promotes people with disabilities making their own decisions on their lives.

Further resources
℘ http://www.unicef.org/crc/
℘ http://www.un.org/disabilities/

Environmental determinants of health

The UK Health Protection Agency uses the following definition; 'environment…includes both the direct and indirect effects of chemical, physical (including ionising and non-ionising radiation, and noise) and biological hazards on health and wellbeing and encompasses some aspects of the physical and social environment that influence health and wellbeing such as housing, urban development, land use and transport'.

Why are children particular susceptible to environmental hazards?

- Children are still growing and developing, so their biological systems are more susceptible to harm than adults and immunity to disease is less well developed.
- They take in more food, water and air/kg body weight than adults and have a different diet than adults (particularly when very young).
- They can absorb some chemicals more easily than adults.
- They are more vulnerable to unintentional injuries because of their exploratory behaviour, play and relative inability to judge risk.

Childhood obesity

- Is a major public health concern (Fig. 14.1) and refer to NICE published guidance in 2006.
- Multicomponent interventions are the treatment of choice. Weight management programmes should include behaviour change strategies to increase people's physical activity, improve eating behaviour and the quality of the diet, reducing energy intake.
- Recommendations were made for the NHS, the LAs (including leisure and planning of the built environment), early years settings, and schools.

Unintentional injury in all environments (Fig. 14.2):
- Leads to more than 2 million visits to accident and emergency departments by children every year, half of these injuries occur in the home.
- Unintentional injury is also a leading cause of death among children and young people with about 200 children dying each year in England and Wales. In 2009, 65 under-15s were killed (and 2267 were seriously injured) in road collisions in Great Britain.
- Other important causes of death are choking, suffocation or strangling, drowning, and fire. In 2010 NICE published 3 pieces of guidance to reduce unintended injuries in children and young people.

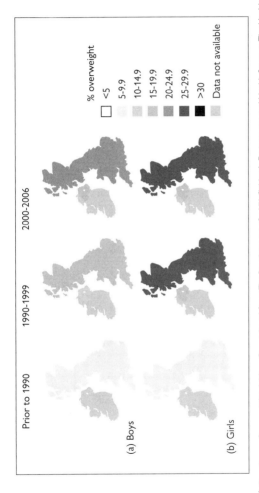

Fig. 14.1 Prevalence of overweight children. Reproduced from *The Development of a UK Children's Environment and Health Strategy*, The Health Protection Agency, Didcot, 2009. Contains public sector information licensed under the Open Government Licence v1.0.

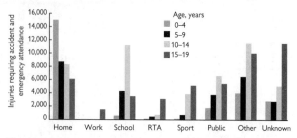

Fig. 14.2 Place and type of unintended injuries by age. Reproduced from *The Development of a UK Children's Environment and Health Strategy*, The Health Protection Agency, Didcot, 2009. Contains public sector information licensed under the Open Government Licence v1.0.

Children's Environment and Health Action Plan for Europe (CEHAPE)

This was developed by the Europe Region of WHO in 2004 and has 4 Regional Priority Goals, based on the main causes of environment related burden of disease. These are described in Table 14.2.

Table 14.2 Summary of children's environment and health strategy priorities according to regional priority goal[a]

	RPG I Water, sanitation and health	RPG II Accidents, injuries, obesity and physical activity	RPG III Respiratory health, indoor and outdoor air pollution	RPG IV Chemical, physical and biological hazards
Preventing harm	Ensure compliance with the lead in drinking water quality standard. Improve documentation and quality of private water supplies. Continue to improve sanitation facilities in schools and childcare settings. Reduce exposure to cryptosporidium in swimming pools.	Ensure a coordinated approach to injury prevention throughout the UK.	Promote awareness of risks associated with carbon monoxide. Educate adults about the effects of environmental tobacco smoke on children. Develop guidance on local air quality management to consider children specifically, where appropriate.	Encourage radon testing and remediation by householders and landlords. Consider applying the radon action level for homes to the school and other childcare environments. Investigate options for reducing or preventing the use of sunbeds amongst children and young people. Identify schools affected by high noise levels and implement protective measures. Continue to consider and involve children and young people in emergency planning and preparedness exercises.
Promoting health	Improve hygiene behaviours in children (e.g. hand-washing).	Continue to encourage physical activity amongst children and young people. Improve access to and strategic planning of green spaces. Greater consideration and inclusion of children and young people in planning urban and residential areas.	Develop a coordinated policy approach to indoor air quality that considers children specifically.	Continue to encourage healthy sun protection behaviour amongst children. Continue to teach children about food hygiene.

(Continued)

Table 14.2 (Cont'd)

Improving understanding	Investigate further the impacts of bathing water quality on child health. Improve understanding of factors involved in disease outbreaks associated with swimming pools. Evaluate the impact of water poverty on child health and well-being.	Investigate further incidence and effects of chronic carbon monoxide poisoning. Review evidence of proximity to major roads and traffic and impact on child health and lung development.	Investigate the non-auditory health and well-being impacts of noise on children. Identify means to further reduce unintentional poisonings. Improve understanding of children's exposure to chemicals. Improve understanding of children's exposure to electromagnetic fields. Improve understanding of neurological developmental and other health effects from chemical exposure in utero or in early life.
Improving intelligence	Improve surveillance of infectious intestinal disease (including waterborne disease) particularly amongst children.	Improve injury surveillance throughout the UK. Monitor success of obesity and physical activity initiatives.	Improve surveillance of biological hazards such as food-borne diseases. Review systems for reporting and surveillance of congenital abnormalities.

ª Reproduced from The Development of a UK Children's Environment and Health Strategy. The Health Protection Agency, Didcot, 2009. Contains public sector information licensed under the Open Government Licence v1.0.

Child poverty and inequalities in health

In 2010, *Fair Society, Healthy Lives*, a review of the social determinants of health chaired by Professor Marmot, was published. This is the latest in a series of reports on inequalities in child health. Some examples of the evidence supporting the social gradient in health and educational outcomes is given in Figs 14.3–14.5. Fig. 14.3 shows the impact on child mortality that would occur if all parts of society experienced the same low death rate as the most wealthy.

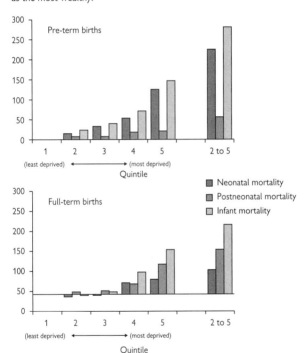

Fig. 14.3 Estimated number of child deaths that could be avoided if all quintiles had the same level of mortality as the least deprived (2005–2006). Reproduced from Oakley L *et al*. Multivariate analysis of infant death in England and Wales in 2005–6, with focus on socioeconomic status and deprivation. *Health Statistics Quarterly* 2009; **42**:22–39, Office for National Statistics. Contains public sector information licensed under the Open Government Licence v1.0.

Fig. 14.4 shows the detrimental impact of low socioeconomic status on learning over the early years to age 10. Children from low socioeconomic groups with high scores at 22 months drift down the learning distribution while those from high socioeconomic groups with low cognitive scores initially, improve over time.

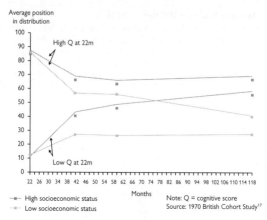

Fig. 14.4 Inequality in early cognitive development of children in the 1970 British Cohort Study, at ages 22 months to 10 years. Reproduced from Feinstein L. Inequality in the early cognitive development of British children in the 1970 cohort. *Economica* 2003; **70**:3–97, with permission of John Wiley & Sons Ltd.

Fig. 14.5 shows the remarkable gradient in road collusion child deaths by socioeconomic class; with at least a 10-fold difference in death rate between group 1 and group 8.

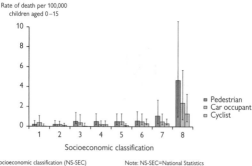

Fig. 14.5 Child deaths by socioeconomic class (NS-SEC), 2001–2003. Reproduced from Edwards P *et al*. Deaths from injury in children and employment status in family: analysis of trends in class specific death rates. *British Medical Journal* 2006; **333** (7559):119–21. With permission from BMJ Publishing Group Ltd.

But this relationship is complex and determined by an interaction of international, national, local, individual level, intergenerational, and life course factors. Models to conceptualize these interactions and their impact have been developed (Fig. 14.6 is an example). Medical interventions play a role but within a social, economic, and political structure beyond the control of the individual patient or doctor. Advocacy is an important tool and health professionals are well placed to press for action on these determinants of child health (see 📖 Advocacy, community resources, and social capital p516), and these are aimed at the primary prevention of child health issues.

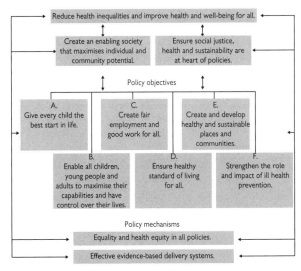

Fig. 14.6 Conceptual framework for reducing health inequalities. Reproduced with permission from the UCL Institute of Health Equity. *'Fair Society, Healthy Lives': The Marmot Review*, UCL, 2010.

Gradients in major child health outcomes reflect inequality across the social spectrum. Gradients are explained by cumulative risk exposures over time and across generations. If inequalities are to be eradicated, a long-term strategy is needed involving investment in families and children to ensure that no child is brought up in poor social circumstances. UNCRC Article 27 says: 'Children have the right to a standard of living adequate for the child's physical, mental, spiritual, moral and social development'.

Two of the policy recommendations in *Fair Society, Healthy Lives* are specifically aimed at children.

1. Giving every child the best start in life.

This includes:

- Reduce inequalities in the early development of physical and emotional health, and cognitive, linguistic, and social skills.
- Ensure high-quality maternity services, parenting programmes, childcare and early years education to meet need across the social gradient.
- Build the resilience and well-being of young children across the social gradient.

2. Enable all children, young people and adults to maximize their capabilities and have control over their lives.

This includes:

- Reduce the social gradient in skills and qualifications.
- Ensure that schools, families, and communities work in partnership to reduce the gradient in health, well-being and resilience of children and young people.

The Marmot review website gives details of innovative examples of implementation to overcome inequalities in health: ℅ http://www.marmotreview.org/implementation.

Further resource

Marmot review: ℅ http://www.marmotreview.org/

Housing and health

Housing is an important determinant of health but the relationship between housing and health is complex and poor housing often coexists with other forms of deprivation such as unemployment, poor education, and social isolation. Nonetheless, specific housing related factors can affect health including:

- Indoor pollutants (e.g. asbestos, carbon monoxide, radon, lead, moulds).
- Cold and damp, infestations, hazardous fixtures or fittings, noise.
- Social and behavioural factors (e.g. overcrowding, sleep deprivation, lack of parks, health centres, neighbourhood safety, and social cohesion).
- Macro-policy environment (e.g. housing allocation, lack of housing, housing tenure and urban planning).

In 2005, NICE published an evidence briefing review of reviews on housing interventions to promote health. This found that:

- There is review level evidence that home visiting in low socioeconomic status areas and advice on home hazards plus health education and media campaigns are effective in encouraging parents to make their homes safer.
- There is review level evidence that provision of free or discounted home safety equipment and/or educational campaigns can lead to behavioural and environmental changes.
- There is review level evidence that physical and chemical interventions can reduce the impact of allergy-related respiratory disease.

Further resources

Housing and public health: a review of reviews of interventions for improving health—Evidence briefing 16 Dec 2005. ℘ www.publichealth.nice.org.uk.

Benefits, allowances, and housing

- Article 26 of the UNCRC says 'Governments must provide extra money for the children of families in need". The UK government does provide access to some benefits for children.
- Families with young children and from economically poor backgrounds are at a higher risk of deprivation and social isolation.
- Raising a child is expensive and it becomes even more challenging if a child has special needs.
- Financial consequences of supporting children may arise due to:
  - Loss of earning.
  - Increased cost of meeting additional needs, e.g. continence aids, mobility appliances, therapy services, child care.
  - Need for a larger house or more reliable transport.
- The benefit and support system across the world is variable. In the UK disadvantaged families have access to many benefits from the state in addition to support from a number of voluntary and charitable organizations.
- The current government is planning to reform the benefit system to make it fairer and financially sustainable in future. Table 14.3 is a brief list of some of the benefits available in the UK currently, although it is likely to change significantly in the near future as a number of different benefits are likely to merge into a single universal credit.

Direct payments for disabled children allow families to arrange care and services themselves instead of receiving them from the council. Direct payments can be made to parents or carers aged 16 or over. Direct payments can be used for a variety of services which offer stimulation, new experiences and independence.

- These may include:
  - Short breaks.
  - Nursery placement providing specialist support.
  - Assistance to attend an activity, e.g. a youth club.
  - Personal care.
- Help can be available to apply for these benefits from local job centre, health visitor, children's centre, and citizen advisory bureau.

Further resources

- http://www.citizensadvice.org.uk
- http://www.dwp.gov.uk
- http://www.dsdni.gov.uk/index
- http:// http://www.direct.gov.uk/en/MoneyTaxAndBenefits/index.htm
- http://www.direct.gov.uk/en/MoneyTaxAndBenefits/BenefitsTaxCreditsAndOtherSupport/index.htm
- http://www.mencap.org.uk
- http://www.nacab.org.uk

Table 14.3 Benefits and allowances (UK)

Disability Living Allowance (DLA)	A tax-free benefit for disabled children and adults who need looking after, or have mobility problems. Includes care and mobility components. 3 tiers of care component and 2 levels of mobility component depending upon level of needs. Affects the level of other benefits if claimed.
Carer's allowance	A taxable benefit to help people who look after someone who is disabled. Claimant does not need to be related to or living with the person caring for.
Tax credit	Payments from the government for people responsible for at least 1 child or young person. Those working on a low income may qualify for Working Tax Credit.
Child benefit	Tax-free payment for families with children. Variable rates for each child. Not means tested. Usually stops when a child reaches age 16 (with some exceptions).
Support for Education and Learning	Statutory obligation on local councils not to discriminate against disabled students. Increasing emphasis on inclusion within mainstream education. Includes providing access, physical environment, appropriate curriculum, technology, and school transport if appropriate. SEN of preschool children are supported by various schemes including Early Support, parent partnership services, and home visiting services. Planning for adult life should start early. Transition planning should include aspirations and aims for future independent life and should address various aspects including education, employment, housing, transport, and health and leisure activities. Disability and extra needs don't stop at exit from school. Universities and colleges should be able to support in number of ways including financial help. These include Disabled Students' Allowances, Access to Learning Fund, DLA, and Employment and Support Allowance.
Housing support	Living with an impairment or disability may necessitate adaptations to the home environment to facilitate independent living and to ensure safety and comfort. It can be in the form of supported housing or to provide financial grant for modification of existing home.
Family fund	Grant available to families of children with disabilities or serious illness living in UK for essential items like washing machine, fridge, clothing and other similar items (℘ http://www.familyfund.org.uk).
Short-term break or respite	Short-term respite care provides a pre-planned placement for a disabled child. Can be institutional (hospice, hospital), family based, breakaway, extra activities, and domiciliary support. Can be short term, one-off or regular, and can last a few hours or a week or more.

Advocacy, community resources, and social capital

- Advocacy means speaking out for a particular issue, idea, or person. Paediatricians advocate for children because they are a vulnerable population and not always able to speak out for themselves.
- The UNCRC is a good starting point for advocacy whether it is for an individual child or family or on a public health issue.
- Box 14.1 explains why advocacy is needed still and Box 14.2 gives some examples of advocacy practised by paediatricians in the past.

Box 14.1 Reasons to practice advocacy[a]

- Interagency work with education, social services, and housing is common and we have a role in promoting children's welfare as we work with other agencies.
- The important role of social determinants in child health means paediatricians should advocate to reduce their impact.
- An approach to paediatrics based on the UNCRC sees advocacy as a key tool for change.
- The environment is a determinant of some common medical conditions in childhood, road traffic accidents and obesity are good examples and so campaigning for environmental change is important.
- Vulnerable children in society such as children in care and unaccompanied asylum seeking children, need advocates to ensure their needs are met.

[a] Reproduced from Waterston T. Teaching and learning about advocacy. *Arch Dis Child Educ Pract Ed* 2009; **94**:24–8. With permission from BMJ Publishing Group Ltd.

Box 14.2 A history of paediatricians as advocates for child health[a]

- James Spence encouraged parents to stay with their children in hospital.
- Donald Court ensured parents were represented on his committee looking into reform of child health services in the early 1970s.
- Murray Katcher campaigned for legislation in the USA to reduce the temperature of water in boilers and so prevent scalds.
- Hugh Jackson brought attention to children accidentally ingesting adult prescribed drugs and fought for child-proof packaging.

[a] Reproduced from Waterston T. Teaching and learning about advocacy. *Arch Dis Child Educ Pract Ed* 2009; **94**:24–8. With permission from BMJ Publishing Group Ltd.

- The skills to practise effective advocacy are different to other paediatric skills and are well described by Waterston (2009).

- There are a wide range of community resources relevant to child health:
  - *Immediate social environment* (family structure, siblings, parenting, socioeconomic class, friends, relatives, type of housing).
  - *Local social fabric* (type of school, social services, neighbourhood, transport facilities, health service delivery, pollution/environment, play facilities).
  - *National and international environment* (gross national product, overall health spending, communication, culture, lifestyle, war/natural disasters).
- It is valuable if paediatricians can access these networks and facilitate provision to children in need.
- Social capital does not have a clear, undisputed meaning. But it describes the pattern and intensity of networks among people and the shared values and support which arise from those networks.
- Greater interaction between people generates a greater sense of community spirit.
- The Office for National Statistics has a Social Capital project 3 which defines social capital as 'networks together with shared norms, values and understandings that facilitate co-operation within or among groups'.
- It is an important concept because higher levels of social capital are associated with better health, higher educational achievement, better employment outcomes, and lower crime rates.

Educational paediatrics

Education is a better safeguard of Liberty than a standing Army.
Edward Everett

Academic failure at school

Introduction
- Academic failure in school has no simple definition and it is often challenging to determine a cause for this.
- It remains an important problem, since it has consequences not only for the individual, but also for the society.

Causes of academic failure
- *Family factors*: parental perception of importance of academic achievement, low socioeconomic status, teenage parent, single-parent family, parental divorce or death, poor parenting.
- *Child factors:* unidentified developmental problems, sensory impairments, unidentified special educational needs (SEN), inadequately managed chronic physical health problem, unidentified/ inadequately managed mental health problems in the child, low self-esteem.
- *School factors:* lack of school resources and appropriately trained staff.
- *Peer factors:* alcohol or substance misuse, bullying.
- *School absenteeism.*

Paediatrician's approach to the child with academic difficulties
- *History*: parental concerns, pregnancy, birth history, past medical history. Family and social history. General health, appetite, and sleep pattern. Early developmental history and developmental progress, behaviour, and social skills
- *Examination*: neurology, dysmorphisms, neurocutaneous stigmata, systems examination, hearing and vision assessments.
- *Assessments*: consider requesting assessments from the following professionals:
  - Educational psychologist.
  - Clinical psychologist.
  - SENCO/ class teacher.
  - SLT.
  - OT.
  - PT.
- *Multiprofessional approach* to identifying 1 or more factors responsible for academic failure and agreeing strategies to support the child.
- *Review* of child's progress after remedial/ support measures have been implemented.

Consequences of academic failure
- Low performing students are less likely to graduate or attend university.
- Academic failure is associated with lower adult wages.
- Adult educational and occupational attainment, in turn, significantly predict adult mental health, longevity and relationship formation, etc.

Prevention of academic failure

- *Primary prevention:* learning difficulties in some children can be prevented by reducing the incidence of alcohol consumption in pregnancy. Further advances in neonatal intensive care could contribute to reducing adverse neurological outcomes in very premature infants. Reducing alcohol or substance misuse in adolescents by appropriate awareness and lifestyle training programmes in school. Prevention programmes for bullying in school are important for an optimal learning environment.
- *Secondary prevention:* diagnosis and management of chronic health problems. Early identification and management of developmental disorders (ADHD, autism, specific learning difficulties). Behaviour support strategies in school for childhood behaviour problems.
- *Tertiary prevention:* specific educational and rehabilitation programmes for sensory impairments and special educational needs

School absence and truancy

- Regular school attendance offers several advantages for the child and allows the best possible start in life.
- Much of the work children miss when they are off school is never made up, leaving these pupils at a considerable disadvantage for the remainder of their school career. Children who miss school frequently have poorer academic outcomes than regular attendees.
  - Of pupils who miss >50% of school, only 3% manage to achieve 5 A* to Cs including English and Maths.
  - Of pupils who miss between 10–20% of school, only 35% manage to achieve 5 A* to C GCSEs including English and Maths.
  - Of pupils who miss <5% of school, 73% achieve 5 A* to Cs including English and Maths.
- Children who attend school regularly are at less risk of getting involved in antisocial behaviour and crime.

School attendance and absence: the law

- All children of statutory school age (5–16 years) must receive a suitable full-time education. For most parents, this means registering their child at a school, although some parents may choose to make other arrangements to provide a suitable full-time education for their child.
- Once a child is registered at a school, parents are legally responsible for making sure the child attends regularly. Parents risk getting a penalty notice or being prosecuted if their child fails to attend school regularly.

Contributory factors for school absence

- *Illness*: this is the commonest recorded cause of school absences. If a child is too ill to return to school or requires hospital admission, the local education authority has a duty to make alternative educational provision.
- *Bullying*: this can exist in several forms (physical, teasing, name-calling and threatening behaviour, cyber bullying). Schools generally have anti-bullying schemes for support.
- *Academic difficulties*: children can struggle academically at school for a variety of reasons and it is not uncommon for adolescents with such difficulties which have been unidentified/ unsupported, to choose not to go to school.
- *Childhood emotional problems*: separation anxiety, school phobia.
- *Family and social factors*: housing or care arrangements, transport to and from school, parental work and financial difficulties.
- *Truancy*.

Truancy

- Truancy is intentional unauthorized absence from school by the pupil. Truants are children who decide not to attend school, generally without the knowledge of their parents.

- Truants have a significantly higher incidence of illegal drug use, underage drinking and smoking, and antisocial behaviours compared to non-truanting pupils.
- The causes of truanting are multifactorial and involve interactions between the child, family, and school which result in the child choosing to do other things than attend school.
- Schools and LAs can issue penalty notices to parents (Education Act 1996), where pupils fail to attend school regularly
- LAs play an important role in supporting schools to tackle high levels of absence. Schools are expected to collect absence data every term, enabling progress to be monitored closely, so that intervention and support can be deployed speedily for those schools which require it.
- Statistics for unauthorized school absences are also influenced by parents taking children out of school during term time for family holidays.

Approach to reducing school absence

Parent responsibilities

- Encouraging a culture of good attendance and punctuality and not promoting an ethos of taking time off from school for minor ailments or holidays.
- Taking an active interest in the education of the child and discussing any problems the child may be having at school with the child and with teaching staff if required.

School responsibilities

Promoting a culture of openness and encouraging communication between parents and school staff for managing issues such as bullying, school phobia, and academic difficulties faced by the child.

Local authority responsibilities

- Supporting home tuition for children with long-term illness.
- Supporting families where children may be assuming the role of carers.
- Establishing parenting contracts to work with the school and parents to improve the child's attendance.

Role of the community paediatrician in reducing school absence

- Identify a medical or developmental cause (where appropriate) for the child's school absence and advise the school and parents about management strategies.
- Consider the whole range of contributory factors for a child's school absence and support the child, family, and school to find a way forward, with the best interest of the child being paramount.

Further resource

Department for Education (Behaviour and attendance): ℘ http://www.education.gov.uk/schools/pupilsupport/behaviour

Special educational needs and educational approach for the disabled child

- The committee of enquiry into 'the education of handicapped children and young people' produced the Warnock Report in 1978.
- This report considered the philosophy that all children are entitled to an education irrespective of their disability and recommended adoption of the term 'special educational need' to take into account a child's abilities as well as disabilities.
- The Education Act 1996 plus the Special Educational Needs and Disability Act 2001 legislate for children with SEN in England and Wales.
- Children have SEN if they have a learning difficulty, which requires special educational provision to be made for them.
- A child has a learning difficulty if they:
  - Have a significantly greater difficulty in learning than the majority of children of the same age, or
  - Have a disability which prevents or hinders the child from making use of educational facilities.
- Although the proportion of pupils with statements of SEN has remained relatively stable over time, there has been a considerable increase in recent years in the number of pupil with SEN without statements, from 10% of all pupils in 1995 to 18.2% or 1.5 million pupils in 2010.

Statutory assessment

- A statutory assessment is a detailed multiagency review to consider a child's special needs and necessary educational provision.
- Please refer to 🕮 Educational psychology p531 for more details.

Statement of SEN

- A Statement of SEN is a legal document detailing a child's special educational needs and setting out the provision the LA considers necessary for the child.
- It forms the basis for the child's future educational plans.
- A medical diagnosis or a disability does not necessarily imply special educational needs. It is the child's educational needs rather than a medical diagnosis that must be considered.
- For the majority of children with SEN, school-based provision without any necessity for statutory assessment is appropriate and in such cases, health professionals should encourage parents to discuss the child's educational needs with the school in the first instance.

Inclusion

- Inclusion in disability rights means removing barriers to participation in society and making sure everyone has the same chance to contribute to it at their own particular level of ability.

- Inclusive Early Years settings provide opportunities for children with and without special needs to learn, play and socialize together. The environment, curriculum, and resources should reflect the ethos that children with special needs are welcomed, cared for, respected, and valued equally with other children.
- Inclusion in Education refers to an approach to educating students with SEN. Inclusive education differs from 'integration' which implied learners becoming 'ready for' accommodation within the mainstream schools. Inclusion is more about the child's right to participate and the school's duty to accept the child.
- Inclusion has 2 subtypes:
  - *Inclusive practice*—which is a form of integration where children with special needs are educated in regular classes at least for more than half the day. Although the student is treated like a full member of the class, most specialized services are provided outside the regular classroom, particularly if these services require special equipment or may be disruptive to the rest of the class
  - *Full inclusion*—where students with special needs are always educated alongside students without special needs
- The Warnock Report recommended integration of children with SEN into mainstream schools whenever possible. 3 forms of integration were envisaged:
  - Location based: special classes in a mainstream school but with little opportunity for contact with other pupils.
  - Social: children from a special class would mix with other pupils at assemblies, playtimes, and mealtimes.
  - Full: children with SEN would be taught in the same classes as other pupils and mix freely with them at all times.
- The majority of children with SEN complete their education in mainstream schools. For children with a Statement of SEN, arrangements are made for the child's education to continue in a mainstream school of the parents' choice.
- For some children with multiple and complex SEN, the facilities, specialist teaching, expertise and adapted environment of a special school may be of greater benefit.

Educational approach for the disabled child

- The medical model of disability focuses on what a disabled person cannot do while the social model sees society as the problem, creating barriers or rejection of the disabled child or adult
- The Equality Act (2010) states that someone is disabled if 'they have a mental or physical impairment which has a substantial and long-term adverse effect on their ability to carry out normal day-to-day activities'.
- Disability is not the same as SEN. Almost half the children with an SEN do not meet the definition of disability.
- Children with SEN experience difficulties in learning in school but may not have an impairment that impacts substantially on their daily life. Similarly, a significant proportion of disabled children do not have special educational needs, including those with health and mental health needs.

- It is not always easy to know whether a child is disabled. Difficulties can vary over time and may depend in part on the specific environment or activities undertaken.
- The Equality Act requires schools to:
  - Promote equality of opportunity.
  - Promote positive attitudes towards disabled people.
  - Assess and monitor the impact of their activities on disabled people.
  - Make reasonable adjustments to ensure disabled children are not disadvantaged.
  - Improve outcomes for disabled people.
- A Disability Toolkit has been developed to help schools in identifying and collecting information on all their disabled pupils.

Future developments

- The UK Department for Education has consulted on a new approach to special educational needs and disability.
- The aim of the proposed new approach is to make the system less stressful for families and less costly to run by giving parents more information and control, making a wider range of short breaks available in all areas and ensuring more choice by allowing parents to name in their child's plan, a preference for any state-funded school.
- A new single assessment process and an 'Education, Health and Care Plan', to replace the statutory assessment and statement by 2014.
- The emphasis is on reinforcing the strong strategic role of Las in working together with health services and with other local areas to secure the right provision for children whilst ensuring that services are cost-effective.

Further resources

Advisory Centre for Education (ACE): ☎ 0808 800 5793 ℘ http://www.ace-ed.org.uk
Independent Parental Special Education Advice (IPSEA): ☎ 0800 018 4016 ℘ http://www.ipsea.org.uk

Writing the SEN report

- The purpose of a statutory assessment of SEN under the Education Act 1996 is to gain a clear picture of the child as a whole person in terms of educational and social strengths as well as educational weaknesses and difficulties
- Health services are expected to normally respond within 6 weeks of the date of receiving the Local Education Authority request for advice
- The SEN toolkit, mainly for schools and LAs, contains practical advice on how to implement the SEN Code of Practice. It was devised in collaboration with professionals and people involved in meeting the needs of children and young people with SEN.
- The toolkit comprises of 12 sections. Section 8 contains guidelines for writing the medical advice.

Points to consider when writing the Medical Advice (also known as Appendix C)

- Write the advice in a manner which can be easily understood by parents and other professionals (avoid medical terminology or explain this where used).
- If there are no medical factors which will affect the child's school performance, state this in the report.
- If there are medical or developmental factors which will require specific medical or therapy support for the child in school, this should be stated.
- If the child's educational needs are known, the doctor's views on this may be included.

Proposed format for writing the report

1. Relevant medical history
- Birth hx, hospitalization, PMHx, prognosis, likely effect on learning, treatments, including medications.

2. Description of the child's physical state and functioning, providing current information on:
- Hearing.
- Vision.
- General health including growth.
- Mobility (locomotor skills).
- Motor control (balance, coordination, and manipulation skills).
- Speech and language.
- Continence.
- Self-care skills.
- Behaviour/emotional state.

3. Consequences for the child's education
- Any aspect of the child's medical condition which may affect their progress in school and advice on managing the condition in school.
- Special aids and equipment.

- The child's welfare and safety especially participation in sport and out-of-school activities and supervision in the playground.
- Physical environment for education and facilities for non-ambulant pupils.
- Other resource implications, continence management, drug administration, supervision requirements, feeding, behaviour management.
- Any special transport arrangements.

4. Implications of the child's medical condition on facilities and services
- Therapies (SLT, OT, PT).
- Nursing.
- CAMHS, clinical psychology
- Medical input and review.
- Advice on special transport requirements.
- Dietary/feeding advice.
- Arrangements to administer medications.

Depending on local agreements, the medical report could contain all the necessary health information (from therapies, nursing, CAMHS) or other reports could be appended to the medical advice.

The report should be signed and dated.

School health promotion

- Schools play an important role in supporting the health and well-being of C&YP.
- In the decades between 1960 and 1990, a range of health services for children were offered in schools. These ranged from screening programmes (school entry, 10-year and school leaving medicals), immunisations, dental and audiology services to the management of medical problems.
- In the last 2 decades, there has been a shift in management of a range of common childhood conditions to primary care, community paediatrics or hospital based outpatient services.
- The concept of the 'school doctor' is now largely limited to a community paediatrician who supports the medical needs of children in special schools in partnership with health and education professionals.

Aims of a school health service

- Early identification and management of health problems that may interfere with the child's learning in school.
- Assessment of children with learning difficulties to exclude health problems as a contributing factor.
- Health promotion—prevention and early intervention services.
- Safeguarding children.
- Support for parents and carers.

Health promotion in schools

Focusing on early intervention and prevention is both socially and economically more effective in the long term.

A needs assessment for a school (or a group of schools) will provide a clear picture of the school community, to enable identified needs to be met.

The key health priorities recommended in the Healthy Child Programme from 5–19 years are:

1. Identification and targeted support for children and young people with particular vulnerabilities:
- C&YP with complex or enhanced needs (illness, disability, complex or long-term health needs including mental health problems).
- C&YP whose family background puts them at higher risk (parents with learning difficulties, serious mental health, drug or alcohol problems).
- C&YP not accessing existing services (refugee and asylum seekers, travellers, living in temporary accommodation).
- C&YP with particular behaviour/lifestyle risks (not in education, employment or training; engaging in risk-taking behaviour).

2. Screening programmes:
- For primary school-aged children:
  - School entry- vision check, hearing test, and height and weight measurement.
- For secondary school-aged young people:

- Universal vision test no longer recommended.
- Chlamydia screening offered to those who may have been sexually active (those under age 16 years need to be Fraser competent to consent).

3. Immunisation programmes:
- BCG, hepatitis B and seasonal Influenza vaccinations for individuals at high risk. HPV vaccination offered to girls aged between 12–13 years (school year 8). Td/IPV booster given between ages 13–18 years.

4. Promoting emotional health, psychological well-being and mental health:
- Early identification of children with emotional distress.
- Improving access to mental health support through universal services.

5. Promoting healthy weight:
- Promoting play and physical activity.
- Good food habits at school and encouraging more children to access the midday school meal.
- Signposting children and families to local weight management services.

6. Teenage pregnancy and sexual health:
- Targeted support for young people most at risk of early sex and teenage pregnancy.
- Information and advice about preventing STIs.

The Department of Education has developed a Healthy Schools Toolkit, designed to help schools to 'plan, do and review' health and well-being improvements for their C&YP and to identify and select activities and interventions effectively.

Educational psychology

- All educational psychologists have a postgraduate degree (Masters/ PHD) in educational psychology.
- Many are qualified and experienced teachers, and all are Chartered Psychologists or eligible for chartering, with the British Psychological Society.
- Educational psychology (EP) services are organized on the basis of geographical areas. These are defined by *school partnerships*, by which is meant a secondary school and its feeder primary schools.
- The age range of the children referred can be from 0–19 years.

Children with the following conditions can be helped by the EP service

- *Physical*, e.g. CP or a child disabled following a road traffic accident.
- *Sensory*, e.g. hearing or visual impairment or a child on the autistic spectrum.
- *Learning*, e.g. children with general learning difficulties or dyslexic type difficulties or children who are gifted and talented and need special support.
- *Behavioural*, e.g. a child with difficulties in anger management or who is withdrawn or who offends in the local community.
- *Emotional*, e.g. a child who has been subject to abuse or has experienced a specific trauma or support for a child who needs to develop emotional literacy.

Work model

- Educational psychologists *always work in conjunction with the staff in the school for the child*. The aim is to help the teachers support the child better on a day-to-day basis in school.
- Key members of staff in school for children are:
  - The class teacher/form tutor in secondary school.
  - The teaching assistant.
  - Special educational needs co-ordinator (SENCo).
  - Designated teacher for safeguarding.
  - Designated teacher for looked after children.
  - School counsellors.
- Educational psychologists *usually work in professional networks* with other professionals/agencies, these can include:
  - Attendance and engagement officers.
  - Behaviour support service.
  - Social workers.
  - School nurses.
  - EYSENIT.
  - Other school advisory services such as the Service for Autism.
  - Community paediatricians.
  - PCAMHS/CAMHS services.
  - Voluntary agencies.
  - Children's centres.

- Referrals can only be made to the EP service *with the agreement of the parent/carer*.
- Parents/carers are encouraged to discuss a child about whom they are concerned with staff who teach their child. However, if a parent/carer is not feeling heard in school, she/he can approach the service directly.

Functions of EP service

- *Assessment* of a child with identified problems.
- Work with teachers to *improve learning programmes*, behaviour plans, and classroom environments to support a child or group of children.
- *Training* for teachers.
- *Advice* to parents/carers with regard to concerns about their children.
- Input to schools with regard to *systemic issues*, such as assessment/ review processes or support for children at transition points.
- *Work in multiprofessional networks*, e.g. when there are safeguarding concerns about a child and family or in special school settings for children with disabilities.
- *Attending meetings* such as annual SEN reviews, meetings where a child's school placement is in jeopardy or reviews by social care colleagues.
- *Offering consultation* to school staff and other professional colleagues.
- Providing *direct work* to child/children, e.g. children with social skills deficits or life story work with an individual child.
- *Evaluating programmes/services* around a child or a group of children.
- Contributing to the work of the LA with regard to *identifying and developing services to meet need*.
- *Direct work with parents* on an individual basis or in groups.

Guiding principles

- All the work of an educational psychologist is within the framework of 'Every Child Matters' (ECM). This is a government initiative which specifies outcomes which require multiagency partnerships.
- The 5 outcomes are:
  - Achieve economic well-being.
  - Be healthy.
  - Enjoy and achieve.
  - Make a positive contribution.
  - Stay safe.
- The work of an educational psychologist with regard to children on the Special Needs Register, is governed by *the SEN Code of Practice* under Part IV, Education Act 1996. The code sets out policies and procedures aimed at helping children with SEN to achieve their potential.

Further resources

British Psychological Society: ஃ http://www.bps.org.uk
Every Child Matters: ஃ http://www.everychildmatters.co.uk
SEN Code of Practice: ஃ http://www.education.gov.uk/childrenandyoungpeople/sen

Educational psychology perspective: supporting children with SEN

SEN tribunal

- When there are differences between the LA and the parents, and agreement cannot be reached, parents have the right to appeal against decisions made by the LA to a SEN tribunal.
- This is an independent body. Tribunal cases are complex, time-consuming, and costly.

Proposed changes to the Code of Practice

- Involve parents in the assessment process and by 2014 give them control of funding for the support their child needs.
- Replace Statements with a single assessment process and a combined education, health, and care plan.
- Ensure assessment and plans run from birth to 25 years old.
- Introduce a new school-based category to help teachers focus on raising achievement.
- Overhaul teacher training and professional development.
- Look at how voluntary groups might coordinate a package of support.
- Give parents a greater choice of schools and community powers to set up special free schools.

Further resources

Advisory Centre for Education (ACE): ☎ 0808 800 5793 🖰 http://www.ace-ed.org.uk
Independent Parental Special Education Advice (IPSEA): ☎ 0800 018 4016 🖰 http://www.ipsea.org.uk

Specialist schooling

Elective home education

- In England, education is compulsory, school is not. Parents can elect to educate their children at home under Section 7, Education Act 1996.
- This may be for a variety of reasons:
  - Distance or access to a local school.
  - Religious or cultural beliefs.
  - Philosophical or ideological views.
  - Dissatisfaction with the system.
  - Bullying.
  - As a short-term intervention for a particular reason.
  - A child's unwillingness or inability to go to school.
  - SEN.
  - Parents' desire for a closer relationship with their children.
- Where a child has a Statement of SEN and is home educated, it remains the LA's duty to ensure that the child's needs are met.

Hospital school

The outreach teaching sector (OTS) or hospital school remit:

- Schools' requests to support the education of pupils who have an illness/diagnosis which indicates prolonged or recurring periods of absence from school.
- Children where there is evidence of need from an appropriate medical professional.
- A reintegration plan is created for a return to school in the context of the child's medical need.
- Pupils receive a minimum entitlement of 5 hours of teaching a week.

Excluded children

- Provision is made for pupils who are permanently excluded or at risk of exclusion by the LA's Pupil Referral Unit and Integration Service.
- Such provisions cater for:
  - Pupil permanently excluded.
  - Pupil on a LA 'planned transfer'.
  - High-level needs pupil moving into county.
  - 'Looked-after' pupil permanently excluded.
  - 'Looked-after' pupil on fixed term exclusion from mainstream school.
  - 'Looked-after' pupil transferring due to change of residential placement.
  - Short-term programmes to support a child with difficulties in school.

Looked-after children/virtual school

- The government is concerned with regard to the under-achievement of children in the looked-after system in terms of their educational achievements. All schools have a designated teacher for looked-after children.
- All children in the looked-after system should have a personal education plan (PEP).

- Psychologists contribute to systems for supporting foster carers and residential staff who care for the children in the looked-after system.

Further resource

⬩ http://www.teachernet.gov.uk

National curriculum

Government national guidelines with regard to what is taught in schools.

Standard Attainment Tests (SATS)

(These are subject to review)

- These are national tests taken by pupils at the end of Key Stages 1, 2, and 3 in core subjects of English, Maths, and Science.
- The target levels are level 2 at the end of KS1, level 4 at the end of KS2 and Level 5/6 at the end of KS3 (Table 15.1).
- Children can achieve at any level in any Key stage.

Table 15.1 Usual bands of attainment

Key stage	Year group	Age	Expected NC level
KS1	1–2	5–7	1–3
KS2	3–6	7–11	2–5
KS3	7–9	11–14	4–8
KS4	10–11	14–16	GCSE/other[a]

([a] GCSE, 14–19 programmes, diplomas, NVQs, Asdan awards)

Each level is subdivided into 3 'steps' which are:

- C: some elements of that level attained.
- B: most elements of that level attained.
- A: level attained—ready to move on to next level.

P scales

- These are used to measure the progress made by children and young people with learning disabilities aged 5–16 who are working below NC level 1.
- The P scales have 8 levels starting at P1 and progressing to P8.

Access arrangements

- These are available for all examinations in line with the Disability Discrimination Act 1995.
- These are pre-examination adjustments which can be applied for, to give all candidates the opportunity to demonstrate in examinations, their skills, knowledge, and understanding of the work they have done.
- Applications for particular access arrangements are made on the basis of evidence of need.
- Need can include a disability, SEN such as dyslexia, a temporary difficulty such as a broken arm, or psychological problems such as bereavement.
- Applications should be applied for as early as possible, with supporting evidence of eligibility provided by a professional whose qualifications are acceptable to the Joint Council for Qualifications.

Various arrangements can be requested to meet individual SEN, such as:
- Alternative accommodation for the exam.
- Braille question papers.
- Extra time up to a maximum of 25%.
- A reader.
- A scribe.
- Supervised rest breaks.
- A word processor etc.

Further resources

British Psychological Society: ℘ http://www.bps.org.uk
Early Bird: email earlybird@nas.org.uk
Education Resources: ℘ http://www.teachernet.gov.uk
Every Child Matters: ℘ http://www.everychildmatters.co.uk
SEN Code of Practice: ℘ http://www.education.gov.uk/childrenandyoungpeople/sen
Access Arrangements. ℘ http://www.jcq.org.uk.

Further education for young adults with disabling long-term conditions

- If there was a 'statement of special educational needs' at school, there should be a 'transition plan' giving details of the level of support that will be needed on leaving school at 16.
- The sixth form or college should pay for the necessary learning support.
- Personal and medical support are arranged through local health and social services.
- Careers advisers should be working with the different agencies to ensure arrangements to support the student into further education are in place.
- Colleges are required to make 'reasonable adjustments' so that disabled people do not suffer a substantial disadvantage.

Educational establishments for young adults with disabling conditions

- There a number of specialist colleges around the UK catering for young people with disabling conditions.
- It is impossible to list them all in the space available. Useful starting points are the livability foundation (formerly the Shaftesbury Society) which lists many specialist colleges and offers to provide advice on suitable colleges.
- Collegenet lists 35 specialist colleges for people with disabilities and or learning difficulties.
- Examples include:
  - Star College (age 16–25) near Cheltenham.
  - Trelaw school (age 9–16) and college (16+) in Hampshire.
  - The Queen Elizabeth Foundation Banstead in Surrey (specializing in brain injury, 16+).

Separation anxiety

- Parents of severely disabled young people have often had to fight for their education, medical care, and social engagement.
- The prospect of the young adult leaving home and moving on to college or independent living is often a highly charged and emotional situation. Parents are torn between pride in, and hope for, their children who are 'moving on', and the pain of letting go.
- It should be approached with great sensitivity, recognizing the needs of the young adult to establish independence, the high degree of emotional investment on the part of parents, and the high potential for very enmeshed relationships.

Further resources

Collegenet: ℘ www.collegenet.co.uk
Directgov: ℘ http://www.direct.gov.uk/en/DisabledPeople/EducationAndTraining/index.htm
livability foundation ℘ http://www.livability.org.uk

Working with partner agencies

Fall seven times, stand up eight.

Asian proverb

Health visitors

- HVs are public health nurses working with young children and families.
- In addition to being a qualified nurse/midwife a HV needs to undertake a specialist community public health nurse training programme.
- As a critical part of integrated children's services they may be based at children's centre or be a part of a primary care team.
- With increasing resource constrains, there has been a shift of emphasis from a 'cradle-to-grave' philosophy to a more family and young children focus.
- Being local and known to families, HVs are in a privileged position to have their trust and confidence.
- Increasingly HVs are providing support with complex issues like managing safeguarding risks (see 📖 p473) and delivering intensive programmes for the most vulnerable children and families.
- With public health issues such as obesity (see 📖 p558) becoming more prevalent, there is an increasing need for preventive strategies and HVs can play a very important role in implementing various public health policies (see 📖 p557).
- HVs role is particularly valuable in socially deprived areas where their input is most likely to make an impact on the overall health of communities (see 📖 p552).

Role of health visitors

In addition to their wide remit to work with families with young children, some HVs have taken upon a specialist role.

General role

- Fundamental role in delivery of:
  - Community Health Programmes.
  - Preventing social exclusion and deprivation.
  - Reducing health inequalities and tackling key health priorities such as obesity, smoking, alcohol abuse, etc.
- Child health promotion, e.g. immunisation, home safety measures and injury prevention, supporting breast feeding, and healthy diet.
- Link with midwifery/social services/mental health teams.
- Source of information about local facilities like parent and toddler groups (see 📖 p29).
- Support to families, parents/carers with young children. It may include:
  - Home visit to families.
  - Running support groups for parents.
  - Working in collaboration with a range of children's agencies and professionals (see 📖 p23).
- Supporting pregnant women.

Specialist role such as:

- Care of next infant (CONI) after a sudden unexpected death in infancy (SUDI, see 📖 p476).
- Stress management.
- Active member of CDT (see 📖 p20).

- Part of multiagency homeless team/supporting travelling families.
- Liaison HV role based at hospital paediatric unit.

Other activities

- Individual case management including identification and referral for postnatal depression,
- Specific health/development concerns (see 📖 p36) e.g. growth monitoring, speech delay, audiology referral etc.
- Identification and support to *families in need*. Quite often HVs take on key worker's role for coordinating various support services for these families (see 📖 p552).

School nursing

- The practice of school nursing and the school nurse's role has changed significantly since 1902 when a school nurse was hired in the United States to reduce absenteeism (see 📖 p522) by intervening with students and families regarding healthcare needs related to communicable diseases.
- School nurses are now considered to be specialist public health practitioners who lead multiskilled teams of nurses, nursery nurses, and support workers using a child-centred (see 📖 p18), public health approach (see 📖 p551).
- They work as part of an integrated universal children's health service with health visiting and bridge health, education, and social care boundaries to help C&YP fulfil their potential within schools (see 📖 p23).

Principles of school nursing

- Focus on health needs of the school-age population.
- Facilitation of health enhancing activities.
- Advocacy for C&YP (see 📖 p516).
- Empowering C&YP in taking control of their health.
- Working in partnership with C&YP, families, and local agencies.

Range of activities of school nurses

The school nurse contributes to the delivery of the 5–19 years Healthy Child Programme (see 📖 p555) in partnership with other school health team members.

- Health assessment at school entry in reception/year 1:
  - Review immunisation status.
  - Measure height and weight for the National Child Measurement Programme (NCMP).
  - Ensure that hearing (see 📖 p299) and vision screening (see 📖 p271) is carried out in line with National Screening Committee guidelines.
  - Provide children, parents, and school staff with information on specific health issues.
- Advise and coordinate healthcare in school for children with medical and complex healthcare needs (see 📖 p524).
- Contribute to the identification of children's special educational needs.
- Provide emotional health and psychological well-being support for C&YP.
- Contribute to and co-deliver the personal, social, and health and citizenship education (PSHCE) programme within schools, to address local public health priorities.
- Contribute to safeguarding children (see 📖 p473) and young persons in partnership with school staff and multiagency colleagues.
- Health review at school transition in year 6/7:
  - Interpreting the BMI score as part of the NCMP and explaining the implications for diet and lifestyle.
  - Responding to health and well-being concerns raised by the young person or parents.

- Immunisations (see ▢ p620):
  - HPV vaccination (for girls aged 12–13).
  - Td/IPV vaccination (for young people between ages 13–18).
- Contraceptives and sexual health advice for young people 11–16 years (see ▢ p101).
- Refer young person to local specialist service for drug and alcohol misuse (see ▢ p367).

Recommended service model for school nursing

- The school nursing service should have a child-centred public health focus and work in partnership with all agencies involved with C&YP and their families.
- Access to the service should be possible in schools, community settings, or in the home.
- Referrals can be accepted from children, young people, parents, carers and other agencies and may be made by telephone, letter, or opportunistic contact.
- The referrals should be assessed and the appropriate package of care offered or the child/young person should be signposted on to the appropriate service.

Future of school nursing

- Healthy children are successful learners. School nursing is now an important public health resource and has a major contribution towards ensuring that C&YP maintain optimum health.
- The school nurse has a multifaceted role within and outside the school setting, one that supports the physical, mental, emotional, and social health of school-age children and facilitates their success in the learning environment.

Portage

- Portage is a *home-visiting educational service* for preschool children with additional support needs and their families. It was developed in an area of Wisconsin, USA called Portage in the early 1970s.
- It is based on the common-sense principle that parents are the key figures in the care and development of their child (see 📖 p18).
- Portage home teachers are drawn from a variety of backgrounds and are trained in the Portage model. They visit the home and plan learning activities and management strategies which parents and child work on during the week.
- Portage-trained teachers have available toys and materials for use in the home. They work in close collaboration with other professionals such as speech therapists, PTs, and OTs, who may be involved with the family (see 📖 p23).
- The emphasis is on finding out the positives and building on what a child can do.
- Activities are designed to boost the child's development in those areas where help is needed-from very early motor skills to the more complex task of using language (see 📖 p36).

Community nursing

The best place to care for a sick child is in his own home among familiar surroundings where the people who normally give him security and affection can attend to his needs.

United Nations, 1955

- Community children nurses (CCN) are specialist nurses who provide quality care and support for children and their families at home.
- They could be a part of:
  - CCN team based in acute service.
  - Team within a general practice.
  - Community-based nurse-led clinic.
  - Palliative or respite care team (see 📖 p105).
  - Support team for children with complex health care as key worker (see 📖 p20).
  - Hospital/ambulatory care outreach.
- CCN can be a generalist or specialist e.g. cystic fibrosis, epilepsy (see 📖 p240), diabetes, etc.

Roles of CCN

- Managing chronic long-term conditions in community, e.g. epilepsy.
- Supporting children in Special Schools (see 📖 p534).
- Supporting children and families with complex healthcare needs including home total parenteral nutrition, stoma, gastrostomy, home ventilation (see 📖 p18), etc.
- Providing support to children with life-threatening/terminal illnesses such as neurodegenerative diseases and cancers (see 📖 p103).
- Providing education and training to carers, e.g. administration of buccal midazolam, care of tracheostomy, etc.
- Liaison role between primary and secondary care.

Potential benefits of CCN support include:

- To provide continuity of care from hospital to home especially in long-term conditions.
- Flexible, individualized, and responsive service.
- Emphasis on family-centred and holistic approach.
- Key worker role to coordinate services for families with multiple and complex needs.
- Avoiding unnecessary hospitalization and better quality of life.
- Easy access to services and information (see 📖 p514).
- Single point of access especially during periods of crises.
- Respite care (see 📖 p104 and p105).

Children and families social work teams

In the UK the children and families assessment teams in SS:
- Facilitate access to range of services to *families in need* including
  - Financial support (see 📖 p514).
  - Parenting skills support.
  - Local support groups.
- Have a statutory duty to protect C&YP from abuse and neglect and work within framework of Children Act 1989 (see 📖 p471 and p473).
- Are responsible for *day care* provisions:
  - Approval and registration of play groups and child minders.
  - Running of day nurseries and quality monitoring of privately run nurseries.
  - Running family centres.
- Provide care to *children in public care* (LAC) and support families and children with additional needs (see 📖 p20).
- *Adoption services* including assessing children and finding families, assessing prospective adopters, and post adoption support (see 📖 p485).
- Provision and maintenance of *Secure units*.
- Provide a range of services especially to *children in need* and those with disability and their families including:
  - Practical assistance in the home including home adaptation (see 📖 p191).
  - Provisions for recreational facilities including holidays and transport arrangements for disabled children. These improve the quality of life for children with disabilities and their family but also provide them with opportunities to meet new people, make new friends (see 📖 p514), etc.
  - Support for young carers.
  - Respite care.
  - Assessment of school leavers to identify their future needs.
- *Joint working* with other agencies including health, education, police and probation services to assess the service needs.
- Other provisions supported by social services department include:
  - Residential care for people not able to live at home independently or with their families.
  - Home care and 'meals on wheels'.
  - Field social work.

Working with voluntary and statutory organizations

(Also see 📖 MDT working p23)

- In order to provide holistic and comprehensive support to children with special needs and their families it is important that various agencies involved work together to deliver effective interventions.
- Health, social care, and education services have a direct role in the delivery of many of these interventions and in other areas, a role in collaborative work with other agencies, in lobbying for policy change and in raising the profile of child health promotion (see 📖 p516 and p557).
- These agencies may represent statutory bodies, public sector, or voluntary organizations.
- Voluntary organizations are not-for-profit organizations set up and run by voluntary unpaid management committees. They differ from private sector which is run for profit and the statutory sector which is set up by statute.

Provision of coordinated and responsive multiagency support to children and families in need

This requires:

- Establishing agreed clear aims, roles, responsibilities, and timetables between partners (see 📖 p23).
- Recognition and acceptance of importance of all the agencies involved working together to achieve a shared goal.
- Commitment to joint working with open and clear communication.
- Acknowledgement of different constraints under which various agencies work.
- Appropriate sharing of information along with respect for each other's confidentiality protocols.
- Mutual respect for each other's roles, and contributions.
- A multiagency steering group and commitment at all levels of the organizations involved.
- Support and training of staff in new way of working.
- Interprofessional programmes of continuing education.

Further resource

National Council for Voluntary Organisations: 🖉 http://www.ncvo-vol.org.uk

Public Health

Acknowledgement: Michele McCoy, Consultant in Public Health, NHS
Dumfries and Galloway, for her support and advice in producing this
chapter

*The superior doctor prevents sickness. The mediocre doctor attends to impend-
ing sickness. The inferior doctor treats actual sickness.*

Chinese proverb

Introduction

This chapter explores various meanings of the term 'public health' and explains how key concepts and tools used in public health (the discipline, including epidemiology, health needs assessment, screening, and surveillance), apply directly to child health.

The Faculty of Public Health in the UK identifies three domains of public health:

1. Health improvement "promotion" (see 📖 p557).
2. Health protection (communicable disease and environmental health) (see 📖 p564).
3. Health service improvement/development (see 📖 p570).

This chapter attempts to describe how the concepts apply to child health across the UK, regardless of the important differences in health policy between nations—it does not, for example, use the term 'Healthy Child Programme' as that term is not used across the whole of the UK. Furthermore, while 'buzz terms' change and date rapidly and are frequently contested (e.g. 'nudging'), the main principles behind public health work remain relatively stable over time and are relevant regardless of healthcare system.

This chapter does not cover clinical treatment of the medical conditions mentioned and nor does it discuss child protection work. These are both discussed in detail in other chapters of this book.

Public Health: an overview

The term 'Public Health' can be used to describe a specialty or discipline, a workforce, and an approach to identifying and addressing health needs.

Public Health (as a discipline) has been described as 'the science and art of preventing disease, prolonging life and promoting health through the organised efforts of society'.[1]

It is consistent with this view of the world that while clinical services often focus on the identification and management of disease, Public Health professionals consider health in its most holistic sense as 'a state of complete physical, mental and social well-being and not merely the absence of disease or infirmity'.[2] Many child health and primary care professionals will also consider health in this way.

The factors affecting health that Public Health attempts to influence are frequently society wide, as demonstrated in Fig. 17.1; this is in contrast to many other clinical specialties that typically work specifically with the individual or the immediate family.

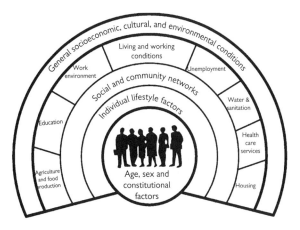

Fig. 17.1 Influences on health. Reproduced with permission from Dahlgren G, Whitehead M. *Policies and Strategies to Promote Social Equity in Health*. Stockholm, Sweden: Institute for Futures Studies, 1991.

1. Acheson ED (1988). *Public health in England. Report of Inquiry into the future development of the public health function*. London: HMSO.
2. Preamble to the Constitution of the World Health Organization as adopted by the International Health Conference, New York, 19 June–22 July 1946.

Public Health is particularly interested in the interplay between all of these influences and how they affect health and wellbeing. There are various models that describe the relationship between the social determinants of health (also known as the broader determinants of health), individual characteristics and healthcare. One simple but widely quoted model is shown in Fig. 17.2. Much more elaborate models are provided in the system maps describing influences on obesity and healthy weight in the Foresight report.

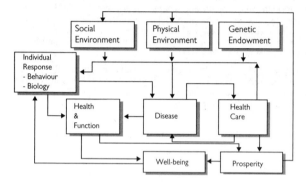

Fig. 17.2 Interconnections between individual factors, broader determinants of health, the health service and outcomes (Evans and Stoddart model). Reproduced with permission of Transaction Publishers from Marmor T et al. Why Are Some People Healthy and Others Not?, 1994.

"Public health work places a central importance on reducing health inequalities. Marmot notes that 'people from different socioeconomic groups experience avoidable differences in health, wellbeing and length of life and that this is unfair and unacceptable'. These differences are mediated by the broad determinants of health (see Fig.17.1) and the structure of society. International comparisons show that such inequalities are not inevitable. Health inequalities in the UK can be observed in the distribution of many diseases and risk factors and, most starkly, in life expectancy. Health inequalities have become more pronounced in the UK over the past thirty years.

The Marmot Review *Fair Society, Healthy Lives* is of particular relevance here as it notes the importance of maternal and child health (the early years), early intervention (see 📖 p59 and p60) and parenting (see 📖 p371). It also notes that 'focusing solely on the most disadvantaged will not reduce health inequalities sufficiently. To reduce the steepness of the social gradient in health, actions must be universal, but with a scale and intensity that is proportionate to the level of disadvantage' referring to this as 'proportionate universalism'. This has clear relevance to child health and debates about universalism versus targeting."

Public Health: the specialty

Public Health is a broad specialty involving a diverse workforce that works with and across a range of different organizations. The specialty can be described as consisting of 3 overlapping domains—health improvement, health protection, and (health) service improvement (see Table 17.1).

Table 17.1 Domains of public health[a]

Health improvement	Health protection	Health service improvement/ development
Inequalities	Infectious diseases	Clinical effectiveness
Education	Chemicals and poisons	Efficiency
Housing	Radiation	Service planning
Employment	Emergency response	Audit and evaluation
Family/community	Environmental health hazards	Clinical governance
Lifestyles		
Surveillance and monitoring of specific diseases and risk factors		
Equity (see 📖 p509 and p522)		

[a] Faculty of Public Health website. Faculty of Public Health of the Royal College of Physicians of the United Kingdom. *What is public health?* Available at: 🔗 http://www.fph.org.uk/ what_is_public_health

A Public Health professional may have responsibilities covering one or more of these domains. Responsibilities may differ during the working week and while on-call, the latter typically including health protection duties.

In the UK, both medical and non-medical specialists can complete the full specialist training for Public Health through the Faculty of Public Health. Public health competencies that are used to guide training, appraisal and revalidation are listed on the Faculty of Public Health website (🔗 http:// www.fph.org.uk).

Screening

Screening is a: 'public health service in which members of a defined population who do not necessarily perceive they are at risk of or already affected by a disease or complications are asked a question or offered a test, to identify those individuals who are more likely to be helped than harmed by further tests or treatments to reduce the risk of a disease or its complications'.[1]

Screening is a whole system or programme of events necessary to achieve risk reduction, not simply a test.

The UK National Screening Committee (NSC) has adapted WHO screening criteria in order to appraise the viability, effectiveness, and appropriateness of a screening programme.

The criteria—which cover the condition, the test, the treatment, and the screening programme overall—are listed in full on the NSC website (℘ http://www.screening.nhs.uk/criteria) and should normally be met in full before introducing a screening programme for a condition.

Screening programmes are commonly coordinated at a regional level by a Public Health consultant or specialist, working closely with clinicians, laboratory/imaging staff, lay representatives and others as required. Careful monitoring and audit of the programme is essential, and screening incidents must be carefully investigated through root cause analysis.

Pregnancy and newborn screening

There have been substantial changes to maternity and child screening in the UK over recent years:

- First trimester DS.
- Fetal anomaly scanning.
- Antenatal and newborn haemoglobinopathy screening.
- MCADD (medium chain acyl dehydrogenase deficiency) screening in newborns have also been introduced in UK.

(MCADD is an error of fat metabolism that can lead to coma and sudden death during periods of fasting/illness.)

The pregnancy and newborn screening programme screens for dozens of different conditions (grouped under DS, communicable disease, haemoglobinopathy, fetal anomaly, newborn hearing, and newborn bloodspot), using several different tests and involving specialist input from a wide range of disciplines, as described more fully on the NSC website.

Therefore, pregnancy and newborn screening is the most complex of all screening programmes currently available in the UK, and has an important impact on child health.

Childhood screening

The number screening of tests offered during childhood has been substantially simplified over time, with only preschool vision (see 📖 p271) and hearing screening (see 📖 p299) remaining in the universal programme in many parts of the UK. The purpose of height and weight measurements is discussed in the following section on screening vs surveillance.

Surveillance versus screening

Health surveillance has been defined as 'the ongoing systematic collection, analysis and interpretation of health data essential for planning, implementing and evaluating public health activities. Surveillance needs to be linked to timely dissemination of the data, so that effective action can be taken to prevent disease. Surveillance mechanisms include compulsory notification regarding specific diseases, specific disease registries (population-based or hospital-based), continuous or repeated population surveys and aggregate data that show trends of consumption patterns and economic activity.'[2] Surveillance and screening are therefore undertaken for different purposes.

Much of the information collected for child health counts as surveillance, including information on:

• Breastfeeding.
• Oral health (see 📖 p165).
• Immunisation (see 📖 p620) (for health improvement purposes).
• Information about notifiable conditions such as measles (see 📖 p566) or meningococcal disease (to inform health protection work).

There is more ambiguity around height and weight measurements. For example, height and weights checks on school entry may be performed in some areas for surveillance purposes, while in others areas they may be classified as screening, with referral of very underweight and obese children and young people for specialist review and referral to the clinical psychology service and/or weight management programme if appropriate. The details will vary by local context and available resources.

Further information on school height and weight measurements is available in England from the National Child Measurement Programme, and in Scotland on the Information Services Division website (see 📖 p600).

Epidemiology

This is of central importance to Public Health. However the full description of 'Epidemiology' is beyond the scope of this chapter/book, but is covered thoroughly in a free to view text on the web: Bonita R, Beaglehole R, Kjellström T. Basic Epidemiology. 2nd edition. World Health Organisation, Geneva. www.academiya.org/sites/default/files/Basic%20Epidemiology.pdf

1. Raffle AE, Gray JAM. Screening: Evidence and Practice. Oxford: Oxford University Press, 2007.
2. Bonita R, et al. Basic Epidemiology. 2nd edition. Geneva: WHO.

A Public Health view of child health

The previous overview has introduced some key terms and concepts in public health work. Arguably child health has embraced its public health role more than any other clinical specialty: school nurses and health visitors are now commonly referred to as public health nurses in the UK, and for over a decade professional and political direction around child health has taken a public health approach even when it is not stated as such. For example, in *Health for All Children* (4th edn, 2006), a key text on child health in the UK, Hall and Elliman note 'the gradual shift from a highly medical model of screening for disorders to a greater emphasis on health promotion, primary prevention and active intervention for children at risk, whether for medical or social reasons. The change results from the increasing interest in social and educational dimensions of child development'.

Hall and Elliman also highlight that increasing prosperity as a society has 'been accompanied by increasing levels of violence, family breakdown, disaffection, and alienation. The gap between rich and poor has widened in many countries including the UK'. A decade on, the economic climate can be expected to exacerbate such problems, reinforcing the importance of taking a public health and holistic view of child health.

Health for All Children also reinforces the importance of considering family health noting that 'a major gap in health care can arise where the adult is the index patient', highlighting the potential role of primary care in assessing and supporting children in such circumstances. The responsibility for children and young people therefore extends beyond child health professionals.

The UN Convention on the Rights of the Child (1989) (see 📖 p502) describes clearly the responsibilities of the statutory sector and wider society to ensure that the needs of children and young people are met, and that children and young people are protected. Achieving the balance between health improvement and child protection (see 📖 p442) is a highly skilled task, relying on the knowledge and experience of the professionals working with the family. Services should guard against orientating services towards child protection to the exclusion of other equally important influences on the health and wellbeing of children, young people and their families, and that requires a clear understanding of public health work.

The following sections consider child health work under the headings of the 3 domains of public health.

Child health promotion and health improvement

Defining health promotion and health improvement

Health promotion has been defined by WHO as 'the process for enabling people to increase control over the determinants of health and thereby improve their health'.[1]

In a more recent definition that provides a useful framework for understanding the importance of health promotion in child health, Tannahill defines health promotion as shown in Box 17.1.

Box 17.1 Tannahill's definition of health promotion[a]

Health education has been defined simply as 'Planned opportunities for people to learn about health and make changes in their behaviour, including:
- Raising awareness of health issues and factors contributing to ill health
- Providing information.
- Motivating and persuading people to make changes in their lifestyle for their health.
- Equipping people with the skills and confidence to make those changes'

[a] Tannahill A. Health promotion: the Tannahill model revisited. *Public Health* 2009; **123**:396–9.

Tannahill's definition of health promotion has a number of merits—it reinforces the positive dimension of health, shifts the responsibility from being solely down to the individual (or what is done to or with the individual), and provides a system-wide view that is consistent with the Dahlgren and Whitehead model (see 📖 Fig. 17.1 p551).

The child health programme in the UK provides valuable opportunities for health promotion. The schedule of visits varies slightly between different parts of the UK and is evolving. The full programme includes screening, surveillance, immunisation and health and development reviews. The Healthy Child Programme in England is described in full in a recent Department of Health publication (🔗 http://www.dh.gov.uk/en/Publicationsandstatistics/Publications/PublicationsPolicyAndGuidance/DH_107563).

Each contact with a midwife, health visitor, or GP provides an opportunity for health promotion, whether it is a planned visit or an extra visit. Examples of health promotion may include:
- Information on infant feeding choices.
- Support to start and continue breastfeeding.
- Nutritional advice for the mother, Child and wider family.
- Discussion about injury prevention (see 📖 p560).
- Advice on smoking, alcohol or substance misuse (see 📖 p367).

It is important, therefore, that all staff understand the theory of behaviour change so that they can take the opportunities to influence behaviour when they arise. The *Stages of Change* model provides a simple but memorable model of the stages towards behaviour change (an individual may go through different stages a number of times and may relapse, so behaviour change needs to be revisited or reinforced):

• Precontemplation (not ready to change).
• Contemplation (thinking of changing).
• Preparation (ready to change).
• Action (making change).
• Maintenance (staying on track).

Health improvement does not have an internationally recognized definition, but is a commonly used term, and is one of the three domains used by the Faculty of Public Health. Simplifying some of Tannahill's arguments, for the purposes of this chapter, health improvement takes the concepts described earlier for health promotion and shifts the focus to population health. Health improvement work stretches beyond the work of a public health nurse team, a public health department or even the healthcare system.

Health improvement in action 1: childhood overweight and obesity

Efforts to tackle childhood obesity provide an example of the scale and nature of health improvement work.

The *National Child Measurement Programme* in England provides up to date information on the epidemiology of obesity in school-age children. The data are reported using epidemiological cut-offs ('overweight' is defined as greater than or equal to the 85th centile but less than the 95th centile; 'obese' is defined as greater or equal to the 95th centile).

For the 09/10 school year:
• 23.1% of 4–5-year-olds were either overweight or obese.
• 33.4% of 10–11-year-olds were either overweight or obese.

The prevalence of obesity (but not overweight) increases with deprivation and varies by ethnicity. The prevalence of childhood obesity has increased dramatically over the past 30 years (see Fig.17.3), and increases throughout childhood, though there are some signs that the figures may have plateaued subsequently in some countries.

The Foresight report 'Tackling Obesities: Future Choices' (Fig. 17.3) notes that by 2050, Britain could be a mainly obese society. If this comes to pass the implications for morbidity, premature mortality and the wider costs to society (estimated at £7 billion for 2002 for England) are almost beyond imagining.

1. First International Conference of Health Promotion (1986). *The Ottawa Charter for Health Promotion*. Geneva: WHO, 1986.

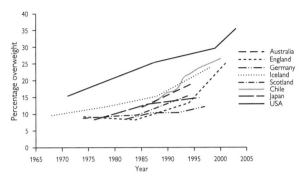

Fig. 17.3 Secular trends for obesity in children. *Tackling Obesities: Future Choices – Project Report*, 2nd Edition. Government Office for Science, 2007 (Contains public sector information licensed under the Open Government Licence v1.0. Reproduced from Foresight).

The Foresight report highlights a number of key components to tackling overweight and obesity, each of which have direct relevance to public health:

- Energy balance (and obesity) is influenced by a *complex multifaceted system* of determinants where no single factor dominates
- We live in an '*obesogenic environment*' that serves to expose the biological vulnerability of human beings with technological change outstripping evolution.
- There is a *life course component*. The risks of becoming obese start at an early stage. Growth patterns in the first few weeks and months of life affect the risk of later obesity and chronic disease.
- There is a *intergenerational dimension* (obesity in a parent increases the risk of childhood obesity by 10%).
- There is a need for a *paradigm shift* in how we address overweight and obesity at a national and global level both in the nature and scale of the intervention.

While the Foresight report covers both prevention and treatment, the report makes clear that the main focus of the report is on prevention (and it can be assumed that any 'paradigm shift' will need to be in this area as well). A particular challenge, however, is that the evidence for success of preventive approaches in the UK is limited. Community-based programmes in France (EPODE) and the United States (Shape Up Somerville) have shown considerable promise. However, cultural differences mean that we cannot simply transfer these programmes to a UK setting and expect success. Indeed, changes in technology (e.g. internet, multichannel television, and an expanding number of digital radio stations) mean that aspects of these programmes may not be achievable in the 21st century.

Overweight and obesity can be seen as an example par excellence of the health improvement challenge. Tackling overweight and obesity requires joined up actions that extend beyond individuals, families, schools, the workplace or communities, and requires the concerted and coordinated action of:

- The public sector (healthcare and local authorities).
- Schools and education authorities.
- The voluntary sector.
- Private sector (retailers, manufacturers, advertisers, and the media).
- Regulators.
- Government (national and supra-national).

Success will rely as much on legislation (e.g. nutritional standards in school catering and prepackaged food) and fiscal measures (e.g. to encourage active travel, or to reduce consumption of sugary drinks or foods high in sugar, fat, and salt) as it will on more local activities and programmes focused around education, prevention and treatment.

Furthermore, as success will require major shifts in physical activity and healthy eating, there would be anticipated wider benefits including:

- *Improvement* in behaviour and educational attainment at school.
- *Improvement* in mental health and emotional well-being.
- *Reductions* in cardiovascular disease and many cancers.

Health improvement in action 2: unintentional injuries

Unintentional injuries represent a challenge of a similar order of magnitude to childhood obesity. Unintentional injuries are common and while most are preventable, success depends on action across society. The epidemiology has been summarized recently in public health guidance issued by NICE. These are summarized as follows. While the figures are mainly for England and Wales, the overall patterns are similar for Scotland.

- Unintentional injury is a leading cause of death among children and young people aged 1–14 years, with 208 deaths in 0–14-year-olds in England and Wales in 2008.
- It is also a leading cause of morbidity with a physical and emotional impact that can extend well beyond the immediate recovery period. In the UK, unintentional injury (in all environments) results in more than 2 million visits to emergency departments by children every year. Half of these injuries occur in the home.
- The rate of deaths and serious injuries from road collisions has been declining over recent decades (by about 4% per year in all ages and 9% in children). Nonetheless, 44% of deaths related to unintentional injury in England and Wales are transport-related.
- In 2009 in the UK, 65 young people aged <15 years were killed and 2267 seriously injured on roads (65% were pedestrians).
- The number of people killed or seriously injured on the road increases with age with a noticeable increase at the transition from primary to secondary school.
- While deaths from unintentional injury have decreased, there are persistent and widening inequalities between socioeconomic groups (see 📖 p510).

- Children of parents who have never worked, or who have been unemployed for a long time, are 13 times more likely to die from unintentional injury than children of parents in higher managerial and professional occupations. The gradient is steepest for deaths due to household fires, cycling, and walking.

The new NICE guidance offers a series of recommendations at a national and local level, both for the health service and partner organizations including local authorities (e.g. environmental health and transport), schools, emergency services and many others. Returning to Tannahill's definition of health promotion/improvement, some of the recommendations are listed in Table 17.2 under his 5 suggested areas of health promotion/improvement activity. As with obesity, coordinated action is required—so for road safety 'engineering, education and enforcement activities are likely to be synergistic' (NICE Guidance).

Table 17.2 Options for reducing unintentional injuries using Tannahill's definition of health promotion/improvement (see 📖 p557)

Health improvement area	Link to NICE recommendation for reducing unintentional injuries
Social, economic, physical environmental, and cultural factors	Consider legislation and regulations where appropriate (e.g. to improve construction of homes). Introduce engineering measures to reduce vehicle speeds, in line with Department for Transport guidance. Make routes commonly used by children and young people safer. This includes routes to schools and parks.
Equity and diversity	In line with 'proportionate universalism', home safety programmes should be accessible to all. However, households at greatest risk should be prioritized for advice and interventions which should be tailored to individual circumstances (e.g. consider disability, literacy, housing type—and rules around home modification in social or rented accommodation).
Education and learning	Home safety assessments and advice have a strong educational component. Education for drivers and cyclists. Workforce training in installation and equipment use/replacement.
Services, amenities, and products	Home safety assessments and advice are provided by a range of providers including fire and rescue services. Safety equipment may include door guards, cupboard locks, safety gates, smoke and carbon monoxide alarms, thermostatic mixing valves, and window restrictors.

(Continued)

Table 17.3 (Continued)

Health improvement area	Link to NICE recommendation for reducing unintentional injuries
Community-led and community-based activity	Establish partnerships with local community organizations.
	Local 'community champions' could help promote home safety interventions and help practitioners gain the trust of householders.
	Early years workers can build on their established links with the community to promote home safety checks (e.g. health visitors, Sure Start, children's centres and nurseries).

Health improvement in action 3: early intervention and parenting

From the Marmot Review, reports on early intervention for the UK and Scottish Parliaments, there is an emerging consensus, across the political spectrum, of the importance of early interventions, early years work and parenting support. The economic case for early intervention is compelling and is summarized in Fig. 17.4.

While recurring investment is yet to follow the promising pilots and rhetoric, the emerging evidence is persuasive. The *Family Nurse Partnership* pilots in parts of England and Scotland, for example, provide an 'intensive, preventive, home-visiting programme delivered by specially trained nurses and

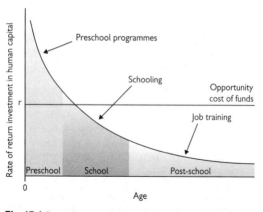

Fig. 17.4 Rates of return to human capital investment. Reproduced from Heckman, James J. and Alan B. Krueger, edited by Benjamin M. Friedman, Inequality in America: What Role for Human Capital Policies?, 'Rates of return to human capital investment', © 2004 Massachusetts Institute of Technology, with permission of the MIT Press.

midwives with experience of working with families in the community. It is a structured programme offered to first-time young parents from early pregnancy until the child is two years old, on the basis that pregnancy and birth are key points when most families are receptive to support and extra help and interventions can have significant impact at these times'.

The *Family Nurse Partnership programme* has health benefits for mother and child during the programme (e.g. reduced maternal smoking and increased breastfeeding) but evidence from delivering this programme over the past 30 years in the USA suggests that there are wider benefits on education, employment, criminal behaviour, child maltreatment and many other areas of life for the mother, child, and the wider family. These benefits come about through strengths/assets-based approach rather than the usual deficits based approach, which makes the reduction in maternal smoking all the more significant.

The Family Nurse Partnership programme has the additional benefit that it is a universal programme, offered to all first time teenage pregnant women in participating areas.

There is also a developing evidence base that shows that well designed parenting programmes have benefits for parents and children, as summarized in the Marmot Review (Box 17.2). Unfortunately, this comes at a time when government spending cuts mean that some of the key interventions appear to be under threat in many parts of the UK. It is clear that the intensity of the support required for many families, and the continuing pressure on health visiting means that early intervention work will require considerable additional new investment.

Box 17.2 Summary of routine support to parents in the preschool years[a]

- Early interventions during pregnancy and ongoing support in early years are critical to the long-term health of the child and other long-term outcomes.
- Universal and proportionately targeted interventions are necessary.
- Emerging evidence shows that Sure Start children's centres have a positive impact on child outcomes.
- Families have the most influence on their children.
- Adequate levels of income and material and psychological support and advice for parents across the social gradient are critical.
- Intensive home visiting is effective in improving maternal and child health.
- Good parent–child relationships in the first year of life are associated with stronger cognitive skills in young children and enhanced competence and work skills in schools.

[a] ℛ http://www.themarmotreview.org

There are, however, grounds for optimism. Recent reports to Scottish Parliament and UK Parliament have repeated the importance of early intervention, including parenting programmes and intensive home visiting. The compelling evidence and long term benefits to society—financial and otherwise—will hopefully prove persuasive to national and local government, particularly at a time of financial austerity.

Health protection

Introduction

Health protection usually refers to communicable disease control, environmental health, and emergency planning. Depending on the health system the professionals who work in this field on a day-to-day basis are typically in a separate team within the public health department, or work in a different organization (e.g. the Health Protection Agency (HPA) in England).

Health protection is the most clinical of subspecialties within public health. However, there are important differences in the duties of health protection professionals and their hospital or community colleagues delivering care to sick patients:

- The attending clinician dealing with a case of infectious disease performs the clinical examination and diagnostic tests, makes the diagnosis, initiates the treatment, and monitors progress.
- The function of health protection teams is 'to protect the community (or any part of the community) against infectious diseases and other dangers to health' (HPA: ℘ http://www.hpa.org.uk/AboutTheHPA/ WhatTheHealthProtectionAgencyDoes/)

This section describes the role of the health protection team and explores the interface between the attending clinician and the health protection team, using the example of meningococcal disease.

The duty of health protection professionals to protect the community can involve a range of different functions that will vary for the specific circumstances. For communicable disease it will typically involve:

- Contact tracing.
- Advising these contacts about necessary prophylactic measures.
- Informing contacts about symptoms and appropriate arrangements for accessing further advice and support in case they become unwell themselves.
- Arranging exclusions from work/school/nursery (may be necessary for case and contacts).
- Keeping a watchful eye for any patterns that may suggest an outbreak or wider threat to public health through surveillance and epidemiological studies.

In addition, it will often be necessary for health protection teams to:

- Communicate with other members of the public identified as directly at risk—e.g. staff and parents at a school.
- Work with NHS and LA communication officers to prepare press releases to inform the wider public.
- Involve other agencies (e.g. colleagues from the appropriate regional or national health protection body, environmental health, environmental protection, water, emergency services, and others as the need arises).

These decisions will often be made by the health protection team after conducting a multidisciplinary problem assessment group. The duty health protection officer will have access to the appropriate guidance, standard operating procedures and plans as well as directories of key professional contacts. However, the list of functions described above can also apply to other disciplines and settings (e.g. the genitourinary medicine clinic's response to a syphilis case or cluster).

It is important that all staff are clear about the division of clinical and health protection responsibilities. Good communication between community/hospital clinical staff, the laboratories, and health protection teams is essential. Paediatricians and general practitioners should know the conditions that are required to be notified by law in their country. Box 17.3 explains the current process for England and Wales. Each step of the process described is essential in communicable disease control. The details may change with the proposed reorganization of the NHS in England.

Box 17.3 Procedure for notification in England and Wales[a]

(Check national health protection website for arrangements in your area.)

Doctors in England and Wales have a statutory duty to notify a 'Proper Officer' of the LA of suspected cases of certain infectious diseases. The attending Registered Medical Practitioner should fill out a notification certificate immediately on diagnosis of a suspected notifiable disease and should not wait for laboratory confirmation of the suspected infection or contamination before notification. The certificate should be sent to the Proper Officer within three days or verbally within 24 hours if the case is considered urgent.

The Proper Officers are required to pass on the entire notification to the HPA within 3 days of a case being notified, or within 24 hours for cases deemed urgent. Health Protection Units (HPU) is the primary recipient within the HPA of clinical notifications from Proper Officers. To contact your local HPU, use the postcode search or browse by region on the HPA homepage.

The Information Management & Technology Department within the HPA Centre for Infections collate the returns at the national level, and publish analyses of local and national trends on a weekly basis.

[a] HPA: ℘ http://www.hpa.org.uk/Topics/InfectiousDiseases/InfectionsAZ/
NotificationsOfInfectiousDiseases/ReportingProcedures

The precise circumstances around reporting cases of infectious disease—and acting on these reports—may also change depending on context. For example:

• The arrangements for reporting influenza cases may change in a pandemic.
• The threshold for acting on reports of measles has reduced with the resurgence in cases over recent years.

Box 17.4 gives a list of notifiable conditions in England and Wales.

Box 17.4 Notifiable conditions in England and Wales

- Acute encephalitis
- Acute meningitis
- Acute poliomyelitis
- Acute infectious hepatitis
- Anthrax
- Botulism
- Brucellosis
- Cholera
- Diphtheria
- Enteric fever (typhoid or paratyphoid fever)
- Food poisoning
- Haemolytic uraemic syndrome
- Infectious bloody diarrhoea
- Invasive group A streptococcal disease and scarlet fever
- Legionnaires' disease
- Leprosy
- Malaria
- Measles
- Meningococcal septicaemia
- Mumps
- Plague
- Rabies
- Rubella
- SARS
- Smallpox
- Tetanus
- Tuberculosis
- Typhus
- Viral haemorrhagic fever
- Whooping cough
- Yellow fever.

As of April 2010, it is no longer a requirement to notify the following diseases: dysentery, ophthalmia neonatorum, leptospirosis, and relapsing fever.

[a] HPA: ℘ http://www.hpa.org.uk/Topics/InfectiousDiseases/InfectionsAZ/
NotificationsOfInfectiousDiseases/ListOfNotifiableDiseases/

Being prepared—and where to find further information

In the UK the national health protection organizations provide information about everyday practice and on-call actions for health protection. The A–Z section on these organizations' websites will take you to information about a specific pathogen. There is also useful generic guidance available on these sites (e.g. how to manage a rash in pregnancy, advice about communicating with public, etc). Many of the conditions are quite uncommon and guidance changes relatively frequently, so it is worth checking that you have the most up-to-date information.

- Health Protection Wales: ✍ http://www.wales.nhs.uk/sites3/home. cfm?orgid=457
- Northern Ireland: Public Health Agency: ✍ http://www.publichealth. hscni.net/
- Health Protection Agency (England): ✍ http://www.hpa.org.uk
- Health Protection Scotland: ✍ http://www.hps.scot.nhs.uk
- European Union Public Health pages: ✍ http://http://ec.europa.eu/ health/index_en.htm
- US Centers for Disease Control and Prevention: ✍ http://www. cdc.gov
- Other clinical guidance and reviews (e.g. NICE, Scottish Intercollegiate Guidelines Network, or Cochrane database).

In addition to these national and international sources of information it is essential to understand local arrangements as well. These will typically be written down in local guidelines/manuals/standard operating procedures. The local context is important as arrangements for testing, treating, and arranging specialist services (e.g. sourcing and administering immunoglobulin) vary from area to area. It is important to understand these local circumstances, and consult with the staff responsible for providing care, to ensure that suspected and confirmed cases are kept away from other vulnerable individuals (e.g. pregnant women and measles). Picking up the telephone and discussing cases with the relevant staff is therefore as important as accessing the appropriate guidance on the internet.

Other useful sources of information for quick reference include:
- Immunisation against infectious disease: 'The Green Book'—2006 updated edition (✍ http://www.dh.gov.uk/en/Publicationsandstatistics/ Publications/PublicationsPolicyAndGuidance/DH_079917)
- A good communicable disease textbook (*Communicable Disease Control Handbook* or *Control of Communicable Diseases Manual*)
- The *British National Formulary* (see also ✍ http://www.bnf.org)

Health protection work can be disruptive to staff, cases, and contacts and potentially involves many different agencies. It is therefore important for the duty health protection officer to consider whether public health action is necessary and, if so, if it is required urgently (e.g. overnight or at the weekend). The duty health protection officer will therefore ask the referring paediatrician questions about the case and their wider circumstances. The preliminary information will be considered along with the knowledge of the natural history of the suspected cause and the up-to-date guidance to work out the next steps.

An example—meningococcal disease

Meningococcal disease is one of the most important health protection emergencies. In the UK, annual rates of invasive disease usually vary between 2–6 per 100,000, with case-fatality rates of about 10%. The epidemiology of meningococcal disease is changing. The current HPA guideline provides a useful summary (see 📖 p555, Epidemiology reference) that is broken down below into time, place and person, adding in 'pathogen':

Time

- The reported incidence of meningococcal disease peaked in 1998/99, particularly associated with serogroup C strains. The introduction of the meningococcal C 'Men C' conjugate vaccination programme in November 1999 was followed by a marked fall in disease caused by serogroup C strains (see Fig. 17.5).
- The highest incidence is seen in the winter months.

Place

- The distribution by serogroup varies across the world. Two national outbreaks of disease due to W135 strains, previously rare in the UK, followed the Hajj pilgrimages in 2000 and 2001.

Person

- Carriage of *Neisseria meningitidis* is common and increases during childhood—from 2% in children <5 years to a peak of 25% in 15–19-year-olds.
- Attack rates are highest in infancy, decline during childhood before a secondary rise in teenagers and young adults.
- Other risk factors include passive smoking, preceding influenza A infection, and overcrowding.

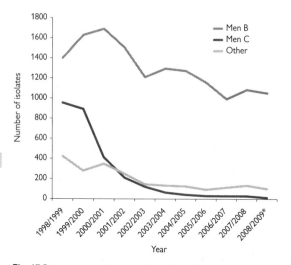

Fig. 17.5 Meningococcal Reference Unit isolates of *Neisseria meningitidis*: England and Wales, by serogroup and epidemiological year, 1998/99–2008/09. *Provisional data. Men B = serogroup B, Men C = serogroup C. The 'other' category includes W135, Y and other serogroups and ungrouped or not serogroupable. (Data from HPA: 🔗 http://www.hpa.org.uk/web/HPAweb&HPAwebStandard/HPAweb_C/1234859711901).

Pathogen
- The mean duration of carriage has been estimated at 21 months, with systemic immunity usually developing within 14 days of acquisition.
- Rarely, acquisition progresses to invasive disease (meningitis and/or septicaemia) before immunity develops, with an incubation period of between 3–5 days.

Despite the reduction in the incidence of meningococcal disease, it is still important to be vigilant for signs and symptoms. The HPA guideline details cases requiring urgent public health action (see Table 17.3).

Table 17.3 Identifying those cases that require public health action and those that do not (meningococcal disease). HPA Guideline.

Cases requiring public health action

Confirmed case: clinical diagnosis of meningitis, septicaemia, or other invasive disease (e.g. orbital cellulitis/septic arthritis)* and microbiological confirmation of *Neisseria meningitidis* (or, in some cases, Gram negative diplococci) from sample from normally sterile site (see guideline for full details)

Probable case: clinical diagnosis of meningitis or septicaemia or other invasive disease where the public health physician, in consultation with the physician and microbiologist, considers that meningococcal infection is the most likely diagnosis

Cases not requiring public health action

Possible case: clinical diagnosis of meningitis or septicaemia or other invasive disease where the public health physician, in consultation with the clinician and microbiologist, considers that diagnoses other than meningococcal disease are at least as likely

Infection in non-sterile sites: isolation of meningococci from sputum or from swabs taken from nasopharynx or genital tract is not by itself an indication for public health action because asymptomatic carriage in the respiratory and genital tract is common—unless other clinical and microbiological parameters suggest that this is a probable case, especially if the isolate is a virulent strain

Meningococcal pneumonia: not an indication for public health action but may carry a low risk of transmission in healthcare settings especially to the immunocompromised

Despite the clarity of the HPA guidance (see Table 17.3), individual cases will not uncommonly have features that make them atypical, or fall between categories. Decisions about the management of these cases requires a judgement call. The guidance makes clear the need for close collaboration between specialties.

The best advice for a junior member of staff is to seek advice from consultant colleagues.

Health service improvement/ development

The third domain of public health work relates to health service improvement/development. In fact, the increasing importance of partnership work means that this type of work extends beyond the health service to include the work of other services and providers. As noted in Table 17.1, the Faculty of Public Health lists the following components to such work (see Table 17.4). The example of introducing a parenting programme is used to illustrate how these components fit together. Similar considerations would apply to an existing programme (e.g. universal newborn hearing screening).

Table 17.4 Some option for health service improvement/ development—using the example of parenting programmes.

Component	Example
Clinical effectiveness and efficiency	Assess the cost-effectiveness of different parenting programmes based on findings from research and pilot studies.
Service planning	Plan for the introduction of the parenting programme(s) that best meets the local population's needs. This may involve: • Health needs assessment. • Securing funding. • Working with colleagues to identify the workforce and training requirements. • Developing quality standards for the ongoing evaluation and monitoring of the programme. • Implementation of the programme. Consider the needs of the whole population and more vulnerable groups (see Proportionate universalism 🕮 p552).
Audit and evaluation	Audit the programme against the agreed quality standards. Evaluate the programme (e.g. using the Donabedian approach of assessing structure, process, and outcome).
Clinical governance	Work with colleagues who deliver the programme and service users, and consider the findings of the audit and evaluation, to develop and improve the quality of the programme (see also section 6.11 in the *Oxford Handbook of Public Health Practice*).

Commonly asked questions concerning immunisation

Parents and health professionals frequently have questions about the need for immunisation, adverse events and concerns generated by media discussion of vaccines. 'The Green Book' is a useful reference for many of these. ℘ http://immunisation.dh.gov.uk/category/the-green-book/

1. My child attends a learning disabilities school and it has been suggested they should be vaccinated against hepatitis B

Hepatitis B vaccination is recommended for individuals with learning difficulties living in residential accommodation and similarly to be considered for adults and children in day care schools and centres for those with severe learning difficulties. The infection risk in these settings arises from the finding of a higher prevalence of hepatitis B infection than in the general population together with close, daily living and behavioural problems such as biting. However, many children in these settings have never been vaccinated and decisions on immunisation need to be made based on a local risk assessment particularly for non-residential settings. Hepatitis B immunisation is routinely given to infants in most countries showing that they consider the benefits justify vaccinating everyone. If there is uncertainty regarding the level of increased risk, vaccination is the safer option.

2. Should all 12–13 year old girls receive the HPV vaccine?

The aim of the national HPV vaccination programme is to protect young girls against their future risk of cervical cancer. It is not always easy to quantify an individual's future risk but the vaccine is safe and effective so all 12–13-year-old girls with or without disabilities should be vaccinated as per the routine schedule. People with, for example, learning difficulties have a poorer outcome for many diseases. This may be due to delays in diagnosis for example and emphasizes the advantages of prevention. Trying to vaccinate later at times outside the programme is possible. It is generally considered easier to vaccinate in line with the national schedule but vaccination will be available up to age 18 and may be available at older ages although this is not currently the case in all areas.

3. The MMR controversy, what was that all about?

There is substantial research evaluating any possible link between the MMR vaccine and autism. This has not shown any evidence for a link. A 2011 *British Medical Journal* editorial by Godlee *et al.* provides a useful overview of the area (℘ http://www.bmj.com/content/342/bmj.c7452. full). However, despite the lack of any evidence some anxiety remains within the population. Although vaccine coverage levels are increasing in infants many older children remain unvaccinated and vulnerable to the diseases which can still circulate in an under-immunised population due to past concerns and residual anxiety. Uptake of MMR vaccine needs to be 95% to be able to stop measles spreading. In the first 5 months of 2011 the

UK reported as many cases of measles as in the whole of the preceding year, so the risk of disease spreading to unvaccinated individuals remains a real one. Unless children are immunocompromised they should receive 2 doses of MMR vaccine.

4. Do children now have so many vaccines that it might 'overload' their immune system?

The ability of a child's immune system to cope with today's multiple vaccines sometimes concerns both parents and some health care workers. The immune system is designed to process and respond to a large variety of different antigens, including micro-organisms, on a daily basis. The vaccines that are used routinely in the UK in 2011 actually contain a smaller variety of antigens than those used prior to 2004 when pertussis vaccine changed from a whole cell vaccine, containing several thousand proteins, to acellular pertussis which contains between 3–5 purified pertussis proteins. These numbers are small compared to the mix of new infections children meet when starting school or nursery.

5. Pertussis vaccination and neurological issues, what's the issue?

Historically public concerns about neurological events after whole-cell pertussis vaccine led to a fall in immunisation coverage with resurgence of disease. The current vaccine is an acellular pertussis vaccine and is less reactogenic than the previous whole-cell vaccine. Children with a stable pre-existing condition can and should be vaccinated against whooping cough. However, any neurological condition that is unstable or deteriorating, including poorly controlled epilepsy should be investigated and immunisation deferred until either: (1) a cause is identified, (2) no cause is identified but the condition has stabilized. This advice, in more detail in 'The Green Book', is given in order to avoid deteriorating neurological conditions being incorrectly attributed to the pertussis vaccine. There is no evidence that vaccine causes neurological deterioration.

6. What constitutes a contraindication to further vaccinations?

There are very few children in whom vaccines are totally contraindicated. Anaphylaxis to any component of the vaccine or a previous dose of the vaccine is an absolute contraindication. However anaphylaxis to vaccines is very rare (estimated at around 1 per million doses in several studies). Anxiety often arises following severe local reactions or mild systemic reactions to a previous dose of vaccine. A carefully taken Hx should elicit the nature of the reaction and if a vaccine may or may not be recommended again. Severe local reactions and non-anaphylactic systemic reactions (e.g. fever, malaise, irritability) are not a contraindication to further doses of vaccines and in many cases will not recur.

7. Incomplete immunisation schedule?

A child's immunisation schedules may not be fully completed for a number of reasons. Ideally they need to be caught up or transferred to the UK schedule from an overseas one using the least amount of vaccines in the shortest amount of time. The HPA immunisation department produces a helpful algorithm to assist in assessing which vaccines to give and when and is at the following link: ℘ http://www.hpa.org.uk/web/HPAwebFile/HPAweb_C/1194947406156

8. Thiomersal, what's the fuss?

Thiomersal is a mercury containing compound used as a preservative in some vaccines. The mercury content of this compound has led to concerns that it may affect brain development. The Committee on Safety in Medicines (2003), European Medicines Agency (2004) and the WHO Global advisory Committee on Vaccine Safety (2002) have all concluded that there is no evidence, including from two large UK-based epidemiological studies, of harm arising from the use of thiomersal containing vaccines. However, as part of a general recommendation to reduce environmental mercury exposure from avoidable sources, many vaccines have had thiomersal content reduced or removed. There are currently no vaccines in the routine immunisation schedule containing mercury. Some influenza vaccines still contain thiomersal. More detailed information can be found at: ℘ http://www.dh.gov.uk/prod_consum_dh/groups/dh_digitalassets/@dh/@en/documents/digitalasset/dh_4070150.pdf

9. Should children with neurodevelopmental and neuromuscular disorders (NNMDs) be offered influenza vaccine?

"Yes". There is evidence of substantial excess risk from influenza in people with these conditions. Data from the USA in 2009, identified that of 36 deaths among children from H1N1, 22 had neurodevelopmental disorders. For children with intact immune systems a good response to vaccination would be expected. Data from England and Wales in the 2010/2011 winter season identified that children in these groups were over 40 times more likely to die after influenza than healthy children.

Vaccine preventable diseases

- Vaccines are a highly effective public health intervention and have had a large impact on the burden of infectious diseases throughout the world.
- In order to discuss the risks and benefits of immunisation with parents it is important to appreciate the severity and pre-vaccine era burden of disease caused by the pathogens for which immunisation is given.
- The number of cases in the UK should be understood in the context of a population in which around 95% of children receive their infant schedule of diphtheria/tetanus/pertussis/polio vaccines by 2 year of age and 88% measles/mumps and rubella (data for England 2009–2010).
- Herd immunity is an important factor for all vaccines except tetanus.

Diphtheria

- An acute bacterial infection of the respiratory tract, or more rarely skin, whose pathogenesis depends on toxin production.
- Complications include upper airway obstruction, cardiomyopathy and polyneuritis.
- Treatment is with antitoxin and antibiotics (penicillin or erythromycin) and the mortality rate is 5–10%.
- Formerly a common disease in the UK (61,000 cases and 3283 deaths in 1940) and now rare due to routine immunisation programme. However, 30% of adults are thought to be non-immune due to lack of natural boosting.
- Cases continue to be reported from South-East Asia, India, Africa, South America, Eastern Europe and travel is a risk both for reintroduction into the UK and for individual exposure to disease.
- Since 2000 there have been 4 cases of disease due to *C. diptheriae* in England and Wales including the death of an unimmunised child in 2008.

Tetanus

- An acute neurological disease due to the production of a neurotoxin by the bacteria *Clostridium tetani* acting on skeletal muscle, spinal cord, brain, and sympathetic nervous system.
- The spores of *C. tetani* are introduced into the body through a contaminated wound.
- Disease manifestations include severe muscle spasms.
- Treatment is antitoxin, antibiotics (penicillin), wound cleaning/debridement, and usually intensive care.
- Mortality 10–30%.
- Disease now rare due to routine immunisation but risk of disease to an individual unchanged from pre-immunisation era as no herd immunity to a disease caused by spores from soil.
- Since 2000 there have been 4 reported cases in children <15 years of age in England and Wales with incomplete immunisation being the primary risk factor.

Pertussis

- A respiatory disease cause by the bacterium *Bordetella pertussis* whose pathogenesis involves production of a toxin.
- A coryzal phase is followed by paroxysms of coughing which can last for several weeks. Post-tussive vomiting and inspiratory whoop are specific features.
- Complications are most common in infants and include weight-loss, hypoxia, apnoea, pneumonia (which can be severe with pulmonary hypertension and requiring intensive care), cerebral haemorrhage.
- Prior to routine immunisation there were >120,000 notified cases annually in the UK.
- A case fatality rate of ~1% is described in settings where intensive care is available and most of this occurs in infants <6 months of age.
- Treatment is with macrolide antibiotics (e.g. erythromycin, azithromycin) but only effective in the coryzal phase.
- Currently in the UK there is significant circulation of *B. pertussis* in the adult population due to a low level of population immunity. The only manifestation of illness in this group may be prolonged cough and these are the most important group for transmission to young infants.
- In 2009 in England and Wales there were 717 laboratory-confirmed cases and estimates from 2003 were that there were 9 deaths/year.

Polio

- A neurological illness caused by one of three serotypes of poliovirus.
- Most infections asymptomatic with a small proportion having symptoms of a non-specific viral illness (sore throat, headache, fever, gastrointestinal symptoms). Some children progress to involvement of the central nervous system with meningeal symptoms and destruction of anterior horn motor neurons causing progressive paralysis.
- Overall 0.1% of all infections result in paralysis with mortality of 5–10% in pre-immunisation era.
- Treatment is supportive.
- In the UK in the last 10 years no case of poliomyelitis has been reported.
- WHO programme of global eradication of poliomyelitis since 1988 (cases reduced from >350,000 to <2000/year). Endemic cases still occurring in Asia (Afghanistan, Pakistan, India) and Africa (Nigeria) with the result that there remains a risk for travellers and potentially imported cases.

Haemophilus influenzae type b (Hib), serogroup C *Neisseria meningitidis* (Nm) and *Streptococcus pneumoniae* (Sp)

- All of these bacteria are common commensals of the nasopharynx but, especially in young children, can also cause severe invasive disease in the form of meningitis, bacteraemia and other suppurative infections (e.g. osteomyelitis).
- In addition Hib and Sp account for a significant proportion of bacterial pneumonia globally.
- While meningitis is more severe (mortality varying from 3–15% and neurological sequelae in 5–30%) pneumonia accounts for a much

greater burden of disease, a fact not always well recognized as an organism is rarely identified.

- In the UK, despite significant herd immunity, induced by routine infant immunisation against Hib, serogroup C Nm, and 13 serotypes of Sp, cases of disease continue to occur with lack of immunisation being the most significant risk factor.
- Infections caused by serogroup B Nm and non-vaccine serotypes of Sp continue to occur as they are not covered by current vaccines.

Measles

- Measles is a respiratory illness characterized by a distinctive syndrome of fever, cough, coryza, conjunctivitis, and rash caused by measles virus.
- Common complications include secondary bacterial infections causing pneumonia, otitis media and diarrhoea. In 1:1000 cases an encephalitis will develop with a 15% mortality rate and 25% left with neurological disability.
- In the UK prior to the introduction of routine immunisation in 1968 there were 160,000–800,000 cases/year with around 100 deaths.
- Measles cases continue to occur in UK with >800 laboratory confirmed cases confirmed in England and Wales in the first 8 months of 2011. The cases occur in clusters within educational institutions or families or associated with travel and the vast majority occur in unimmunised individuals.
- Measles is highly infectious and current immunisation coverage in many areas of the UK is not sufficient to induce full herd immunity. The last death from acute measles in the UK was in 2006.

Mumps

- Mumps virus causes a non-specific febrile illness with a distinctive (but not universal) parotitis.
- Complications include orchitis in males, with some suffering subsequent impaired fertility, aseptic meningitis, deafness and encephalitis.
- Prior to immunisation mumps was the commonest cause of viral meningitis and resulted in 1200 hospital admissions/year in England and Wales. In 2010 there were 3857 cases of mumps confirmed in the same regions.

Rubella

- Rubella virus causes a mild, often subclinical illness. When symptomatic this consists of fever, cervical lymphadenopathy, and rash.
- Complications include a postviral arthritis.
- The major concern is rubella in pregnancy which may result in congenital rubella syndrome in the child involving hearing loss, mental retardation, cardiovascular defects, and ocular defects.
- <50 cases of rubella are confirmed annually in England and Wales.
- Between 1997–2007 there were 15 cases of confirmed congenital rubella in UK with 10 of the mothers having acquired infection abroad, emphasizing the risk of travel if unimmunised.

Cervical cancer

- Cervical cancer is estimated to affect 1:116 women over the course of a lifetime and there were 2253 cases in England in 2005.

- The causative agent is infection with human papilloma virus. Of more than 40 types of human papilloma virus infecting the genital tract, types 16 and 18 cause ~65% of disease.
- Vaccines available include Cervarix® (types 16/18) and Gardasil® (HPV 6/11/16/18) which includes the two additional serotypes responsible for >90% of the more than 80,000 cases of genital warts detected annually in the UK.

Hepatitis B

- A viral infection of the liver initially causing asymptomatic infection or flu-like illness with symptomatic jaundice in 30–50% of adults and ~10% of children.
- The virus is transmitted through contact with bodily secretions and blood and major routes of transmission are sexual, blood contact, and perinatal. Hepatitis B is 50–100 times more infectious than HIV.
- Chronic infection succeeds acute infection in 90% of perinatal transmission falling to ~5% for adult transmission. Around 1/4 of those with chronic infection will develop progressive liver disease with an increased risk of hepatocellular cancer.
- The current UK seroprevalence is ~0.14% (higher in certain risk groups) but is around 10% of the population in some areas of the world (e.g. China).
- In 2008 177 countries had already introduced hepatitis B vaccine into routine immunisation programmes. The UK is not one of these countries. This reflects the importance of a disease which causes chronic liver disease in an estimated 360 million individuals globally and is responsible for around 600,000 deaths annually.

Influenza

- Influenza virus causes an infection of the respiratory tract ranging from coryza and cough through to marked fever, malaise, and myalgia.
- Complications include secondary bacterial pneumonia and otitis media and encephalitis.
- Severe illness is more common in the young, old, and those with underlying health problems.
- Most cases occur over a 2–3 months period each winter in UK.
- Treatment with neuraminidase inhibitors (oseltamivir and zanamivir), particularly when given within the first 48 hours of symptoms, has been shown to reduce shedding of virus and lead to more rapid recovery but there is less data on treatment related reductions in complications.
- The predominant strains of influenza virus change over time (genetic drift and shift) requiring new vaccines to be produced annually.
- The recent H1N1 swine flu pandemic disproportionately affected young children and those with pre-existing neurological comorbidity and this virus is likely to continue circulating in future 'flu' seasons.

Further resource

Information on diseases and their epidemiology in England and Wales: ✆ http://www.hpa.org.uk/

Conclusions

This chapter has provided an introduction to key concepts in public health, illustrating simple ways to conceptualize complex topics, and explains how they relate to child health.

- Child health professionals have a key role in improving and protecting the health and well-being of children, young people, and families, so they make a key contribution to public health.
- Their work cannot, however, be in isolation. Successful child public health work relies on
  - Collaboration (e.g. with local authority and voluntary sector colleagues).
  - Coordinated action at all levels (national, regional, local, and individual).
  - Careful planning and clear accountability at each of these levels.
- The current focus on early years and early intervention is a great opportunity, but also a major challenge. The current interest at government level needs to be translated into programmes that meet local needs. That will require the technical and professional knowledge of child health and public health professionals working in collaboration with other organizations and the communities themselves. That requires adaptability, imagination, and long-term thinking and perhaps, therefore, a different relationship with government, local authorities, and the voluntary/third sector.
- At a time of substantial change in healthcare in many parts of the UK (some ideological, some evidence based) it is important to continue delivering the basics as well. Good care, communication, surveillance, and assessment of need are every bit as important as expensive new programmes.

Support organizations and information resources for parents and carers

Education is an ornament in prosperity and refuge in adversity.

Aristotle

Support organizations and information resources for parents and carers

Contact a Family (CaF)

Provide advice, information, and support to:
• Families with disabled children.
• Local parent groups.
• UK-wide groups for specific conditions and rare disorders.

CaF have a network of UK offices and individual representatives. Further details can be found at ✒ http://www.cafamily.org.uk
• UK Office ☎ 0808 808 3555 (Mon–Fri) Email: info@cafamily.org.uk
• Should be your first port of call if you cannot find any info or support organization
• Northern Ireland office ☎ 028 9262 7552 Email: nireland.office@ cafamily.org.uk
• Scotland office ☎ 0131 659 2930 Email: scotland.office@cafamily.org.uk
• Wales office ☎ 029 2039 6624 Email: wales.office@cafamily.org.uk
• CaF has produced >20 *guides for parents and families* bringing up disabled children on diverse topics such as 'Aids & equipment' to 'Working tax credit'.
• Parents can access these guides free of charge. The guides are also available online. Professionals have to pay a very small fee, but they are worth every penny!
• In addition to these guides the CaF website has *downloadable medical information leaflets* on >400 conditions.

Abuse and neglect
• *Barnardos:* ✒ http://www.barnardos.org.uk. Projects for children across the UK.
• *Child Exploitation and Online. Protection centre (CEOP):*
• 0870 000 3344 ✒ http://www.ceop.gov.uk & ✒ http://www. thinkuknow.co.uk. Guide to internet safety for children.
• *National Society for the Prevention of Cruelty to Children (NSPCC):* ✒ http://www.nspcc.org.uk Services to protect children.
• *Stop it now!:* ☎ 0808 1000 900. ✒ http://www.Stopitnow.org.uk
• Prevent child sexual abuse.

Adolescents
• *Brook Advisory Service* Tel: 0808 802 1234. ✒ http://www.brook.org.uk
• *Connexions* ☎ 0808 001 3219. ✒ http://www.connexions.com
• *Family Planning Association:* ☎ 0845 122 8690. ✒ http://www.fpa.org.uk

- *National Youth Agency:* ✍ http://www.nya.org.uk
- *Sexwise:* for under 19s. ☎ 0800 28 29 30

Adoption

- *Adoption UK:* Linden House, 55 The Green, South Bar Street, Banbury, OX16 9AB. ☎ 01295 752240
- *British Agencies for Adoption and Fostering:* Saffron House, 6–10 Kirby Street, London, EC1N 8TS. ☎ 020 7421 2600, Email: mail@baaf.org.uk
- *National Children's Bureau:* 8 Wakley Street, London, EC1V 7QE. ☎ 020 7843 6000. Email: enquiries@ncb.org.uk
- *The Who Cares? Trust:* Kemp House, 152–160 City Road, London EC1V 2NP. ☎ 020 7251 3117. Email: mailbox@thewhocarestrust.org.uk

Advocacy/children's rights

- *Council for Disabled Children:* http://✍ http://www.ncb.org.uk/cdc
- *Child Rights Information Network:* ✍ http://www.crin.org
- *Child Poverty Action Group:* ✍ http://www.cpag.org.uk
- *The Children's Society:* ✍ http://www.childrenssociety.org.uk
- *National Children's Bureau (NCB):* ✍ http://www.ncb.org.uk
- *NCH Action for Children:* ✍ http://www.actionforchildren.org.uk
- *Royal College of Paediatrics and Child Health:* ✍ http://www.rcpch.ac.uk
- *Save the Children:* ✍ http://www.savethechildren.org.uk

Alcohol

- *FASawareUK:* ☎ 01942 223780. ✍ http://www.fasaware.co.uk
- *NOFAS-UK:* ☎ 0870 033 3700. ✍ http://www.nofas-uk.org

Autism

- National Autistic Society: 393 City Road London EC1V 1NG. Helpline ☎ 0845 070 4004. ✍ http://www.autism.org.uk

Bereavement

- *Child Bereavement Charity:* ☎ 01494 568900
- ✍ http://www.childbereavement.org.uk

Breast feeding

- *Baby Café:* ✍ http://www.thebabycafe.co.uk
- *Breast feeding network:* ☎ 0300 100 0212. ✍ http://www. breastfeedingnetwork.co.uk.

Cancer

- *CLIC Sargent:* ☎ 0800 197 0068. ✍ http://www.clicsargent.org.uk

Child death

- *Child Death Helpline:* ☎ 0800 282 986. ✍ http://www. childdeathhelpline.org.uk
- *Foundation for the Study of Infant Deaths:* ☎ 0808 802 6868. ✍ http:// www.fsid.org.uk

Communication

- *Ace (Aiding Communication in Education) Centre Advisory Trust:*
- ☎ 01865 759800. ✍ http://www.ace-centre.org.uk

- *1 Voice:* ℘ http://www.1voice.info. Network and support for C & YP using communication aids.
- *Speakability:* ☎ 0808 808 9572. ℘ http://www.speakability.org.uk

Congenital malformations

- *Changing Faces:* ☎ 0845 450 0275. ℘ http://www.changingfaces.org.uk
- *VACTERL Association Support Group:* ☎ 01752 482 568.
  ℘ http://www.vacterl-association.org.uk

Difficulty

- *Childline:* ☎ 0800 1111. ℘ http://www.childline.org.uk.
  24h counselling service.
- *Samaritans:* ☎ 08457 909090. ℘ http://www.samaritans.org.uk.
  Emotional support 24 hours a day.

Disability—general

- *Cerebra:* ℘ http://www.cerebra.org.uk. Support, advice, grants, library.
- *Directgov:* ℘ http://www.direct.gov.uk/en/DisabledPeople.
- *MENCAP:* ☎ 0808 808 1111. ℘ http://www.mencap.org.uk.
- *Powerpack* ℘ http://www.powerpack.uk.com. Create opportunities for disabled children in wheelchairs.
- *Radar key* ℘ http://www.radar.org.uk. Access into all locked disabled access toilets in UK. Need to apply for a key.
- *Riding for the disabled:* ☎ 0845 241 4393. ℘ http://www.rda.org. uk. Provision of opportunities for riding and/or carriage driving for disabled.
- *Walks with wheelchairs:* ℘ http://www.walkswithwheelchairs.com. Free information on routes that are suitable for wheelchair users.
- *Whizz-Kidz:* ☎ 020 7233 6600. ℘ http://www.whizz-kidz.org.uk. Provide help and funding with mobility.

Education

- *National Portage Association* ℘ http://www.portage.org.uk Home-visiting educational service.

Entertainment and leisure

- *Merlins Magic Wand:* ℘ http://www.merlinsmagicwand.org. A free ticket once a year to any of the Merlin Group Theme Parks.
  - Many theme parks offer an 'exit pass' for children who find it hard to queue.
- *National Association of Toy and Leisure Libraries:* ℘ http://www.natll. org.uk.
- *Special Needs Family Fun:* ℘ http://www.family-friendly-fun.com
- *Tourism for all:* ☎ 0845 124 9971. ℘ http://www.tourismforall.org.uk. Holidays for families with disabled child.

Funding/grants

- *Family Fund Trust* ℘ http://www.familyfund.org.uk. Grants to low-income families raising disabled and seriously ill C&YP.
- *Grant Search Engine:* ℘ http://www.grants.net. Grant Finder.

Growth disorders
- *Child Growth Foundation* Tel: 020 8995 0257. ✆ http://www.childgrowthfoundation.org.

Hearing
- *Cochlear Implanted Children's Support Group:* ✆ http://www.cicsgroup.org.uk.
- *Hearing & Disabilities:* http://hald.org.uk. website for people with hearing loss.

Heart
- *Children's Heart Federation:* ☎ 0808 808 5000. ✆ http://www.children's-heart-fed.org.uk

Information resources
- *Caring for someone or disabled people:* http://✆ http://www.direct.gov.uk
- *Families Online:* ✆ http://www.familiesonline.co.uk
- *For mothers:* ✆ http://www.mumsnet.co.uk. Just Mums. Section on Special Needs—chat forum.
- *Patient stories* describing their care journeys are available at 'Healthtalkonline' from DIPEx at ✆ http://www.healthtalkonline.org.
- *Special Families:* ✆ http://www.specialfamilies.org. Online forum for families of disabled children.

Limbs
- *Limbless Association:* ☎ 01277 725 182. ✆ http://www.limbless-association.org.
- *Steps:* ☎ 01925 750271. ✆ http://www.steps-charity.org.uk

Medical conditions
- *The Anaphylaxis Campaign:* ☎ 01252 542 029. ✆ http://www.anaphylaxis.org.uk.
- *Coeliac UK:* ☎ 0845 305 2060. ✆ http://www.coeliac.org.uk.
- *Cystic Fibrosis Trust:* ☎ 0300 373 1000. ✆ http://www.cftrust.org.uk.
- *Diabetes UK:* ☎ 0845 120 2960. ✆ http://www.diabetes.org.uk.
- *Kidney Research UK:* ☎ 0845 300 1499. ✆ http://www.kidneyresearch.org.
- *Mental Health:* ☎ 0845 766 0163. ✆ http://www.mind.org.uk.
- *National Eczema Society:* ☎ 0800 0891 122. ✆ http://www.eczema.org.

Mobility
- *Motability Scheme:* ☎ 0845 456 4566 / 0845 050 7666. ✆ http://www.motability.co.uk.

Premature and sick babies
- *BLISS:* ✆ http://www.bliss.org.uk.
- *Premature babies UK:* ✆ http://www.premature-babies.co.uk.

Respiratory
- *Mechanical/long-term ventilation:* ☎ 01258 820715. ✆ http://www.breatheon.org.uk.

Social skills

- *Social Skills:* ☏ http://www.do2learn.co.uk. Social skills tools box.

Parents/parenting

- *Parentline:* ☎ 0808 800 2222. ☏ http://www.parentlineplus.org.uk.
- *Cry-sis:* ☎ 08451 228 669. ☏ http://www.cry-sis.org.uk.
- *National Family and Parenting Institute:* ☏ http://www.nfpi.org.

Parents with disability

- *Disabled Parents Network:* ☏ http://www.disabledparentsnetwork. org.uk.
- *Disability, Pregnancy and Parenthood International:* ☏ http://www.dppi.org.uk.

Speech and language

- *Afasic:* ☎ 0845 355 5577. ☏ http://www.afasic.org.uk.
- *I CAN Charity:* ☎ 0845 225 4073 ☏ http://www.ican.org.uk.
- *The British Stammering Association:* ☎ 0845 603 2001 ☏ http://www. stammering.org.

Syndromes

- *Hypermobility Syndrome Association:* ☏ http://www.hypermobility.org.
- *Turner Syndrome Support Society:* ☎ 0845 230 7520 ☏ http://www.tss. org.uk.

Therapy

- *Bobath Centre:* ☏ http://www.bobath.org.uk. Individually tailored therapy for children with neurological conditions.
- *The Movement Centre:* ☏ http://www.the-movement-centre.co.uk. Physiotherapy centre to help children with CP and movement disorder.
- *Whoopsadaisy:* ☏ http://www.whoopsadaisy.org. Conductive Education for children with CP and motor disorders.

Vision

- *Ability website:* ☏ http://www.lookupinfo.org. For people experiencing vision problems.
- *Sparklebox:* ☏ http://www.sparklebox.co.uk. For visual aids.

Further information and reading

Sources of further information

Disclaimer
The information in this chapter has been collated and compiled over the years by the editor. Neither the editor nor the OUP accept any responsibility of the accurancy of the information or the integrity of the websites.

Medline Plus

ADAM Medical Encyclopedia hosts thousands of articles about various medical and surgical conditions, tests, drugs, supplements, etc. verified by medics. The service/site is provided by US National Library of Medicine, National Institute of Health. This can be accessed at: ℘ www.nlm.nih.gov/medlineplus/encyclopedia.html.

NHS Choices

This website provides Health encyclopaedia under A–Z Health conditions. The website also has tabs for 'Symptom Checker', 'Medicines Information A–Z', 'Healthy Living', Finding health services near you e.g. 'Nearest GP, Dentist, Hospital etc.' This can be accessed at: ℘ http://www.nhs.uk/Pages/HomePage.aspx.

Patient UK

A comprehensive and popular, website which provides information checked by health professionals. The website hosts information on: lets Medical conditions, Medicines (side effects, benefits), Directory of UK Health websites, Find a…therapist/doctor/nurse function, Benefits and finances, Carers and support, Patientline Plus (for professionals, contains guidelines, evidence based medical information, etc.). The website can be accessed at: ℘ http://www.patient.co.uk.

Children First for Health

A very reliable source of information on a wide range of health conditions for children, young people, families, and allied health professionals. The site is a service provided by Great Ormond Street Hospital, London. The website also provides information on a range of procedures, treatments, medicines information, general health advice on mental health, sexual health, healthy eating etc. The website address is: ℘ http://www.childrenfirst.nhs.uk/medical-conditions/.

Literature searches

℘ http://www.ncbi.nlm.nih.gov/PubMed.
℘ http://www.embase.com.

Guidelines

SIGN: ℘ http://www.sign.ac.uk.
NICE: ℘ http://www.nice.org.uk.
National Guideline Clearinghouse ℘ http://www.guideline.gov/.
A very useful public resource for evidence-based clinical practice guidelines provided by US Department of Health & Human Services.

Skin

Electronic Dermatology Atlas: ℘ http://www.dermis.net.

Dysmorphology information sources

Online Mendelian Inheritance in Man: ℘ http://www.ncbi.nlm.nih.gov/omim.

London Dysmorphology Database: ℘ http://www.lmdatabases.com.

Growth charts

RCPCH growth charts: ℘ http://www.growthcharts.rcpch.ac.uk.

Child health and development

NHS. Birth to Five Development Timeline: ℘ http://www.nhs.uk/Tools/Pages/birthtofive.aspx?Tag=Interactive+timelines.

Mental health

Information and leaflets on various conditions: ℘ http://www.rcpsych.ac.uk.

Understanding your tests

Explanations of clinical laboratory tests are available at ℘ http://labtestonline.org.uk.

Other resources for medical information

(These require individual/organizational subscription.)

UpToDate®

℘ http://www.uptodate.com.

A US website provides up-to-date/current medical information on over 9000 clinical conditions written by doctors and directed at medical professionals.

Emedicine Medscape Reference

℘ http://emedicine.medscape.com.

A US website provides comprehensive information on drugs, diseases, procedures classified under individual specialties in an A-Z format. There are peer reviewed CME modules on a wide range of clinical conditions.

Neurological and developmental disorders

℘ http://www.simulconsult.com.

Further reading

NOTE: This chapter contains a selection (key) of references and recommendations for sources of further reading. This is not an exhaustive list.

Chapter 1: Introduction to community paediatrics

Roles of a community paediatrician

American Academy of Paediatrics (Committee on Community Health Services). The Paediatrician's Role in Community Paediatrics. *Paediatrics* 1999; **103**:1304–7.

Royal College of Paediatrics and Child Health. *Strengthening the care of children in the community.* London: RCPCH; 2002.

Ukpeh H. Community Paediatrics: Ideas for the way forward. *Paediatr Child Health* 2009; **14**:299–302.

Consultation in the community

Kurtz SM, Silverman JD. The Calgary-Cambridge Referenced Observation Guide. An aid to defining the curriculum and organising the teaching in communication training programmes. *Med Educ* 1996; **30**:83–9.

History taking

Horridge KA. Assessment and investigation of the child with disordered development. *Arch Dis Child Educ Pract Ed* 2011; **96**:9–20.

Kurtz SM, Silverman JD. The Calgary-Cambridge Referenced Observation Guide: An aid to defining the curriculum and organising the teaching in communication training programmes. *Med Educ* 1996; **30**:83–9.

Child development

Illingworth RS. *The Development of the Infant & Young Child – Normal & Abnormal*, 9th edn. Edinburgh: Churchill Livingstone, 1997.

Luiz D et al. *GMDS-ER Two to Eight years, Administration Manual.* Oxford: Hogrefe –The Test Agency, 2006: ℘ http://www.aricd.org.uk

Chapter 2: Working with child and family

Communicating with children

Hockenberry MJ. Communication and physical assessment of the child. In: Hockenberry MJ, Wilson D (eds) *Wong's Nursing care of infants and children*, 9th edn. St Louis, MO: Elsevier Mosby, 2010.

Child- and family-centred care

American Academy of Pediatrics. Committee on Hospital Care. Institute for family-centred care. Policy statement. Organizational Principles to Guide and Define the Child Health Care System and/or Improve the Health of All Children. Family-Centered Care and the Pediatrician's Role. *Pediatrics* 2003; **112**(3):691–6.

Jolley J, Shields L. The evolution of family-centered care. *J Pediatr Nurs* 2009; **24**(2):164–70.

Child development team

Court SDM. *Fit for the future. Report of the Committee on Child Health Services.* London: HMSO, 1976.

Multidisciplinary working

Sloper P. Facilitators and barriers for co-ordinated multi-agency services. *Child Care Health Dev* 2004; **30**(6):571–80.

Providing information, support, and advice

Scope. *Right From the Start Template: Good practice in sharing the news.* 2003. Available from: ℘ http://rightfromthestart.org.uk

The Foundation for People with Learning Disabilities. *First Impressions: Emotional and practical support for families of a young child with a learning disability.* 2005. Available from: ℘ http://www.learningdisabilities.org.uk

Pain H. Coping with a child with disabilities from the parents' perspective: the function of information. *Child Care Health Dev* 1999; **25**(4):299–312.

Care of siblings

O'Brien I et al. Impact of childhood chronic illnesses on siblings: a literature review. *Br J Nurs* 2009; **18**(22):1358.

Chapter 3: Development

Principles of neurodevelopmental testing

Luiz D et al. GMDS-ER Two to Eight years, Administration Manual. Oxford: Hogrefe –The Test Agency, 2006: ℘ http://www.aricd.org.uk

Tips on 'real-world' developmental testing

Luiz D et al. GMDS-ER Two to Eight years, Administration Manual. Oxford: Hogrefe –The Test Agency, 2006: ℘ http://www.aricd.org.uk

℘http://www.psychcorp.co.uk/Psychology/ChildCognitionNeuropsychologyandLanguage/ ChildNon-verbalAbilities/Goodenough-HarrisDrawingTest/Goodenough-HarrisDrawingTest. aspx#top

℘ http://www.sdqinfo.com

Fine motor skills

Sheridan MD. From Birth to Five Years Children's Developmental Progress. London: Routledge, 1997.
Erhardt RP. Developmental Hand Dysfunction Theory, Assessment, and Treatment 2nd edn. Texas: Therapy Skill Builders, 1994.

Chapter 4: Neurodevelopmental disorders

ICF-CY and application to childhood disability

Msall ME, Msall ER. Functional Assessment in Neurodevelopmental Disorders. Vol I. Capute & Accardo's Neurodevelopmental Disabilities in Infancy & Childhood, 3rd edn. Baltimore, MD: Paul H Brooks Publishing Co., 2008.
Rosenbaum P. Childhood disability & social policies. BMJ 2009; **338**:bmj.b1020.
World Health Organization. International Classification of Functioning, Disability and Health for Children and Youth. Geneva: WHO, 2007.

Cerebral palsy

Gupta R, Appleton RE. Cerebral palsy: not always what it seems. Arch Dis Child 2001; **85**:356–60.
Johnson MW et al. Neurobiology, Diagnosis & Management of Cerebral Palsy. In Accardo PJ (ed) Capute & Accardo's Neurodevelopmental Disabilities in Infancy & Childhood, Vol II: The Spectrum of Neurodevelopmental Disabilities, 3rd edn. Baltimore, MD: Paul H Brooks Publishing Co., 2008.
Krageloh-Mann I, Bax M. Cerebral Palsy. p 210–242. Clinics in Developmental Medicine. Diseases of the Nervous System in Childhood. 3rd edn. London: Mac Keith Press. 2009.
Miller G et al. Clinical Manifestations; Diagnosis of Cerebral Palsy. ℘ http://www.uptodate.com Accessed 18 Nov 2011. UpToDate©

Gastroenterological care of a child with disability

Sullivan PB. Gastrointestinal disorders in children with neurodevelopmental disabilities. Dev Disabil Res Rev 2008; **14**(2):128–36.
Sullivan PB. Feeding and Nutrition in Children with Neurodevelopmental Disability. London: Mac Keith Press, 2009.

Respiratory care of a child with disability

Hull J et al. Paediatric Respiratory Medicine. Oxford: Oxford University Press, 2008.
Marks JH. Pulmonary care of children and adolescents with developmental disabilities. Pediatr Clin N Am 2008; **55**:1299–314.

Bone health in children with disability

Bachrach LK. Biphosphonates use in childhood osteoporosis. Clinical review. J Clin Endocrin Metab 2009; **94**(2):400–9.
Hough et al. Systemic review of interventions for low bone mineral density in children with cerebral palsy. Pediatrics 2010; **125**:e670
Houlihan CM, Stevenson RD. Bone density in CP. Phys Med Rehab Clin N Am 2009; **20**(3):493–508.
Ward L et al. Bisphosphonate therapy for children and adolescents with secondary osteoporosis. Cochrane Database Syst Rev 2007; Issue 4.

Gynaecological care of the child disability

Greydanus DE, Omar HA. Sexuality issues and gynaecologic care of adolescents with developmental disabilities. Pediatr Clin N Am 2008; **55**:1315–35.

Hospice and care of the dying child

Amery J. *Children's palliative care handbook for GPs* (Woodhead S, ed). Bristol: ACT, Association for Children's Palliative Care, 2011, ⅋ http://www.act.org.uk

Bennett H, Ilic M. Care of the child after death: guidance for children's hospice services. Children's Hospices UK, 2011.

Helen and Douglas House Palliative Care Toolkit 2010, available on the Helen and Douglas House website: ⅋ http://www.helenanddouglas.org.uk/

Hindmarsh C. *On the Death of a Child*, 3rd edn. Abingdon: Radcliffe Publishing, 2000.

Autistic spectrum disorders

Ministry of Health and Education. *New Zealand Autism Spectrum Disorder guideline*, 2008. www.moh.govt.nz/autismspectrumdisorder

Ministry of Health Singapore. *Autism Spectrum Disorders in preschool children.* Available at: M www.moh.gov.sg/cpg 2010.

Missouri Autism Guidelines Initiative. *Autism Spectrum Disorders: Missouri Best Practice Guidelines for screening, diagnosis and assessment.* Available at: ⅋ www.autismguidelines.dmh.mo.gov 2010.

National Autism Plan for Children (2003). Available at: ⅋ www.autism.org.uk

New York State Department of Health. *Report of the Guideline Recommendations Autism / Pervasive Developmental Disorders. Assessment and Intervention for Young Children (Age 0–3 Years).* New York State Department of Health Early Intervention Program. Available at: ⅋ http://www.health.state.ny.us/community/infants_children/early_intervention/disorders/autism/index.htm#Table_of_Contents 2005.

NICE. *Autism: recognition, referral and diagnosis of children and young people on the autism spectrum. NICE clinical guidelines 128*, 2011. Available at: ⅋ http://www.nice.org.uk/nicemedia/live/13572/56428/56428.pdf

Ohio Developmental Disabilities Council. *Service guidelines for individuals with autism spectrum disorder/ pervasive developmental disorder (ASD/PDD).* Available at: ⅋ http://www.asgc.org/downloads/autismbook.pdf

Scottish Intercollegiate Guideline Network. *Assessment, diagnosis and clinical interventions for children and young people with autism spectrum disorders, a national clinical guideline, number 98.* July 2007. Available at: ⅋ http://www.sign.ac.uk/pdf/sign98.pdf

Intellectual disability/LD

Learning Disabilities – Suspected & Multidisciplinary Management. Contributors invited by Map of Medicine Ltd. Published 26 Apr 2011. Available at: ⅋ http://mapofmedicine.com/map/legal

Kruti Acahrya et al. The spectrum of cognitive-adaptive developmental disorders in intellectual disabilities. In Accardo PJ (ed) *Capute & Accardo's Neurodevelopmental Disabilities in Infancy & Childhood, Vol II: The Spectrum of Neurodevelopmental Disabilities*, 3rd edn, pp. 241–59. Baltimore, MD: Paul H Brooks Publishing Co., 2008.

Pivalizza P et al. Intellectual disability in children: definition, causes, diagnosis/evaluation/management. January 2011 Literature review, *Up-To-Date®*.

Shevell M. Global developmental delay and mental retardation or intellectual disability: Conceptualisation, evaluation & aetiology. *Pediatr Clin N Am* 2008; **55**:1071–84.

Investigation of developmental delay

Horridge KA. Assessment & investigation of the child with disordered development. *Arch Dis Child Educ Pract Ed* 2011; **96**:9–20.

McDonald L et al. Investigation of global developmental delay. *Arch Dis Child* 2006; **91**:701–5.

Shevell M. Global developmental delay & mental retardation or intellectual disability: conceptualization, evaluation & etiology. *Pediatr Clin N Am* 2008; **55**:1071–84.

ADHD

American Psychiatric Association. *Diagnostic and Statistical Manual of Mental Disorders (DSM-IV)*, 4th edn. Washington DC: APA, 1994.

NICE. *ADHD: Diagnosis and management of ADHD in children, young people and adults. Clinical guideline 72.* London: NICE; 2008.

Taylor E (ed). *People with Hyperactivity: Understanding and managing their problems. CDM 171.* London: Mac Keith Press, 2007.

SIGN. *Management of attention deficit and hyperkinetic disorders in children and young people. A national clinical guideline. SIGN publication no.122.* Edinburgh: SIGN, 2009.

World Health Organization. *International Statistical Classification of Diseases and Related Health Problems*, 10th rev edn. Geneva: WHO, 1994.

DCD

Gibbs J et al. Dyspraxia or Developmental Coordination Disorder? Unravelling the enigma. Review article. *Arch Dis Child* 2007; **92**:534.

Sugden D. Current approaches to intervention in children with developmental coordination disorder. *Dev Med Child Neurol* 2007; **49**:467.

Sutton Hamilton S et al. Overview of developmental coordination disorder. *UpToDate©*. ℘ http:// www.uptodate.com. Accessed 18 Nov 2011.

The 2006 Leeds Consensus statement. Available at: ℘ http://www.dcd-uk.org/diagnosis_c-d.html

Apraxia of speech

ASHA Practice Policy. *Childhood Apraxia of Speech. Ad Hoc Committee on AOS in Children. Technical Report 2007.* Available at: ℘ http://www.asha.org/docs/html/TR2007-00278.html

Simms MD. Language disorders in children: Classification and clinical syndromes. *Pediatr Clin N Am* 2007; **54**:43–67.

Developmental dyslexia

Grizzle KL.. Developmental dyslexia. *Pediatr Clin N Am* 2007; **54**:507–23.

Shaywitz SE et al. Management of dyslexia, its rationale, and underlying neurobiology. *Pediatr Clin N Am* 2007; **54**:609–23.

Developmental dysgraphia and dyscalculia

Von Hahn LK et al. Specific learning Disabilities in Children: Clinical features. ℘ http://www.uptodate.com. Accessed 18 May 2011. *UpToDate®*

Von Hahn LK et al. Specific learning Disabilities in Children: Educational management. ℘ http:// www.uptodate.com. Accessed 18 May 2011. *UpToDate®*

Inherited metabolic disorders

Cleary MA et al. Developmental Delay: when to suspect and how to investigate for an inborn error of metabolism. *Arch Dis Child* 2005, **90**:1128–32.

Emergency management guidelines for IMDs. Available at: ℘ http://www.bimdg.org.uk

Green A et al. National Metabolic Biochemistry Network. Best Practice Guidelines for the Biochemical Investigation of Global Developmental Delay for Inborn Errors of Metabolism (IMD). Available at: ℘ http://www.metbio.net.

Kamboj M. Clinical approach to the diagnoses of inborn errors of metabolism. *Pediatr Clin N Am* 2008; **5**:1113–29.

Incontinence in children with DD

Rogers J. One step at a time: how to toilet train children with learning disabilities. *Nursing Times* 2010; **106**:47

Sleep disorders and management

American Academy of Sleep Medicine. Practice parameters for behavioural treatment of bedtime problems & night wakings in infants & young children. *Sleep* 2006; **29**:1263–76.

Galland BC, Mitchell EA. Helping children sleep. *Arch Dis Child* 2010; **95**:850–3.

Nutter DA, Pataki C. Pediatric sleep disorders. Available at: ℘ http://emedicine.medscape.com. Accessed 20 Aug 2011.

Phillips L, Appleton RE. Systematic review of Melatonin in children with neurodevelopmental disabilities. Cochrane Database (Accessed 19 August 2011).

Chapter 5: Consults with allied professionals

Physiotherapy: approaches to treatment

Green EM et al. *The Chailey Approach to Postural Management: An Explanation of the Theoretical Aspects of Posture Management and Their Practical Application Through Treatment and Equipment,* 2nd rev edn. East Sussex: Chailey Heritage Clinical Services, 2004.

Sheridan M et al. *From Birth to Five Years: Children's Developmental Progress,* 3rd rev edn. London: Routledge, 2007.

Staheli LT, Song KM. *Pediatric orthopaedic secrets,* 3rd edn. Philadelphia, PA: Hanley & Belfus, Inc, 2007.

GMFCS and GMFM

Palisano R et al. Content validity of the expanded and revised Gross Motor Function Classification System. *Dev Med Child Neurol* 2008; **50**:744–50.

Rosenbaum P et al. Prognosis for gross motor function in cerebral palsy: Creation of motor development curves. *JAMA* 2002; **288**:1357–63.

Posture management and special seating

Pope P. *Severe and Complex Disability: Management of the Physical Condition.* London: Butterworth Heinemann, 2006.

Occupational therapy: principles and assessment

Case-Smith J, O'Brien JC. *Occupational Therapy for Children*, 6th edn. St Louis, MO: Mosby, 2009.

Occupational therapy: aids and adaptations

Case-Smith, J., O'Brien, J.C. (2009). *Occupational Therapy for Children* 6th edn. St Louis, MO:. Mosby, 2009.

Oxfordshire Grant-aided. *Home Adaptations bringing independence to people with disabilities who live in privately-owned of rented housing.* Oxford: Oxfordshire County Council, 2009.

Occupational therapy: enabling hand function

Case-Smith J, O'Brien JC. *Occupational Therapy for Children*, 6th edn. St Louis, MO: Mosby, 2009.

Erhardt RP. *Developmental Hand Dysfunction Theory, Assessment, and Treatment,* 2nd edn. Austin, TX: Therapy Skill Builders, 1994.

Poutney TE et al. *The Chailey Approach to Postural Management: An Explanation of the Theoretical Aspects of Posture Management and Their Practical Application Through Treatment and Equipment.* East Sussex: Chailey Heritage Clinical Services, 2004.

Occupational therapy: sensory integration

Bundy, AC et al. *Sensory Integration Theory and Practice,* 2nd edn. Philadelphia, PA: F.A Davis, 2002.

Case-Smith J, O'Brien JC. *Occupational Therapy for Children*, 6th edn. St Louis, MO: Mosby, 2009.

Kranowitz CS. *The Out-of-Sync Child Has Fun Activities for Kids with Sensory Processing Disorder (revised edition).* New York: Perigee Trade, 2006.

Miller LJ *Sensational Kids Hope and Help for Children with Sensory Processing Disorder (SPD).* London: Penguin Group, 2006.

Speech and language therapy

Bercow J. *The Bercow Report. A review of services for children and young people 0-19 with speech, language and communication needs.* London: Department for Children, Schools and Families, 2008.

Buckley B. *Childrens' communication skills from birth to 5 years.* London: Routledge, 2003.

Crystal D. *Listen to your child, a parent's guide to children's language.* London: Penguin Health Books, 1989.

Neuropsychology

Davis A. *The Handbook of Pediatric Neuropsychology.* Springer, 2010.

Flanagan DP, Kaufman AS. *Essentials of WISC-IV Assessment. Essentials of Psychological Assessment,* 2nd edn. Hoboken, NJ: Wiley, 2009.

Rutter M et al. *Rutter's Child and Adolescent Psychiatry,* 5th edn. Oxford: Blackwell, 2008.

Orthoses

Gage JR et al. *The identification and treatment of Gait Problems in Cerebral Palsy,* 2nd edn. London: Wiley, Mac Keith Press.

Hsu JD, et al. *AAOS Atlas of Orthoses and Assistive Devices,* 4th ed. Philadelphia, PA: Mosby, 2008

Morris C, Dias L. (eds) *Paediatric Orthotics.* London: Mac Keith Press, 2007.

Morris C et al. *ISPO Cerebral Palsy Consensus Conference Report,* 2009 (available free at ℘ http://www.ispoint.org).

Chapter 6: Neurology

Aicardi J. *Diseases of the Nervous System in Childhood,* 3rd edn. London: Mac Keith Press, 2009.

Appleton R, Boudewyn Peters AC. *Common Neurological Problems in General Paediatrics,* London: Martin Dunitz, 2003.

Cohen M, Duffner P. *Weiner and Levitt's Pediatric Neurology,* 4th edn. Philadelphia, PA: Lippincott Williams and Wilkins, 2003.

Forsyth R, Newton R.. *Paediatric Neurology*. Oxford: Oxford University Press, 2007.

Lindsay K, Bone I. *Neurology and Neurosurgery Illustrated*, 3rd edn. London: Churchill Livingstone, 1999.

Fenichel GM. *Clinical Paediatric Neurology. A Signs and Symptoms Approach*, 6th edn. Philadelphia, PA: Elsevier Saunders, 2009.

Chapter 7: Vision

Denniston AKO, Murray PI (eds). *Oxford Handbook of Ophthalmology*, 2nd edn. Oxford: Oxford University Press, 2009.

James B, Benjamin L. *Ophthalmology: Investigation and Examination Techniques*. London: Butterworth-Heinemann, 2007.

Taylor D, Hoyt C. *Pediatric Ophthalmology*, 4th edn. Philadelphia, PA: Elsevier, 2011.

Chapter 8: Hearing

American National Standards Institute. *Acoustical performance criteria, design requirements and guidelines for schools*. Washington DC: ANSI S12.60, 2002.

Auditory Processing Disorder (APD) Steering Committee, British Society of Audiology. *Interim position statement on APD*, 2007. Available at: ℅ www.thebsa.org.uk/apd/BSA_APD_Position_statement_Final_Draft _Feb_ 2007.doc

BAAP/BAPA. *Guidelines for aetiological investigation of infants with congenital hearing loss identified through newborn hearing screening. Best practice guidelines*, 2009. Available at: ℅ http://www.baap.org.uk.

Bamiou D-E, et al. Aetiology and clinical presentations of auditory processing disorders – a review. *Arch Dis Child* 2001; **85**:361–5.

Bamiou D-E, Luxon LM. Auditory processing disorders. *BMJ 2008*; **337**:1306–7.

Browning GG et al. Grommets (ventilation tubes) for hearing loss associated with otitis media with effusion in children. *Cochrane Database Syst Rev* 2011; **10**:CD001801.

Griffin G et al. Antihistamines and/or decongestants for otitis media with effusion (OME) in children. *Cochrane Database Syst Rev* 2006; **4**:CD003423.

Kimberling WJ. Genetic hearing loss associated with eye disorders. In: Toriello HV et al. (eds) *Hereditary Hearing Loss and its Syndromes*, 2nd edn. Oxford: Oxford University Press, 2004.

Luxon LM, et al. (eds). *Textbook of Audiological Medicine*. London: Martin Dunitz, 2003

Moore DR, et al. Effects of otitis media with effusion (OME) on central auditory function. *Int Jl Pediatr Otorhinolaryngol* 2003; **67**(Suppl. 1):S63–S67.

Newton VE (ed). *Paediatric Audiological Medicine*, 2nd edn. Chichester: John Wiley & Sons, Ltd., 2009.

Niemensivu R et al. (2006). Vertigo and balance problems in children – an epidemiological study in Finland. *Int J Pediatr Otorhinolaryngol* **70**(2):259–65.

Russel G, Abu-Arafeh I. Paroxysmal vertigo in children – an epidemiological study. *Int J Pediatr Otorhinolaryngol* 1999; **49**(Suppl 1):S105–S107.

Simpson SA et al. Oral or topical nasal steroids for hearing loss associated with otitis media with effusion in children. *Cochrane Database Syst Rev* 2011; **5**:CD001935.

Stephens D et al. Audiological, epidemiological and genetic definitions. In: Martini A et al. (eds) *Definitions, protocols & guidelines in genetic hearing impairment*. London: Whurr, 2001.

Wiener-Vacher SR. Vestibular disorders in children. *Int J Audiol* 2008; **47**:578–83.

Chapter 9: Mental health

Introduction

American Psychiatric Association. *DSM-IV-TR: Diagnostic and statistical manual of mental disorders*, 4th ed. Text revision. Washington DC: American Psychiatric Press Inc., 2000.

Garralda ME, Bailey D. Psychiatric disorders in general paediatric referrals. *Arch Dis Childhood* 1989; **64**:1727–33.

World Health Organization. *ICD-10: The ICD-10 classification of mental and behavioural disorders: clinical descriptions and diagnostic guidelines*. Geneva: WHO, 1992.

Working with CAMHS

Graham P. Paediatric referral to a child psychiatrist. *Arch Dis Child* 1984; **59**:1103–5.

The psychiatric evaluation

Rutter M et al. *Rutter's child and adolescent psychiatry*. Oxford: Wiley-Blackwell, 2008.

Psychological aspects of LD

Allington-Smith P. Mental health of children with learning disabilities. *Adv Psychiatr Treat* 2006; **12**:13–8.

ASD-CAMHS aspects

Attwood T. Asperger's Syndrome: a guide for parents and professionals. London: Jessica Kingsley Publishers, 1997.

Dunn Buron K., Curtis M. *The incredible 5-point scale: assisting children with ASDs in understanding social interactions and controlling their emotional responses.* Shawnee Mission KS: Autism Asperger Publishing Co, 2003.

Elvins R, Green J. Pharmacological management of core and comorbid symptoms in autism-spectrum disorders. *Advances Psychiatric Treat* 2010; **16**:349–60.

McPheeters ML *et al.* A systematic review of medical treatments for children with autism spectrum disorders. *Pediatrics* 2011; **127**(5):e1312–21.

Myers SM, Johnson CP. Management of children with autism spectrum disorders. *Pediatrics* 2007; **120**:1162–82.

Scottish Intercollegiate Guidelines Network. *Assessment, diagnosis and clinical interventions for children and young people with autism spectrum disorders, Guideline No. 98.* Edinburgh: SIGN, 2007. Available at: ℘ http://www.sign.ac.uk/guidelines/fulltext/98/index.html

Asperger syndrome

Attwood T. *Asperger's Syndrome: a guide for parents and professionals.* London: Jessica Kingsley Publishers, 1997.

Gallo DP. Diagnosing autism spectrum disorders: a lifespan perspective. London: Wiley-Blackwell, 2010.

NICE. *Autism spectrum disorders in children and young people: full guideline.* London: NICE. Available at: ℘ http://www.nice.org.uk/

Scottish Intercollegiate Guidelines Network. *Assessment, diagnosis and clinical interventions for children and young people with autism spectrum disorders, Guideline No. 98.* Edinburgh: SIGN, 2007. Available at: ℘ http://www.sign.ac.uk/guidelines/fulltext/98/index.html

Tic disorder

Cath D *et al.* European clinical guidelines for Tourette Syndrome and other tic disorders. Part I: assessment. *Eur Child Adolesc Psychiatry* 2011; **20**:155–71.

Roessner V *et al.* European clinical guidelines for Tourette Syndrome and other tic disorders. Part II: pharmacological treatment. *Eur Child Adolesc Psychiatry* 2011; **20**:173–96.

Conduct disorder and ODD

Keen D. Conduct disorders and us: from heart sink to heart warming? *Arch Dis Child* 2007; **92**:838–41.

Webster-Stratton C. *The incredible years.* Seattle, WA: Incredible years, 2006.

Enuresis

NICE. *Nocturnal enuresis – the management of bedwetting and nocturnal enuresis in children and young people.* London: NICE, 2010. Available at: ℘ http://guidance.nice.org.uk/CG111

Preschool behaviour problems

Gardner F, Shaw D. Behavioral problems of infancy and preschool children (0–5). In Rutter M *et al.* (eds) *Rutter's Child and Adolescent Psychiatry,* pp. 882–93. London: Blackwell Publishing Limited, 2008.

School refusal

Creswell C, Willetts L. *Overcoming your child's shyness and social anxiety: a self-help guide using cognitive behavioral techniques.* London: Robinson Publishing, 2007.

Heyne D, Rollings S. *School refusal (parent, adolescent and child training skills 2).* London: Wiley-Blackwell, 2002.

Kearney C, Silverman W. Measuring the function of school refusal behavior: the school refusal assessment scale. *J Clin Child Psych* 1993; **22**(1):85–96.

Attachment disorders

Rees CA. Thinking about children's attachments. *Arch Dis Child* 2005; **90**:1058–65.

Consequences of child abuse

American Academy of Paediatrics. Understanding the behavioral and emotional consequences of child abuse. *Pediatrics* 2008; **122**(3):667–73.

Depression

Chrisman A et al. Assessment of childhood depression. *Child Adoles Mental Health* 2006; **11**:111–16.

Gilbert P. Overcoming depression: a self-help guide using cognitive behavioral techniques. Robinson, 2009. Adult book suitable for older adolescents.

NICE. *Depression in children and young people: identification and management in primary, community and secondary care.* London: NICE, 2005. Available at: ℘ http://www.nice.org.uk/CG28

Suicide and deliberate self-harm

NICE. *Clinical guideline CG 16, Self-harm: The short-term physical and psychological management and secondary prevention of self-harm in primary and secondary care.* London: NICE, 2004. Available at: ℘ http://guidance.nice.org.uk/CG16

Wood A. Self-harm in adolescents. *Adv Psychiatr Treat* 2009; **15**:434–41.

Anxiety disorders

AACAP Official Action. Practice parameters for the assessment and treatment of children and adolescents with anxiety disorders. *J Am Acad Child Adoles Pscyhiat* 2007; **46**:267–83.

Creswell C, Willetts L. *Overcoming your child's shyness and social anxiety: a self-help guide using cognitive behavioral techniques.* London: Robinson Publishing, 2007.

Rapee R, et al. *Helping your anxious child: a step-by-step guide for parents.* Oakland, CA: New Harbinger Publications, 2008.

Eating disorders

American Academy of Pediatrics, Rosen D. Clinical report: identification and management of eating disorders in children and adolescents. *Pediatrics* 2010; **126**:1240–53.

National Institute for Health and Clinical Excellence. *Eating disorders: Core interventions in the treatment and management of anorexia nervosa, bulimia nervosa and related eating disorders.* London: NICE, 2007. Available at: ℘ http://guidance.nice.org.uk/CG9

Treasure J, Smith G, Crane A. *Skills-based Learning for Caring for a Loved One with an Eating Disorder: The New Maudsley Method.* London: Routledge, 2007.

Somatizing disorders

Leary P. Conversion disorder in childhood – diagnosed too late, investigated too much? *J R Soc Med* 2003; **96**:436–8.

Sibler T. Somatization disorders: diagnosis, treatment, and prognosis. *Pediatr Rev* 2011; **32**:56–64.

CFS and ME

NICE. *Chronic fatigue syndrome/myalgic encephalomyelitis (or encephalopathy): diagnosis and management of CFS/ME in adults and children.* London: NICE, 2007. Available at: ℘ http://guidance.nice.org.uk/CG53

Royal College of Paediatrics and Child Health. *Evidence based guideline for the management of CFS/ME in children and young people.* London: RCPCH, 2004. Available at: ℘ http://www.rcpch.ac.uk/rcpch-guidelines

Chronic illness and mental health

American Academy of Child and Adolescent Psychiatry Official Action. Practice parameter for the psychiatric assessment and management of physically ill children and adolescents. *J Am Acad Child Adolesc* 2009; **48**:213–33.

PTSD

American Academy of Child and Adolescent Psychiatry. Practice parameter for the assessment and treatment of children and adolescents with posttraumatic stress disorder. *J Am Acad Child Adolesc Psychiat* 2010; **49**:107–25.

Dyergrov A and Yule W. A Review of PTSD in Children. *Child Adolesc Mental Health* 2006; **11**(4):176–84.

National Institute for Health and Clinical Excellence. *CG26 Post-traumatic stress disorder (PTSD): The management of PTSD in adults and children in primary and secondary care.* London: NICE, 2005. Available at: ℘ http://www.nice.org.uk/CG26.

Taureen A et al. Best practice: Post-traumatic stress disorder in childhood. *Arch Dis Child, Ed Prac Ed* 2007; **92**:ep1–ep6.

Alcohol and substance use

Jones R et al. What paediatricians should know about young people and drugs in the UK. *Arc Dis Child Educ Pract Ed* 2006; **91**:81–6.

Parenting

Royal College of Psychiatrists. *CR 164. Parents as patients: supporting the needs of patients who are parents and their children.* London: RCP, 2011. Available at: ℘ http://www.rcpsych.ac.uk/publications/collegereports

Webster-Stratton C. *The incredible years.* Seattle WA: Incredible years.

Treatment non-adherence

La Greca A, Mackey E. Adherence to pediatric treatment regimens. In Roberts M, Steele R (eds) *The Handbook of Pediatric Psychology,* 4th edn, New York: The Guildford Press, 2009.

McNamara E. Motivational interviewing: theory, practice and applications in children and young people. Merseyside: Positive Behaviour Management (PBM), 2009.

NICE. *Medicines adherence: involving patients in decisions about prescribed medicines and supporting adherence. Clinical guideline CG76.* London: NICE, 2009. Available at: ℘ http://guidance.nice.org.uk/CG76

World Health Organization. *Adherence to long-term therapies: evidence for action.* Geneva: WHO, 2003. Available at: ℘ http://www.who.int/chp/knowledge/publications

Chapter 10: Genetics

Gorlin RJ et al. (eds.) *Syndromes of the head and neck,* 4th edn. Oxford: Oxford University Press, 1989.

Harper PS. *Practical Genetic Counselling,* 6th edn, revised reprint. London: Arnold, 2004.

Jones KL (ed.) *Smith's recognisable patterns of human malformations,* 5th edn. Philadelphia, PA: W.B. Saunders, 1997.

Rimoin DL et al. *Emery and Rimoin's principles and practices of medical genetics,* 4th edn. Edinburgh: Churchill Livingstone, 2002.

Strachan M, Read AP. *Human Molecular Genetics,* 3rd edn. Philadelphia, PA: Garland Science, 2003.

Winter RM, Barraister M (eds.) *London Dysmorphology Database 2003.* ℘ http://www.lmdatabses.com

Chapter 11: Orthopaedics

Bevan WP et al. Arthrogryposis multiplex congenital (amyoplasia): an orthopaedic perspective. *JPO* 2007; **27**:594–600.

Cornell MS. The hip in cerebral palsy. *Dev Med Child Neurol* 1995; **37**:3–18.

Davids et al. Validation of the Shriners Hospital for Children Upper Extremity Evaluation (SHUEE) for children with hemiplegic cerebral palsy. *JBJS* 2006; **88**:326–33.

Dobson F et al. Hip surveillance in children with cerebral palsy. *JBJS* 2002; **84-B**:720–6.

Gage JR. *The Treatment of Gait Problems in Cerebral Palsy.* London: Mac Keith Press distributed by Cambridge University Press, 2004.

Krumlinde-Sundholm L et al. The Assisting Hand Assessment: current evidence of validity, reliability, and responsiveness to change. *Dev Med Child Neurol* 2007; **49**(4):259–64.

Smith R et al. *Clinical and Biochemical disorders of the skeleton.* Oxford: Oxford University Press, 2005.

Spranger JW et al. *Bone Dysplasias.* Oxford: Oxford University Press, 2002.

Staheli L. *Clubfoot: Ponseti Management,* 3rd edn. Global Help, 2007. Available at: ℘ http://www.global-help.org/publications/books/help_cfponseti.pdf

Ward L et al. Bisphosphonate therapy for children and adolescents with secondary osteoporosis. *Cochrane Database Syst Rev* 2007; **4**:CD005324.

Chapter 12: Child abuse

Epidemiology

NSPCC. *Child Cruelty in the UK 2011 An NSPCC study into child abuse over the past 30 years.* London: NSPCC.

Bruises

Maguire S. Which injuries may indicate child abuse? *Arch Dis in Child*, 2010; **95**(6):170–7.

Sugar NF *et al*. Bruises in infants and toddlers: those who don't cruise rarely bruise. *Arch Pediatr Adolesc Med* 1999; **153**:399–403.

Stephenson T, Bialas Y. Estimation of the age of bruising. *Arch Dis Child* 1996; **74**(1):53–5.

Fractures

Maguire S. Does cardiopulmonary resuscitation cause rib fractures in children? A systematic review. *Child Abuse Negl* 2006; **30**(7):739–51.

CSA

Berenson A *et al*. Appearance of the hymen in prepubertal girls. *Pediatrics* 1992; **89**(3):387–94.

Hobbs C *et al*. *Child Abuse and Neglect. A Clinician's Handbook*, 2nd edn, pp.196–7. London: Churchill Livingstone, 1999.

Heger A *et al*. *Evaluation of the Sexually Abused Child*, 2nd edn. Oxford: Oxford University Press, 2000.

Heger AH *et al*. Appearance of the genitalia in girls selected for nonabuse: review of hymenal morphology and nonspecific findings. *J Pediatr Adolesc Gynecol* 2002; **15**(1):27–35.

NICE. When to suspect child maltreatment. London: NICE, 2009.

Ofsted. Learning the lessons from serious case reviews 2009-10. London: Ofsted, 2010. Available at: ℘ http://www.ofsted.gov.uk/publications/100087.

Offiah AC, Hall CM. *Radiological Atlas of Child Abuse*. Oxford: Radcliffe Publishing, 2009.

RCPCH. *Child Protection Companion*. London: RCPCH, 2006.

RCPCH. *Child Protection Reader*. London: RCPCH, 2007.

RCPCH. *The Physical Signs of Child Sexual Abuse*. London: RCPCH, 2008.

RCPCH. *Fabricated or Induced Illness by Carers (FII). A practical Guide For Paediatricians*. London: RCPCH, 2009.

Other resources

Local OSCB guidelines/procedures.

HM Government. *Working Together to Safeguard Children*. London: Department for Education, 2010.

HM Government (16 November 1989). Children Act.

Chapter 13: Adoption, fostering, and looked-after children

Department for Education and Skills. *Care Matters: Transforming the Lives of Children and Young People in Care*. London: The Stationery Office 2006.

Department of Health. *Promoting the health and wellbeing of looked after children*. London: Department of Health, 2009.

National Institute for Health and Clinical Excellence. *NICE Public health Guidance 4: Community based interventions to reduce substance misuse among vulnerable and disadvantaged children and young people*. London: NICE, 2007.

National Institute for Health and Clinical Excellence. *NICE Public Health Guidance 24: Alcohol use disorders: Preventing the development of hazardous and harmful drinking*. London: NICE, 2010.

National Institute for Health and Clinical Excellence. *NICE Public Health Guidance 28: Promoting the quality of life for looked after children and young people*. London: NICE, 2010.

Wade J *et al*. (ed) *Unaccompanied asylum seeking children: the response of social work services*. London: British Agencies for Adoption and Fostering, 2005.

Adolescents in public care

Meltzer H *et al*. *Mental health of children and adolescents in Great Britain*. London: The Stationary Office, 2000.

Meltzer H *et al*. *The mental health of young people looked after by local authorities in England*. London: The Stationary Office, 2003.

Vinnerljung B, *et al*. Teenage parenthood among child welfare clients: A Swedish national cohort study of prevalence and odds. *J Adolescence* 2007; **30**(1):97–116

Vinnerljung B, Sallnäs M. Into adulthood: a follow-up study of 718 young people who were placed in out-of-home care during their teens. *Child Family Social Work* 2008; **13**(2):144–55.

Intercountry adoption

British Agencies for Adoption and Fostering produces a practice note on '*Health screening of children adopted from abroad*'.

Selman P (ed). *Intercountry adoption; developmental, trends and perspectives.* London: British Agencies for Adoption and Fostering, 2000.

Chapter 14: Social paediatrics

UNCRC

Royal College of Paediatrics and Child Health. *Not just a phase – a guide to the participation of children and young people in health services.* London: RCPCH, 2010.

Toward Equity in Health: A Joint Meeting of the Royal College of Paediatrics and Child Health and the American Academy of Pediatrics September 2000. *Pediatrics* 2003; **12**(Suppl):700–72.

Environmental determinants of health

Health Protection Agency. *A Children's Environment and Health Strategy for the UK.* Health Protection Agency, Didcot, 2009.

National Institute for Health and Clinical Excellence. *Obesity; guidance on the prevention, identification, assessment and management of overweight and obesity in adults and children.* London: NICE: 2006.

National Institute for Health and Clinical Excellence. *Strategies to prevent unintentional injuries among children and young people aged under 15.* London: NICE: 2010.

National Institute for Health and Clinical Excellence. *Preventing unintentional injuries in the home among children and young people aged under 15: home safety assessments and providing safety equipment.* London: NICE: 2010.

National Institute for Health and Clinical Excellence. *Preventing unintentional injuries among children and young people aged under 15: road design and modification.* NICE, London, 2010.

World Health Organization. *Children's Environment and Health Action Plan for Europe.* Fourth Ministerial Conference on Environment and Health. Budapest 23–25 June, 2004.

Child poverty and inequalities in health

Acheson D. *Independent Inquiry into Inequalities in Health Report.* London: The Stationery Office, 1998.

Black D et al. *Report of the Working Party on Inequalities in Health.* London: DHSS, 1980.

Marmot M. *Fair Society, Healthy Lives:* London: UCL, 2010

Spencer N. Social, economic, and political determinants of child health. *Pediatrics* 2003; **112**(3): 704–06.

Spencer N. *Poverty and Child Health.* Oxford: Oxford: Radcliffe Medical Press, 1996.

Whitehead M. *The Health Divide.* London: Health Education Council, 1987.

Housing and health

Braubach M et al. Summary report: Environmental burden of disease associated with inadequate housing. Geneva: WHO, 2011. Available at: ℘ http://www.euro.who.int/__data/assets/pdf_file/0017/145511/e95004sum.pdf.pdf

Taske N et al. *Housing and Public Health: a review of reviews of interventions for improving health; Evidence Briefing.* London: NICE, 2005.

Wilkinson P et al. *Cold comfort. The social and environmental determinants for excess winter death in England, 1986–96.* Bristol: The Policy Press for Joseph Rowntree Foundation, 2001.

Advocacy, resources, and social capital

Cote S, Healy T. *The Well Being of nations. The role of human and social capital.* Paris: Organisation for Economic Co-operation and Development, 2001.

Office for National Statistics. The Social Capital Project. ℘ http://www.ons.gov.uk/about-statistics/user-guidance/sc-guide/the-social-capital-project/index.html

Unicef. Convention on the Rights of the Child ℘ http://www.unicef.org/crc/

Waterston T. Teaching and Learning about advocacy. *Arch Dis Child Educ Pract Ed* 2009; **94**:24–8.

Chapter 15: Educational paediatrics

Academic failure

Slavin RE (ed). *Preventing early school failure: Research, policy, and practice.* Boston, MA: Allyn & Bacon, 1994.

Menzies HM, Lane, KL. Using self-regulation strategies and functional assessment-based interventions to provide academic and behavioral support to students at risk within three-tiered models of prevention. *Preventing School Failure* 2011; **55**:181–91.

Neitzel, J. Positive behavior supports for children and youth with autism spectrum disorders. *Preventing School Failure* 2010; **54**:247–55.

SEN and educational approach to disabled child

Dare A et al. *Good Practice in Caring for Children with Special Needs*, 3rd edn. Cheltenham: Nelson Thornes, 2009.

Department for Education. *Support and aspiration: A new approach to special educational needs and disability.* London: Department for Education, 2011

Department for Education. *Disability Toolkit.* London: Department for Education, 2011

Department for Education and Skills. *SEN Code of Practice.* London: Department for Education and Skills. 2001

Special Educational Needs and Disability Act 2001. ✍ http://www www.legislation.gov.uk

The Equality Act (2010) Disability Regulations. ✍ http://www www.legislation.gov.uk

Writing the SEN report

Department for Education. *SEN Toolkit 8. Guidelines for writing advice.* London: Department for Education. Available at: ✍ http://www.Education.gov.uk

School health promotion

Croghan E. *Promoting Health in Schools: A practical guide for teachers and school nurses working with children aged 3 to 11.* London: Sage Publications, 2007.

Department for Education. *Pupil health and wellbeing.* ✍ http://www.education.gov.uk/schools/pupilsupport/pastoralcare/health

Department of Health. *Healthy Child Programme from 5 to 19 years.* London: Department of Health.

Chapter 16: Working with partner agencies

Health visitor

Department of Health. *Facing the Future: A review of the role of health visitors.* London: DH, 2007. Available at: ✍ http://www.dh.gov.uk/en/Publicationsandstatistics/Publications/PublicationsPolicyAndGuidance/DH_075642

School nurses

Department of Health. *Healthy Child Programme: From 5–19 years.* London: Department of Health, 2009.

Royal College of Nursing. *An RCN toolkit for school nurses.* London: RCN, 2008.

Community nursing

Sidey A. Competences for community health care nursing (children). In: Sines D (ed) *Community health care nursing.* Oxford: Blackwell Science, 1995.

Chapter 17: Public health

Acheson ED. *Public health in England. Report of Inquiry into the future development of the public health function.* London: HMSO, 1988.

Allen G. *Early Intervention: Smart Investment, Massive Savings. The Second Independent Report to Her Majesty's Government.* London: HM Government, 2011. Available at: ✍ http://www.cabinet-office.gov.uk/sites/default/files/resources/earlyintervention-smartinvestment.pdf

Allen G. *Early Intervention: The Next Steps. An Independent Report to Her Majesty's Government.* London: HM Government, 2011. Available at: ✍ http://www.dwp.gov.uk/docs/early-intervention-next-steps.pdf

Audit Commission. *Better safe than sorry. Preventing unintentional injury to children.* London: Audit Commission, 2007.

Dahlgren G, Whitehead M. *Policies and strategies to promote social equity in health.* Stockholm: Stockholm Institute of Future Studies, 1991.

Department of Health. *Immunisation against infectious disease. The 'Green Book'.* Check website for chapter updates. Available at: ✍ http://www.dh.gov.uk/en/Publicationsandstatistics/Publications/PublicationsPolicyAndGuidance/DH_079917

Department of Health. *Healthy Child Programme: Pregnancy and the first five years of life.* London: Department of Health, 2009. Available at: ✍ http://www.dh.gov.uk/en/Publicationsandstatistics/Publications/PublicationsPolicyAndGuidance/DH_107563

Department of Health. *The Family Nurse Partnership Programme*. Available at: ✍ http://www.dh.gov.uk/en/Publicationsandstatistics/Publications/PublicationsPolicyAndGuidance/DH_118530 (See also references to peer reviewed academic publications in the evaluation reports available at this site.)

Economos CD *et al.* A community intervention reduces BMI z-score in children: Shape Up Somerville first year results. *Obesity* 2007; **15**:1325–36.

Evans RG, Stoddart GL. Producing health, consuming health care. *Soc Sci Med* 1990; **31**:1347–63.

Faculty of Public Health of the Royal College of Physicians of the United Kingdom. *What is public health?* Available at: ✍ http://www.fph.org.uk/what_is_public_health

First International Conference of Health Promotion. *The Ottawa Charter for Health Promotion*. Geneva: WHO, 1986.

Foresight. *Tackling Obesities: Future Choices - Project Report*, 2nd edn. London: Government Office for Science, 2007.

Hall DMB, Elliman D. *Health for all Children*, 4th rev edn. Oxford University Press, Oxford, 2006.

Hawker J et al. *Communicable Disease Control Handbook*, 2nd edn. Oxford: Wiley-Blackwell, 2005.

Health Protection Agency Meningococcus and Haemophilus Forum (2011). Guidance for public health management of meningococcal disease in the UK. ✍ http://www.hpa.org.uk/web/HPAwebFile/HPAweb_C/1194947389261

Health Protection Agency website. List of notifiable diseases. ✍ http://www.hpa.org.uk/Topics/InfectiousDiseases/InfectionsAZ/NotificationsOfInfectiousDiseases/ListOfNotifiableDiseases

Health Protection Agency website. Reporting procedures. ✍ http://www.hpa.org.uk/Topics/InfectiousDiseases/InfectionsAZ/NotificationsOfInfectiousDiseases/ReportingProcedures

Health Protection Agency website. What the health protection agency does. ✍ http://www.hpa.org.uk/AboutTheHPA/WhatTheHealthProtectionAgencyDoes

Health Protection Agency website. Meningococcal Reference Unit isolates of *Neisseria meningitidis*: England and Wales, by serogroup & epidemiological year, 1998/99-2008/09. ✍ http://www.hpa.org.uk/web/HPAweb&HPAwebStandard/HPAweb_C/1234859711901

Heymann DL. *Control of Communicable Diseases* manual. Washington, DC: American Public Health Association, 2008.

Information Services Division of National Services Scotland website. Child Weight & Growth. ✍ http://www.isdscotland.org/Health-Topics/Child-Health/Child-Weight-and-Growth

Information Services Division of National Services Scotland website. Unintentional Injuries. http://www.isdscotland.org/Health-Topics/Emergency-Care/Publications

Killoran A et al. NICE Update. NICE public health guidance update. *J Public Health* 2011; **33**:151–2.

Kipping RR et al. Obesity in children. Part 1: Epidemiology, measurement, risk factors, and screening. *BMJ* 2008; 337:a1824.

Marmot M, Friel S. Global health equity: evidence for action on the social determinants of health. *J Epidemiol Community Health* 2008; **62**:1095–7.

Naidoo J, Wills J. *Foundations for Health Promotion*. London: Bailliere Tindall, 2000.

National Patient Safety Agency website. Root cause analysis. ✍ http://www.nrls.npsa.nhs.uk/rca

National Screening Committee website. Programme appraisal criteria. www.screening.nhs.uk/criteria

National Screening Committee. Screening in England. ✍ http://www.screening.nhs.uk/england (access condition specific mini-sites, also available for other UK countries).

NICE. *Preventing unintentional injuries in the home among children and young people aged under 15: home safety assessments and providing safety equipment. NICE Public Health Guidance 30*. London: NICE, 2010.

NICE. *Preventing unintentional road injuries among under-15s: road design and modification. NICE Public Health Guidance 31*. London: NICE, 2010.

Preamble to the Constitution of the World Health Organization as adopted by the International Health Conference, New York, 19 June–22 July 1946.

Raffle AE, Gray JAM. *Screening: Evidence and Practice*. Oxford: Oxford University Press, 2007.

Romon M et al. Downward trends in the prevalence of childhood overweight in the setting of 12-year school- and community-based programmes. *Public Health Nutr* 2009; **12**:1735–42.

Scottish Parliament website. Finance Committee – Inquiry into preventative spending. ✍ http://www.scottish.parliament.uk/s3/committees/finance/inquiries/preventative.htm

Tannahill A. Health promotion: the Tannahill model revisited. *Public Health* 2009; **123**:396–9.

The Health and Social Care Information Centre. *National Child Measurement Programme: England, 2009/10 school year*. London: Department of Health, 2010. (Information is updated regularly, so check website for most recent publication: ✍ http:// www.ic.nhs.uk/)

Appendix

Growth chart: boys 0–1 years

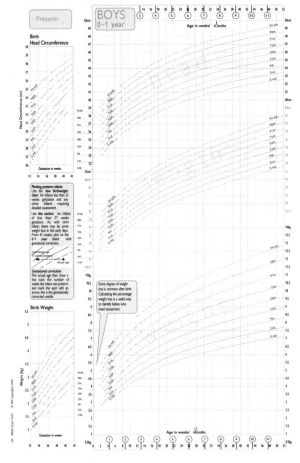

UK-WHO 0–1 (boys) © DH Copyright 2009.

Growth chart: boys 1–4 years

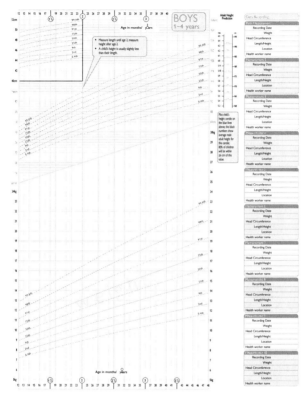

UK-WHO 0–4 (boys) © DH Copyright 2009.

Growth chart: girls 0–1 years

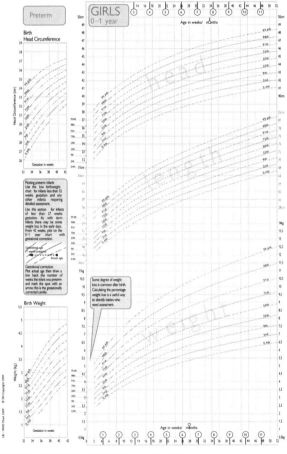

UK-WHO 0–1 (girls) © DH Copyright 2009.

Growth chart: girls 1–4 years

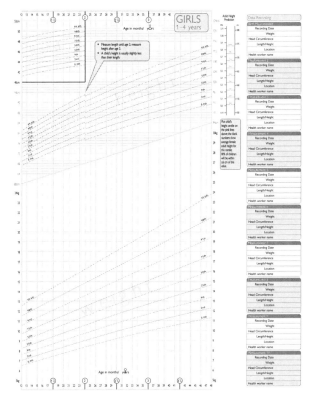

UK-WHO 0–4 (girls) © DH Copyright 2009.

Growth chart: boys height 5–18 years

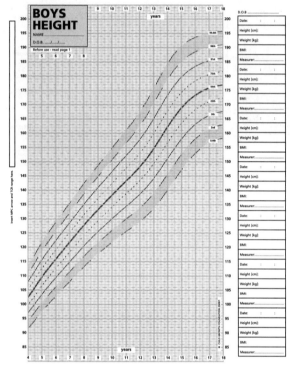

UK 1990 4–18 (boys) © Child Growth Foundation 2009/10.

Growth chart: boys weight 5–18 years

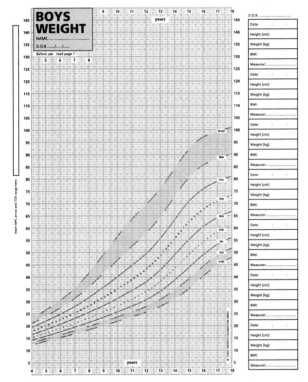

UK 1990 4–18 (boys) © Child Growth Foundation 2009/10.

Growth chart: girls height 5–18 years

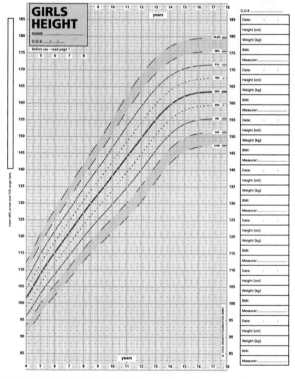

UK 1990 4–18 (girls) © Child Growth Foundation 2009/10.

Growth chart: girls weight 5–18 years

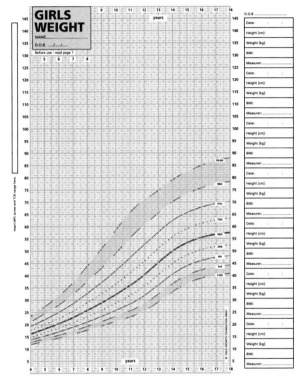

UK 1990 4–18 (girls) © Child Growth Foundation 2009/10.

Down syndrome: boys 0–4 years

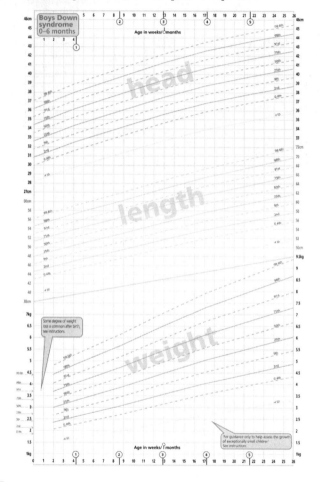

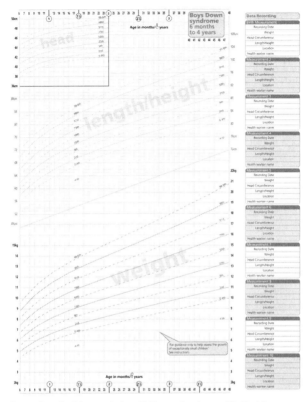

Reproduced with permission, © Down Syndrome Medical Interest Group.

Down syndrome: boys 4–18 years

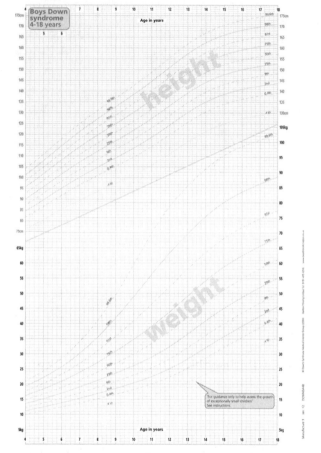

Reproduced with permission, © Down Syndrome Medical Interest Group.

Down syndrome: girls 0–4 years

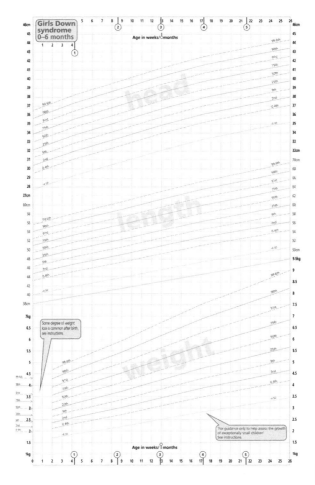

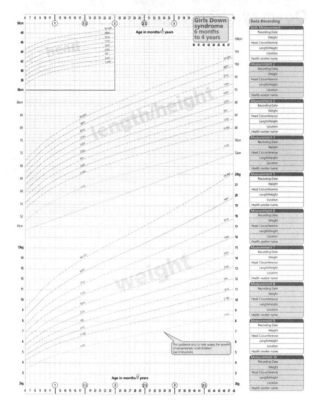

Reproduced with permission, © Down Syndrome Medical Interest Group.

Down syndrome: girls 4–18 years

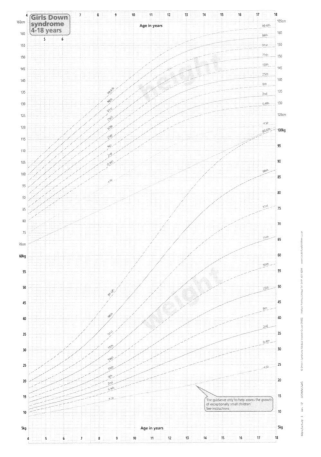

Reproduced with permission, © Down Syndrome Medical Interest Group.

Head circumference: boys

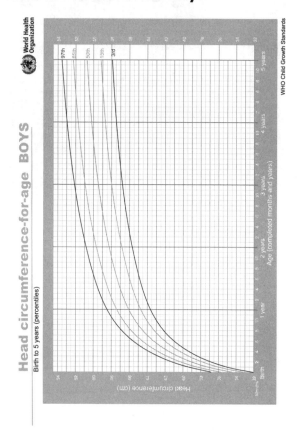

Reproduced from The WHO Child Growth Standards © World
Health Organization.

Head circumference: girls

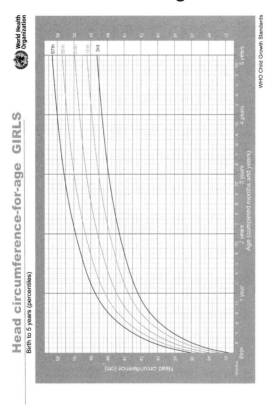

Reproduced from The WHO Child Growth Standards © World
Health Organization.

BMI centile charts: boys

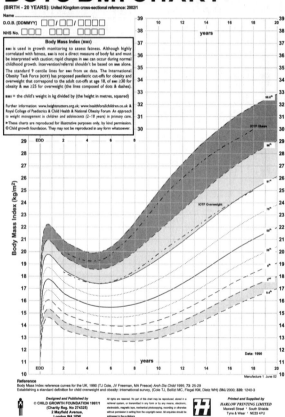

BMI (boys) © Child Growth Foundation.

BMI centile charts: girls

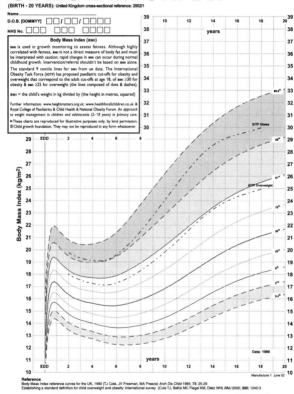

GIRLS BMI CHART

(BIRTH - 20 YEARS): United Kingdom cross-sectional reference: 2002/1

Name ....

D.O.B. [DDMMYY] □□ / □□ / □□□□

NHS No. □□□ □□□ □□□□

Body Mass Index (BMI)

BMI is used in growth monitoring to assess fatness. Although highly correlated with fatness, BMI is not a direct measure of body fat and must be interpreted with caution; rapid changes in BMI can occur during normal childhood growth. Intervention/referral shouldn't be based on BMI alone.

The standard 9 centile lines for BMI from UK data. The International Obesity Task Force (IOTF) has proposed paediatric cut-offs for obesity and overweight that correspond to the adult cut-offs at age 18, of BMI ≥30 for obesity & BMI ≥25 for overweight (the lines composed of dots & dashes).

BMI = the child's weight in kg divided by (the height in metres, squared)

Further information: www.heightmatters.org.uk; www.healthforallchildren.co.uk & Royal College of Paediatrics & Child Health & National Obesity Forum An approach to weight management in children and adolescents (2–18 years) in primary care.

► These charts are reproduced for illustrative purposes only, by kind permission.
© Child growth foundation. They may not be reproduced in any form whatsoever.

Reference
Body Mass Index reference curves for the UK, 1990 (TJ Cole, JV Freeman, MA Preece) Arch Dis Child 1995; 73: 25-29
Establishing a standard definition for child overweight and obesity: international survey (Cole TJ, Bellizi MC Flegal KM, Dietz WH) BMJ 2000; 320: 1240-3

Designed and Published by
© CHILD GROWTH FOUNDATION 1997/1
(Charity Reg. No 274325)
2 Mayfield Avenue,
London W4 1PW

Printed and Supplied by
HARLOW PRINTING LIMITED
Maxwell Street ' South Shields
Tyne & Wear ' NE33 4PU

BMI (girls) © Child Growth Foundation.

UK routine immunisations: 2012

Table A.1 Routine childhood immunisation programme

Age	Diseases or pathogens for which immunisation given	Vaccine given in UK 2011
2 months	Diphtheria, tetanus, pertussis, polio, Hib (DTaP/IPV/Hib)	Pediacel®
	Streptococcus pneumoniae (PCV13)	Prevenar13®
3 months	DTaP/IPV/Hib	Pediacel®
	Serogroup C *N. meningitidis* (MenC)	Menjugate®, NeisVac-C®, Meningitec®
4 months	DTaP/IPV/Hib	Pediacel®
	MenC	Menjugate®, NeisVac-C®, Meningitec®
	PCV13	Prevenar13®
Between 12–13 months	Hib/MenC	Menitorix®
	Measles, mumps, rubella (MMR)	MMR vax PRO®, Priorix®
	PCV13	Prevenar13®
3 years 4 months–5 years	DTaP/IPV	Repevax® or Infanrix IPV®
	MMR	MMR vax PRO®, Priorix®
12–13 years (or year 8) Girls	Human papilloma virus (3 injections over 6 months)	Gardasil
13–18 years	dT/IPV	Revaxis®

Table A.2 Infant immunisation given to risk group

Tuberculosis	In at-risk groups	BCG vaccine
Hepatitis B	Infant of infected mother (or other household member with infection) neonatal programme	Hepatitis B vaccine at 0, 1, 2, and 12 months

Antibiotic regimens

(Also see 📖 p94)

Clinical syndrome of infection	1st choice	Penicillin allergy. If known anaphylactic reaction to penicillin then avoid cephalosporins and meropenem. Consult microbiologist for further advice.
Sepsis if meningitis ruled out >3 months old	ceftriaxone iv 80mg/kg once daily	
	Severe allergy to penicillin: chloramphenicol 25mg/kg iv as a single dose PLUS gentamicin 7mg/kg as a single dose and then consult microbiology for further advice	
Meningitis >3 months old	ceftriaxone iv 80mg/kg daily Consider need for aciclovir and corticosteroids	
	Severe allergy to penicillin: chloramphenicol 25mg/kg iv as a single dose and then consult microbiology for further advice	
Urinary tract infection Give for 5-10 days	Oral: co-amoxiclav oral (see BNF for dose by weight/age)	Oral: cephalexin 25mg/kg bd oral
	IV: co-amoxiclav 30mg/kg tds iv +/- gentamicin 7mg daily iv	IV: ceftriaxone 80mg/kg daily iv +/- gentamicin 7mg/kg daily iv
Pneumonia: mild/moderate, community acquired	amoxicillin 30mg/kg tds oral for 5 days	azithromycin 10mg/kg oral for 3 days once daily
Pneumonia: severe, community acquired	amoxicillin 30mg/kg tds iv	ceftriaxone 80mg/kg once daily iv
Tonsillitis	Consider no antibacterial for 24-48 hours	
	penicillin V 15mg/kg qds oral for 10 days	azithromycin 10mg/kg once daily for 3 days, oral
Otitis Media	Consider no antibacterial for 24-48 hours	
	amoxicillin 30mg/kg tds oral for 5 days	azithromycin 10mg/kg once daily for 3 days, oral
Cellulitis	flucloxacillin 25mg/kg qds oral If severe flucloxacillin 25mg/kg iv PLUS clindamycin 6mg/kg qds oral	cephalexin 25mg/kg bd oral If severe ceftriaxone 80mg/kg daily IV PLUS clindamycin 6mg/kg qds oral
Wound infection	flucloxacillin 25mg/kg qds oral	cephalexin 25mg/kg bd oral
	Consider anaerobic cover if relevant	
Dog/human bites Give for 5 days	Oral: co-amoxiclav oral (see BNF for dose by weight/age)	ceftriaxone 80mg/kg once daily iv PLUS metronidazole 7.5mg/kg tds oral (max 400mg)
Clostridium difficile colitis Give for 14 days	vancomycin 5mg/kg qds oral Stop all other antibacterials if possible	

With permission of the Medicines Advisory Committee, Oxford University Hospitals NHS Trust.

Drug dosages: BNF for children 🕭 www.bnf.org.

❶ Does change by weight and age.

Normal development milestones (average age)

Table A.3

Age	Gross motor	Fine motor and vision	Speech, language, and hearing	Personal and social
5 years	Jumps lightly on toes Skips Walk heel to toe Can catch a ball	Draws triangle Draws house Builds 3 steps with 6 cubes Recognize and copy alphabets	Names colours Counts 10 pennies Repeats sentence of 10 syllables Grammatical speech	Dresses/undress alone, Uses knife Ask Q about meaning of words Domestic role-playing
4 years	Hops on 1 foot Throws ball over arm Uses scissors to cut Stairs up/down 1 foot per step	Copies square, cross Draws a man with 3–4 parts	Counts 20 or more Counts 4 pennies Tells a story	Plays with other children Social interaction Goes to toilet alone
3 years	Throws over arm Stands briefly on 1 foot Climbs stairs 1 foot per step Rides tricycle	Tower of 9 cubes Copies a circle Cuts with scissors	Talks in sentences Names 4 pictures Knows age and sex Repeats 3 numbers	Eats with fork and spoon, washes hands Puts on clothing Names friend Dry by day and night Plays in parallel
2 years	Kicks ball Climbs stairs 2 feet per step Can squat, run	Tower of 6–7 cubes Circular scribble Imitates horizontal stroke	Joins 2–3 words Knows 5–6 body parts, Knows 50 words Identifies 2 pictures	Removes a garment e.g. a sock Mainly dry by day Listens to stories Helps to undress

Table A.3 (Continued)

18 months	Walks well Runs Sits on small chair Explores	Tower of 2–4 cubes Scribble Imitates vertical strokes	6–12 words Knows some body parts	Uses spoon Helps in house Symbolic play Tells mum when s/he needs potty
1 year	Pulls to stand Cruises Stands alone(briefly) Walks alone 13 months	Puts block in a cup Casting	One or two words with meaning Jargon	Imitates activities Plays ball Object permanence established
9 months	Crawls Sits steadily and pivots	Pincer grasp Index finger approach Bangs 2 cubes	Can perform Distraction hearing test (7–8 months) 2-syllable babble	Waves bye bye Understands 'no' Plays pat a cake Indicate wants
6 months	No head lag Sits with support Up on forearms when prone May roll front to back	Reaches with Palmer grasp Transfers objects from hand to hand	Babbles	Works for toy May finger feed Chews

Paediatric reference intervals

Paediatric reference intervals
p=plasma; s=serum; f=fasting; B=boy; G=girl; EDTA=edetic acid

Biochemistry (1mmol = 1mEq/L)

Albumin[P]	36–48g/dL
Alk phos[P] (depends on age)	see below
α1-antitrypsin[P]	1.3–3.4g/dL
Ammonium[P]	2–25μmL/L; 3–35μg/dL
Amylase[P]	70–300u/L
Aspartate aminotransferase[P]	<40u/L
Bilirubin[P]	2–16μmol/L; 0.1–0.8mg/dL
Blood gases, arterial	pH 7.36–7.42
P[a]CO₂	4.3–6.1kPa; 32–46mmHg
P[a]O₂	11.3–14.0kPa; 85–105mmHg
Bicarbonate	21–25mmol/L
Base excess	–2 to +2mmol/L
Calcium[P]	2.25–2.75mmol/L; 9–11mg/dL
Neonates:	1.72–2.47; 6.9–9.9mg/dL
Chloride[P]	98–105mmol/L
Cholesterol[Pf]	≤5.7mmol/L; 100–200mg/dL
Creatine kinase[P]	<80u/L
Creatinine[P]	25–115μmol/L; 0.3–1.3mg/dL
Glucose[f]	2.5–5.3mmol/L; 45–95mg/dL
	(lower in newborn. Fluoride tube)
IgA[S]	0.8–4.5g/L (low at birth,
	rising to adult levels slowly)
IgG[S]	5–18g/L (high at birth, falls
	and then rises slowly to adult level)
IgM[S]	0.2–2.0g/L (low at birth, rises to
	adult level by one year)

IgE[S]	<500u/mL
Iron[S]	9–36μmol/L; 50–200μg/dL
Lead[EDTA]	<1.75μmol/L; <36μg/dL
Magnesium[P]	0.6–1.0mmol/L
Phenylalanine[P]	0.04–0.21mmol/L
Potassium[P] mean mmol/L	Day 1: 6.4
	Day 2: 5.9; Day 3: 5.9 (later 4–5.5)
Protein[P]	63–81g/L; 6.3–8.1g/dL
Sodium[P]	136–145mmol/L
Transferrin[S]	2.5–4.5g/L
Triglyceride[fs]	0.34–1.92mmol/L
	(=30–170mg/dL)
Urate[P]	0.12–0.36mmol/L; 2–6mg/dL
Urea[P]	2.5–6.6mmol/L; 15–40mg/dL
Gamma-glutamyl transferase[P]	<20u/L

Hormones—a guide. ► Consult lab

Cortisol[P]	9am 200–700nmol/L
	midnight <140nmol/L, mean
Dehydroepiandrosterone sulfate[P]:	
Day 5–11	0.8–2.8μmol/L (range)
5–11yrs	0.1–3.6μmol/L
17α-Hydroxyprogesterone[P]:	
Days 5–11	1.6–7.5nmol/L (range)
4–15yrs	0.4–4.2nmol/L
T₄[P]	60–135nmol/L (not neonates)
TSH[P]	<5mu/L (higher on day 1–4)

Alk phos range u/L: 0–½yr 150–600; ½–2yr 250–1000; 2–5yr 250–850; 6–7yr 250–1000; 8–9yr 250–750; 10–11yr G = 259–950, B ≤ 730; 12–13yr G = 200–750, B ≤ 785; 14–15yr G = 170–460, B = 170–970; 16–18yr G = 75–270, B = 125–720; >18yr G = 60–250, B = 50–200.

Haematology mean ±1 standard deviation. Range × 10⁹/L (median in brackets)

Day	Hb g/dL	MCV fl	MCHC%	Retic%	WCC	Neutrophils	Eosins	Lymphs	Monos
1	19.0 ± 2	119 ± 9	31.6 ± 2	3.2 ± 1	9–30	6–26 (11)	2–.8	2–11	0.4–3.1
4	18.6 ± 2	114 ± 7	32.6 ± 2	1.8 ± 1	9–40				
5	17.6 ± 1	114 ± 9	30.9 ± 2	1.2 ±0.2					
Weeks									
1–2	17.3 ± 2	112 ± 19	32.1 ± 3	0.5 ± 0.03	5–21	1.5–10 (5)	0.07–0.1	2–17	0.3–2.7
2–3	15.6 ± 3	111 ± 8	33.9 ± 2	0.8 ± 0.6	6–15	1–9.5 (4)	0.07–0.1	2–17	0.2–2.4
4–5	12.7 ± 2	101 ± 8	34.9 ± 2	0.9 ± 0.8	6–15	(4)		(6)	
6–7	12.0 ± 2	105 ± 12	33.8 ± 2	1.2 ± 0.7	6–15	(4)		(6)	
8–9	10.7 ± 1	93 ± 12	34.1 ± 2	1.8 ± 1	6–15	(4)		(6)	
Months—all the following Hb values are Medians/Lower limit for normal									
3	11.5/9	88/88			6–15	(3)		(6)	
6	11.5/9	77/70			6–15	(3)		(6)	
12	11.5/9	78/72			6–15	(3)		(5)	
Year									
2	11.5/9	78/74			6–15	(3)		(5)	
4	12.2/10	80/75			6–15	(4)		(4)	
6	13/10.4	82/75			5–15	(4.2)		(3.8)	
12	13.8/11	83/76			4–13	(4.9)		(3.1)	
14B	14.2/12	84/77			4–13	(5)		(3)	
14G	14/11.5								
16B	14.8/12	85/78	30–36	0.8–2	4–13	2–7.5	(5)0.04–.4	1.3–3.5	0.2–.8
16G	14/11.5								
18B	15/13								

Note Basophil range: 0–0.1 × 10⁹/L; B[S][12]; ≥150ng/L
Red cell folate[EDTA] 100–640ng/mL.

Platelet counts do not vary with age; range: 150–400 × 10⁹/L.
From the *Oxford Handbook of Clinical Specialties 7e*, edited by Collier J, Longmore M, and Brinsden M (2006) by permission of Oxford University Press.

Pharmacological treatment by epilepsy syndrome

Table A.4 provides a summary reference guide to pharmacological treatment.

Table A.4 Antiepileptic drug (AED) options by epilepsy syndrome

Epilepsy syndrome	1st-line AEDs	Adjunctive AEDs	Other AEDs that may be considered on referral to tertiary care	Do not offer AEDs (may worsen seizures)
Childhood absence epilepsy or other absence syndromes	Ethosuximide Lamotrigine[a] Sodium valproate	Ethosuximide Lamotrigine[a] Sodium valproate	Clobazam[a] Clonazepam Levetiracetam[a] Topiramate[a] Zonisamide[a]	Carbamazepine Gabapentin Oxcarbazepine Phenytoin Pregabalin Tiagabine Vigabatrin
Juvenile absence epilepsy or other absence syndromes	Ethosuximide Lamotrigine[a] Sodium valproate	Ethosuximide Lamotrigine[a] Sodium valproate	Clobazam[a] Clonazepam Levetiracetam[a] Topiramate[a] Zonisamide[a]	Carbamazepine Gabapentin Oxcarbazepine Phenytoin Pregabalin Tiagabine Vigabatrin

Table A.4 (Continued)

Juvenile myoclonic epilepsy	Lamotrigine[a] Levetiracetam Sodium valproate Topiramate[a]	Lamotrigine[a] Levetiracetam Sodium valproate Topiramate[a]	Clobazam[a] Clonazepam Zonisamide[a]	Carbamazepine Gabapentin Oxcarbazepine Phenytoin Pregabalin Tiagabine Vigabatrin
Epilepsy with generalized tonic–clonic seizures only	Carbamazepine Lamotrigine Oxcarbazepine[a] Sodium valproate	Clobazam[a] Lamotrigine Levetiracetam Sodium valproate Topiramate		
Idiopathic generalized epilepsy	Lamotrigine[a] Sodium valproate Topiramate[a]	Lamotrigine[a] Levetiracetam[a] Sodium valproate Topiramate[a]	Clobazam[a] Clonazepam Zonisamide[a]	Carbamazepine Gabapentin Oxcarbazepine Phenytoin Pregabalin Tiagabine Vigabatrin
Infantile spasms not due to tuberous sclerosis	Discuss with, or refer to, a tertiary paediatric epilepsy specialist Steroid (prednisolone or tetracosactide) or vigabatrin			

Infantile spasms due to tuberous sclerosis	Discuss with, or refer to, a tertiary paediatric epilepsy specialist Vigabatrin or steroid (prednisolone or tetracosactide[a])		
Benign epilepsy with centrotemporal spikes	Carbamazepine[a] Lamotrigine[a] Levetiracetam[a] Oxcarbazepine[a] Sodium valproate	Carbamazepine[a] Clobazam[a] Gabapentin[a] Lamotrigine[a] Levetiracetam[a] Oxcarbazepine[a] Sodium valproate Topiramate[a]	Eslicarbazepine acetate[a] Lacosamide[a] Phenobarbital Phenytoin Pregabalin[a] Tiagabine[a] Vigabatrin[a] Zonisamide[a]
Panayiotopoulos syndrome	Carbamazepine[a] Lamotrigine[a] Levetiracetam[a] Oxcarbazepine[a] Sodium valproate	Carbamazepine[a] Clobazam[a] Gabapentin[a] Lamotrigine[a] Levetiracetam[a] Oxcarbazepine[a] Sodium valproate Topiramate[a]	Eslicarbazepine acetate[a] Lacosamide[a] Phenobarbital Phenytoin Pregabalin[a] Tiagabine[a] Vigabatrin[a] Zonisamide[a]
Late-onset childhood occipital epilepsy (Gastaut type)	Carbamazepine[a] Lamotrigine[a] Levetiracetam[a] Oxcarbazepine[a] Sodium valproate	Carbamazepine[a] Clobazam[a] Gabapentin[a] Lamotrigine[a] Levetiracetam[a] Oxcarbazepine[a] Sodium valproate Topiramate[a]	Eslicarbazepine acetate[a] Lacosamide[a] Phenobarbital Phenytoin Pregabalin[a] Tiagabine[a] Vigabatrin[a] Zonisamide[a]

Table A.4 (Continued)

Dravet syndrome	Discuss with, or refer to, a tertiary paediatric epilepsy specialist Sodium valproate Topiramate[a]	Clobazam[a] Stiripentol		Carbamazepine Gabapentin Lamotrigine Oxcarbazepine Phenytoin Pregabalin Tiagabine Vigabatrin
Continuous spike and wave during slow sleep Lennox–Gastaut syndrome	Refer to a tertiary paediatric epilepsy specialist Discuss with, or refer to, a tertiary paediatric epilepsy specialist Sodium valproate			Carbamazepine Gabapentin Oxcarbazepine Pregabalin Tiagabine Vigabatrin
Landau–Kleffner syndrome	Refer to a tertiary paediatric epilepsy specialist	Lamotrigine	Felbamatea Rufinamide Topiramate	
Myoclonic-astatic epilepsy	Refer to a tertiary paediatric epilepsy specialist			

a At the time of compilation (January 2012), this drug did not have UK marketing authorization for this indication and/or population (please see table 3 in appendix E of the NICE guideline for specific details about this drug for this indication and population). Informed consent should be obtained and documented.

A consistent supply of a particular manufacturer's AED preparation is recommended, unless the prescriber, in consultation with the child, young person, adult and their family, and/or carers as appropriate, considers that this is not a concern. Different preparations of some AEDs may vary in bioavailability or pharmacokinetic profiles and care needs to be taken to avoid reduced effect or excessive side effects. Please see recommendation 1.9.1.4 of the NICE guideline for further information.

Reproduced with permission from 'The epilepsies: the diagnosis and management of the epilepsies in adults and children in primary and secondary care' (NICE clinical guideline 137). The guideline and implementation tools are available from: www.nice.org.uk/CG137.

Pharmacological treatment by seizure type

Table A.5 provides a summary reference guide to pharmacological treatment.

Table A.5 Antiepileptic drug (AED) options by seizure type

Seizure type	1st-line AEDs	Adjunctive AEDs	Other AEDs that may be considered on referral to tertiary care	Do not offer AEDs (may worsen seizures)
Generalized tonic–clonic	Carbamazepine Lamotrigine Oxcarbazepine[a] Sodium valproate	Clobazam[a] Lamotrigine Levetiracetam Sodium valproate Topiramate		(If there are absence or myoclonic seizures, or if juvenile myoclonic epilepsy suspected) Carbamazepine Gabapentin Oxcarbazepine Phenytoin Pregabalin Tiagabine Vigabatrin

Table A.5 (Continued)

Tonic or atonic	Sodium valproate	Lamotrigine[a]	Rufinamide[a] Topiramate[a]	Carbamazepine Gabapentin Oxcarbazepine Pregabalin Tiagabine Vigabatrin
Absence	Ethosuximide Lamotrigine[a] Sodium valproate	Ethosuximide Lamotrigine[a] Sodium valproate	Clobazam[a] Clonazepam Levetiracetam[a] Topiramate[a] Zonisamide[a]	Carbamazepine Gabapentin Oxcarbazepine Phenytoin Pregabalin Tiagabine Vigabatrin
Myoclonic	Levetiracetam[a] Sodium valproate Topiramate[a]	Levetiracetam Sodium valproate Topiramate[a]	Clobazam[a] Clonazepam Piracetam Zonisamide[a]	Carbamazepine Gabapentin Oxcarbazepine Phenytoin Pregabalin Tiagabine Vigabatrin

Seizure type			
Focal	Carbamazepine Lamotrigine Levetiracetam Oxcarbazepine Sodium valproate	Carbamazepine Clobazam[a] Gabapentin[a] Lamotrigine Levetiracetam Oxcarbazepine Sodium valproate Topiramate	Eslicarbazepine acetate[a] Lacosamide Phenobarbital Phenytoin Pregabalin[a] Tiagabine Vigabatrin Zonisamide[a]
Prolonged or repeated seizures and convulsive status epilepticus in the community	Buccal midazolam[b] Rectal diazepam[b] Intravenous lorazepam		
Convulsive status epilepticus in hospital	Intravenous lorazepam Intravenous diazepam Buccal midazolam	Intravenous phenobarbital Phenytoin	
Refractory convulsive status epilepticus	Intravenous midazolam[b] Propofol[b] (not in children) Thiopental sodium[b]		

a At the time of publication (January 2012) this drug did not have UK marketing authorization for this indication and/or population (please see table 3 in appendix E of the NICE guideline for specific details about this drug for this indication and population). Informed consent should be obtained and documented.

b At the time of publication (January 2012), this drug did not have UK marketing authorisation for this indication and/or population (please see table 3 in appendix E of the NICE guideline for specific details about this drug for this indication and population). Informed consent should be obtained and documented in line with normal standards in emergency care.

Reproduced with permission from 'The epilepsies: the diagnosis and management of the epilepsies in adults and children in primary and secondary care' (NICE clinical guideline 137). The guideline and implementation tools are available from: www.nice.org.uk/CG137

Accidental/abusive bruise patterns

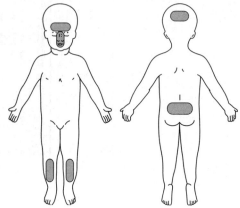

Accidental bruising patterns.

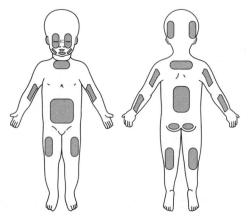

Abusive bruising patterns.

Above diagrams Reproduced from Education and practice, an edition of Archives of Disease in Childhood, Maguire S, 95, 171, 174. 2010 with permission from BMJ Publishing Group Ltd.

Abusive scald patterns

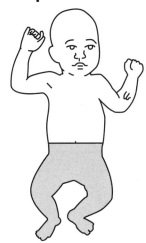

Abusive scald immersion pattern.

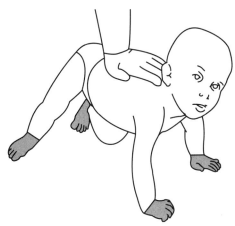

Abusive scald "glove and stocking" pattern.

Consent form for Child Protection Medical Examination

Consent form for Child Protection Medical Examination.

Name: .... DOB: ....

NHS No: ....

Address: ....

....

Post Code: ....

Permission must be gained from parent(s) or other(s) with responsibility for the child, and from the child where appropriate.

I give permission for:

1.	Medical Examination	Yes	No	NA
2.	Photography of clinical/genital findings	Yes	No	NA
3.	Collection of specimens for laboratory tests	Yes	No	NA

Photographs may be used to support clinical evidence of injury and may need to be shared with another doctor involved in any court proceedings, or may be used for teaching and training other professionals.

I give permission for photographs to be used:

1.	To support clinical evidence in court proceedings	Yes	No
2.	For teaching/training purposes	Yes	No
3.	For peer review	Yes	No

I give permission for a report/letter/summary on the medical examination of my child to be shared with:

Social Care	Yes	No
Police	Yes	No
GP/Health Visitor/School Nurse	Yes	No

Other (specify)

A report from the doctor may be requested by the Court.
The doctor may have to give evidence in Court regarding the medical findings.
The procedure has been fully explained to me by the doctor, and I understand that at any stage of the examination I may withdraw my consent.

Signed: .... Date: ....

Name: .... **Parent/Carer/Professional with parental responsibility**

Signed: .... Date: ....

Name: ....**Child/Young Person**

Signed: .... Date: ....

Doctor(s): ....

Body maps to document injuries

Body maps

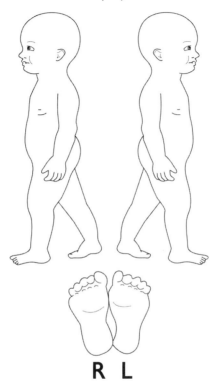

R L

Body maps

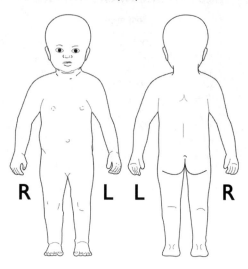

R   L   L   R

Prepubertal female genital anatomy

Prepubertal female genital anatomy

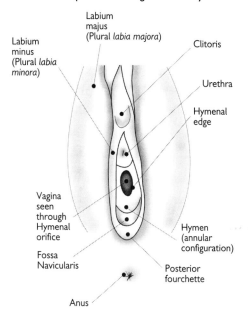

Female genital examination, labial traction

Labial Traction

Hold labia majora between thumb and
forefinger and apply gentle traction in
downward and outward direction

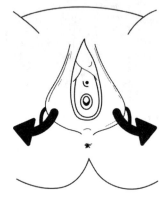

Female genital examination, clockface

Clock face position as used for
describing genital findings

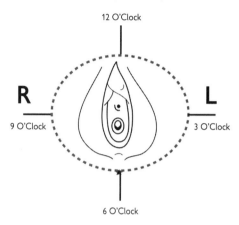

12 O'Clock

R

9 O'Clock

L

3 O'Clock

6 O'Clock

Male genitalia, anatomy

Male genitalia

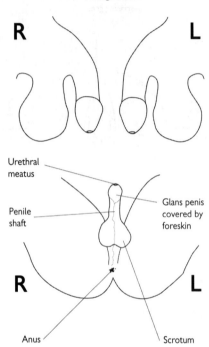

Urethral meatus

Glans penis covered by foreskin

Penile shaft

Anus

Scrotum

Index